E. Meani · C. Romanò · L. Crosby · G. Hofmann (Eds.)

Infection and Local Treatment in Orthopedic Surgery

E. Meani · C. Romanò · L. Crosby · G. Hofmann (Eds.)

Editorial Coordinator: G. Calonego

Infection and Local Treatment in Orthopedic Surgery

With 173 Figures in 317 Parts and 49 Tables

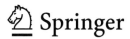 Springer

Editors:

ENZO MEANI, MD
Istituto Ortopedico G. Pini
Centro per il Trattamento delle Complicanze
Ortopediche Settiche (COS)
Piazza Cardinal Ferrari 1
20122 Milano, Italy

CARLO ROMANÒ, MD
Istituto Ortopedico G. Pini
Centro per il Trattamento delle Complicanze
Ortopediche Settiche (COS)
Piazza Cardinal Ferrari 1
20122 Milano, Italy

LYNN CROSBY, MD
Department of Orthopaedic Surgery
30 East Apple Street
Dayton, Ohio 45409, United States

GUNTHER HOFMANN, MD
BG-Klinikum Bergmannstrost Halle
Department of Traumatology
Merseburger Straße 165
06112 Halle a. d. Saale, Germany

Editorial Coordinator:
GIOVANNI CALONEGO
Scientific Coordinator
Tecres S.p.A.
Via A. Doria, 6
37066 Sommacampagna/VR, Italy

ISBN 978-3-540-47998-7   Springer-Verlag Berlin Heidelberg New York

Library of Congress Control Number: 2006939134

Springer is a part of Springer Science+Business Media
http://www.springer.com

© Springer-Verlag Berlin Heidelberg 2007

Printed in Germany

Editor: Gabriele Schröder
Desk Editor: Irmela Bohn
Copy-editing: WS Editorial Ltd, Shrewsbury, UK
Production Editor: Joachim W. Schmidt

Cover design: eStudio Calamar, Spain

Typesetting: FotoSatz Pfeifer GmbH, D-82166 Gräfelfing
Printed on acid-free paper – 24/3151 – 5 4 3 2 1 0

Preface

Bone infections involve enormous social, economic and human impact.

Despite improvements in surgical techniques, asepsis and prevention, the increasing use of surgery in orthopaedics and trauma means that the absolute number of bone infections is progressively increasing in western countries.

The work of orthopaedic surgeons is increasingly assisted by industrial innovation designed to meet new requirements and achieve what clinical and scientific evidence indicates in terms of prevention and treatment of bone and joint infections.

In particular, new technologies in recent years, such as those allowing local treatment with antibiotic-loaded cements and preformed spacers, have made it possible to improve substantially the effectiveness of infection treatment in orthopaedics.

This book collects the scientific contributions of eminent European and International scientists, which were presented during the International Congress organized by Tecres Spa (Verona, Italy) and held in Verona at the "Palazzo della Gran Guardia" (7–9 September 2006).

Specialists of surgery and medicine (orthopaedic, trauma and infection surgeons, microbiologists and pharmacologists) from all over the world met to exchange the latest information. This is a collection of their personal clinical experience in the treatment of orthopaedic implant infections.

With the hope that this book may represent a useful tool for updating those who dedicate themselves to the difficult art of treating osteo-articular infections, we wish a good reading!

Enzo Meani
Carlo Romanò
Lynn Crosby
Gunther Hofmann

Table of Contents

Clinical Applications: Knee

Novel Applications and Perspectives

Corresponding Authors

Dr. Jordi Asuncion Márquez
Department of Orthopaedics
Hospital Mutua de Terrassa
Plaza Dr. Robert 5
08221 Terrassa, Spain

Eng. Massimiliano Baleani
Medical Technology Laboratory
Rizzoli Orthopaedic Institutes
Via di Barbiano 1/10
40136 Bologna, Italy

Prof. Elisa Bertazzoni Minelli
Department of Medicine
and Public Health
Pharmacology Section
Policlinico "G.B. Rossi"
P.le L.A. Scuro, 10
37134 Verona, Italy

Dr. Pia Baiocchi
Department of Clinical Medicine
Policlinico Umberto I
University "La Sapienza"
Viale del Policlinico 155
00161 Roma, Italy

Ass. Prof. R. Stephen J. Burnett
Department of Orthopaedic Surgery
Washington University School of Medicine
Barnes-Jewish Hospital
Barnes-Jewish, Barnes-Jewish West Count
& St. Luis VA Medical Center Hospitals
One Barnes-Jewish Hospital Plaza
Suite 11300
Saint Louis, MO 63110, USA

Prof. Claudio Carlo Castelli
Department of Orthopaedics and
Traumatology
Ospedali Riuniti of Bergamo
Largo Barozzi 1
24100 Bergamo, Italy

Prof. Alberto Cigada
Department of Applied Physical
Chemistry
Politecnico di Milano
Via Mancinelli 7
20131 Milan, Italy

Prof. Ercole Concia
Department of Infectious Disease
University of Verona
Policlinico "G.B. Rossi"
P.le L.A. Scuro, 10
37134 Verona, Italy

Prof. Lynn A. Crosby
Department of Orthopaedic Surgery
Wright State University Boonshoft
School of Medicine
30 E. Apple Street, Suite 5250
Dayton, Ohio, USA

Dr. Michael Diefenbeck
Berufsgenossenschaftliche Kliniken
Bergmannstrost
Klinik für Unfall- und
Wiederherstellungschirurgie
Merseburgerstr. 165
06112 Halle/Saale

Dr. Costantino Errani
5th Department of Oncologic
Orthopaedics and Traumatology
Rizzoli Orthopedic Institutes
Via Pupilli 1
40136 Bologna, Italy

Dr. Xavier Flores Sánchez
Hospital Universitari Vall d'Hebron
Passeig de la Vall d'Hebrón, 119–129
08035 Barcelona, Spain

Dr. Mauro Battista Gallazzi
Service of Radiodiagnostic
"G. Pini" Orthopaedic Institute, Milan
Piazza Cardinal Ferrari 1
20142 Milan, Italia

Prof. Giorgio Gasparini
Orthopaedic department
Catholic University
Largo Francesco Vito 8
00128 Rome, Italy

Dr. Thorsten Gehrke
Medical Director
Endo-Klinik
Holstenstrasse 2
22767 Hamburg, Germany

Prof. Roberto Giardino
Department of Experimental Surgery
Rizzoli Orthopaedic Institutes
Via Di Barbiano, 1/10
40136 Bologna, Italy

Prof. Federico A. Grassi
Department of Orthopaedics and
Traumatology "Mario Boni"
University of Insubria
Ospedale di Circolo – Fondazione
Macchi
Viale Borri, 57
21100 Varese, Italy

Dr. Giovanni Gualdrini
7th Division of Orthopaedics and
Traumatology
Rizzoli Orthopaedics Institutes
Via Pupilli 1
40136 Bologna, Italy

Prof. Reinhold Alexander Laun
Head of Department of Trauma and
Reconstructive Surgery
General Hospital Centre Neukölln of
Capital Berlin
Rudower Str. 48
12351 Berlin, Germany

Prof. Christoph H. Lohmann
Department of Orthopaedics
University of Hamburg-Eppendorf
Martinistr. 52
20246 Hamburg, Germany

Dr. Arne Lundberg
Department of Orthopaedics,
Karolinska University Hospital
Huddinge, SE-141 86 Stockholm,
Sweden

Dr. Bruno Magnan
Department of Orthopaedics
University of Verona
Policlinico "G.B. Rossi"
P.le L.A. Scuro, 10
37134 Verona, Italy

Prof. Konstantinos N. Malizos
Department of Orthopaedic Surgery
University of Thessalia
41110 Mezourlo
Larissa, Greece

Prof. Enzo Meani
Center for Treatment of Septic
Complications (COS)
"G. Pini" Orthopaedic Istitute
Via G. Pini 9
20122 Milan, Italy

Dr. Vito Pavone
Department of Surgical Medical
Sciences
Section of Orthopaedics and
Traumatology
University of Catania
Via Plebiscito 628
Catania, Italy

Dr. Antonio Pellegrini
Center for Treatment of Septic
Complications (COS)
"G. Pini" Orthopaedic Istitute
Piazza Cardinal Ferrari 1
20122 Milan, Italy

Prof. William Petty
Professor (ret.)
University of Florida
Chairman
Exactech, Inc.
Gainesville, Florida USA

Prof. Rocco P. Pitto
Professor of Orthopaedic Surgery
Bioengineering Institute
Symonds St. 70, Level 5
Auckland, New Zealand

Prof. Carlo L. Romano
Center for Treatment of Septic
Complications (COS)
"G.Pini" Orthopaedic Istitute
Piazza Cardinal Ferrari 1
20122 Milan, Italy

Dr. Clemente Sandrone
Department of Osteo-articular
Inflammatory Disease
Santa Corona Hospital
Via XXV Aprile 38
17027 Pietra Ligure (SV), Italy

Dr. Renzo Soffiatti
Technical Director
Research & Development
Tecres Spa
Via A. Doria 6
37066 Sommacampagna (VR), Italy

Dr. Alex Soriano
Department of Infectious Deseases
Hospital Clínic
C / Villarroel 170
08036 Barcelona, Spain

Dr. Stephan Tohtz
Charité – Universitätsmedizin Berlin
Centrum für Muskuloskeletale
Chirurgie
Klinik für Orthopädie
Charitéplatz 1
10117 Berlin, Germany

Prof. Luca Vaienti
Unit of Plastic and Reconstructive
Surgery
Department of Surgical Medical
Sciences, University of Milan
Istituto Policlinico San Donato
Via Morandi, 30
20097 San Donato Milanese (MI), Italy

Dr. Ernesto Valenti
Orthopaedic and Traumatologic Unit
Buccheri La Ferla Fatebenefratelli
Hospital
Via Messina Marine 197
90123 Palermo, Italy

Eng. Tomaso Villa
Laboratory of Biological Structure
Mechanics
Department of Structural Engineering
Politecnico di Milano
Piazza Leonardo da Vinci 32
20133 Milano, Italy

Prof. Christof von Eiff
Institute of Medical Microbiology
University Hospital of Münster
Domagkstrasse 10
48149 Münster, Germany

Ass. Prof. Geert H.I.M. Walenkamp
Department of Surgery and
Orthopaedics
University Hospital Maastricht
Post Box 5800
NL 6202-AZ Maastricht
The Netherlands

Dr. Heinz Winkler
Osteitis Center Privatklinik Döbling
Heiligenstaedterstrasse 57–63
1190 Wien, Austria

Prof. Eivind Witsø
Department of Orthopaedic Surgery
St. Olavs University Hospital
Norwegian University of Science and
Technology
N-7006 Trondheim, Norway

Dr. Giorgio Zappalà
Department of Orthopaedic and
Traumatology "Mario Boni"
University of Insubria
Ospedale di Circolo – Fondazione Macchi
Viale Borri, 57
21100 Varese, Italy

The Socio-economic Burden of Musculoskeletal Infections

K.N. Malizos, L.A. Poultsides

Department of Orthopaedic Surgery, University of Thessalia, Larissa, Greece

Magnitude and Predicted Trends of Burden

Musculoskeletal disorders are the most common cause of severe chronic pain and physical disability affecting many millions of people. Their impact on the health related quality of life of the individual, the society and the health care systems is enormous [45]. This trend will increase dramatically over the next years as the population is ageing and the lifestyle is changing towards more mobility and recreational activities. These parameters have brought up musculoskeletal disorders as the most expensive disease category, requiring 23 % of the total cost of illness treatment as the Swedish "cost of illness" study has indicated. The indirect costs related to morbidity and disability are the greatest in most European Union countries and in the United States, while in both the total Health Expenditures are increasing in relation with the respective gross domestic products [45]. For example, since 1965, the percentage of the United States gross domestic product spent on health care has increased from 5 % to 13.4 %, a figure that is expected to continue to rise to 15.9 % by 2010 [75]. However, the disorders of the bone and the joints have not yet been addressed as health care priorities. The established market economies allocate less than 5 % of their national spending on research related to these conditions.

The burden stemming from Musculoskeletal Infections escalates due to new surgical innovations, the increasing life expectancy, urbanization and motorization, expanding application of implants while the number of operated patients at risk of infection and other adverse outcomes is increasing, as well as lack of training in their management.

The most commonly occurring Orthopaedic infections are Soft Tissue infections, Necrotizing fasciitis, Hematogenous Osteomyelitis, Septic Arthritis, Post-traumatic Osteomyelitis and/or Septic Non-union, as well as infections around Arthroplasties and Internal Fixation devices. They have a devastating effect on the patient as they may lead to temporary impairment, long lasting disability or even permanent handicap, inevitably incurring social and economic isolation [25]. The importance of infections in the musculoskeletal system lies in the fact that the application of implants is continuously expanding and more operated patients are at risk of developing infection. Nowadays, antibiotic overuse makes bacteria more resistant to antibiotics. Bacteria spread through patients' transfer among hospitals, making nosocomial infections a major threat for the hospitalized patients. On the other hand, surgeons are not always adequately trained to manage musculoskeletal infections. All these factors result in increasing burden placed upon the patient, health services or the society as a whole, which may be of a medical, economic or social nature, depending on the viewpoint adopted.

The Need for Estimating the Burden

The number of reports examining the cost of musculoskeletal infections in the last two decades is small in comparison with the unanimous recognition that bone and joint infections induce major financial cost, and more severely, great human suffering. Raising awareness of the patient, the physician and the society in general is of paramount importance. Recognition of the burden of the musculoskeletal infections will result in greater awareness of the pervasive effect they have on the individual and of their cost to society. So estimating the burden will facilitate the process of setting appropriate priorities and adopting relevant strategies towards its reduction.

The cost-of-illness (COI) studies provide a most comprehensive methodology to assess the scale and nature of musculoskeletal infections as a health problem, and raise the profile of the patient group who suffer from them. Through identification of the three basic components of the burden, i.e. the direct costs, the costs due to loss of productivity (indirect costs) and the psychosocial or intangible costs [34], the COI studies may assist the decision-making process at policy and planning levels, and reveal where the major burden of cost might lie in the treatment and care of these patients [13, 35].

Direct medical and non-medical costs [2, 3, 66], for which actual payments are made, have an impact on both the patient and health services. They include treatment costs, hospital and medication costs, which can be divided into fixed and variable ones. Control of variable costs such as implants and supplies plays a predominant role in cost-containment programmes. Personal payments such as the cost of transport to the health provider and specialist aids, as well as the building's opportunity cost consist the direct non-medical costs.

As for the costs due to loss of productivity [2, 3, 66] no direct payment is actually made. They include morbidity costs, which consist of lost resources due to the patient's or a relative's absence from work, less production during the work shift, and early retirement due to illness. The mortality costs also reflect lost production (potential years of life loss and loss of productive years) due to premature death caused by a lethal infection.

The third category refers to psychosocial or intangible costs [2, 3, 66], which represent deterioration in the quality of the patient's life, as well as their families' and friends'. People with musculoskeletal infections suffer from disability, pain, reduced self-esteem, and feelings of non-well-being, those being factors extremely difficult to quantify.

Inevitable Burden of Orthopaedic Infections

Data examining deep-space Orthopaedic Infections provide a glimpse of the patient population where the infection is more severe, the direct and indirect financial costs and the sequelae on their functional ability and quality of living. The majority of relevant studies are made on heterogenous groups of patients and infections. Whitehouse et al [77], studied surgical site infections after orthopaedic surgery and reported dramatically greater financial costs for the infected patients. They had twice as many hospitalizations and operative procedures as those of matched uninfected control patients, fourteen days longer hospital stay and four times higher median hospital costs. Infected patients also reported greater physical limitation and greater reduction in health-related quality of life. In a similar study conducted in the United Kingdom concerning infections occurring after elective orthopaedic surgery the results indicated a seventeen-day increase in length of hospitalization [61].

It has been shown that joint replacement is among the most successful surgical procedures performed in terms of consistent improvement of the patient's quality of life [65, 78]. As stated above, due to expanded indications for total joint arthroplasties and the growth and ageing of the population, the number of primary total joint arthroplasties performed each year is increasing in the United States and in Europe, resulting unfortunately in a proportionate increase in the absolute number of infected total joint arthroplasties [38, 56]. The estimated prevalence of infection following total joint arthroplasty has been reported to range from 0.5 % to 7.5 % [4, 31]. Risk factors for infection are influenced by many variables that include the patient, the procedure, the surgeon, and the hospital characteristics.

Infection often results in the need for multiple reoperations, prolonged use of intravenous and oral antibiotics, extended inpatient and outpatient rehabilitation, and frequent follow-up visits. Furthermore, clinical outcomes following single-stage and two-stage revision total joint arthroplasty have been less favourable than those after revision for other causes of failure not associated with infection [10]. In a study of infected total knee replacements [33], the infected patients who underwent revision arthroplasty averaged thirty-two hospitalization days, which are significantly more than nine and thirteen days utilized for primary and aseptic revision respectively. Infected patients required more operative procedures, were re-hospitalized more often and received more units of blood. Hospital charges were more than four times higher for the patients undergoing arthroplasty secondary to infection of a primary knee procedure and nearly three times higher compared to an aseptic knee revision. Surgeons' billed charges were 50 % more for the infected revisions than for the non-infected revision cohort.

For an infected knee arthroplasty there was an average of 3.4 more operations and 2.4 more hospitalizations, with 3.7 times longer stay than that required for the primary total knees and 2.7 longer stay than that necessary for an aseptic revision. The total operative time required for a two-stage revision of an infected knee is 3.4 times more than that required for a primary total knee replacement and 1.8 times more than that of an aseptic revision [7, 11]. Bozic et al. [16] found that the total direct medical costs associated with revision total hip arthroplasty because of an infection are 2.8 times higher than the direct medical costs associated with revision total hip arthroplasty because of aseptic loosening and 4.8 times higher than the direct medical costs associated with primary total hip arthroplasty. Furthermore, revision of a total hip arthroplasty because of infection was associated with significantly more hospitalizations, total days in the hospital, number of operations, outpatient visits, outpatient charges, and complications than was revision because of aseptic loosening or primary total hip arthroplasty [68].

Several other studies have further reiterated that the human work and the system resources required for the treatment of an infected arthroplasty is three to four times more than those necessary for the treatment of a primary total joint replacement, and two to three times more than work and resources for an aseptic revision [7 – 12]. Some groups propose the single-stage exchange revision of an infected joint arthroplasty as a means to decrease costs and rehabilitation time and possibly to reduce the mechanical complications, however, the method is less likely to be more cost-effective than the two-stage exchange because of the higher probability for re-infection it carries, where the overall financial and emotional cost must also be added [39].

The lost opportunity for patients suffering from other health disorders which results from bad resource utilization in the management of musculoskeletal infections is another important parameter. Referring to the experience reported for the United Kingdom (UK), it has been estimated that in 2003 there have been performed 75,000 total joint replacements. At a mean follow-up of five to seven years, the infection rate was approximately 3 %, which means that 2250 arthroplasties probably became infected in the same period of time. With a mean direct cost of 75,000 pounds per patient, a crude estimation indicated that the total direct cost of management for the infected joint arthroplasties comes up to 170 million pounds, while the total health expenditure in the UK for 2003 reached 93 billion pounds [45]. That means that the treatment cost for the infected arthroplasties exceeded 0.18 % of the total health expenditures for that particular year. However, the percentage of those who are provided with the corresponding health services comprises only the 0.0037 % of the total UK population.

Except for the financial costs the infected joints impose on patients and their families, there is the emotional burden as well. Even in patients whose treatment was successful, 6 – 18 months are necessary in order to be able to regain function similar to the one they had prior to the infection [1]. Moreover some patients may never return to pre-infection levels of function.

In the case of life threatening systemic sepsis and when local tissue conditions or the host's general health status became severely impaired, a percentage of 5.7 % of 1058 total knee arthroplasties (a combined series) resulted in amputation. Besides, the periprosthetic infections, although rare, may become lethal with an overall mortality rate ranging from 1 to 2.7 % concerning patients around 65 years of age, but in patients older than 85 years it escalates from 2 to 7 %. In the first three months after rejection arthroplasty, the probability of death increases twofold [17, 23, 27, 37, 39, 73].

Malpractice

Malpractice insurance is most often obligatory, further increasing treatment costs. Because the presentation, diagnosis, treatment, and sequelae of poor treatment are well established, lawyers find that it is possible to prove that there was a deviation from care standards and that the actions of the physician were the proximate cause, scenario easily reproduced in case of infections [29]. Financial incentive may be a significant motivation for malpractice suits in certain populations, or in areas with high concentrations of attorneys. A 1997 review of a New York State malpractice database concluded that the incidence of malpractice claims correlated with the number of law firms filing malpractice claims, rather than the number of practising board-certified orthopaedic surgeons [54, 64]. Besides the factors that are beyond the control of the orthopaedic surgeon, malpractice claims can be broken down into two broad categories: technical errors and problems with communication. Although at times this is unavoidable, the literature is replete with various examples of the importance of strong physician-patient interaction and communication skills as a prophylaxis against unwarranted litigation [5, 76].

The surgeon's liability is based on number of procedures, complications and legal claims. Finally, the opportunity cost of specialized training for each physician specialized in infectious diseases, although hard to quantify, it must be identified and calculated as well.

Is There a Solution to the Problem?

It is obvious that the treatment of an infected total joint arthroplasty necessitates a team approach and especially the cooperation of specialized surgeons in musculoskeletal infections and in reconstructive orthopaedic surgery, microbiologists, pathologists, radiologists and physiotherapists, in order to accomplish a functional outcome to this devastating complication. In the process of cost identification, it is imperative to have a better insight on the considerable burden of the surgeon or the physicians managing bone and joint infections. Firstly, we have to take into consideration the total work of treating and especially the time spent, mental effort, judgement, technical skill, physical effort, stress and preoperative planning. Secondly, the relative specialty practice cost is of paramount importance. According to Barrack et al [11], revision procedures require significantly more from the surgeon in terms of time, mental and physical effort, stress, and exposure to liability. This is not reflected in the differential in reimbursements that are currently received as the amount reimbursed to the surgeon represented only 18 % of the total amount collected for the procedure. Surgeons, however, have not fared as well. Decreasing the length of stay and decreasing operative time requires more effort and probably a certain amount of increased risk on the part of the surgeon. All surgeons must conduct quality improvement as an integral part of patient care rather than viewing it as an externally-imposed burden unrelated to our practice goals. We should never hesitate to diagnose an infectious complication in one surgical procedure we have been involved, by developing a high index of suspicion and proceeding with the appropriate diagnostic approach and prompt management.

Reducing the Burden and Future Directions

Although, several investigators have demonstrated a direct association between hospital and surgeon procedure volume and better clinical outcomes in terms of readmissions, reoperations, complications, and mortality rates [41, 43, 69], the economic burden that results from the disproportionate resource utilization and the concomitant lack of incremental reimbursement will further contribute to the financial problems that currently plague many tertiary-care referral centers [14, 41, 43]. Due to these strong financial disincentives that have been created under current reimbursement patterns, certain high-volume joint replacement centers have already considered restricting access for patients with an infected total joint arthroplasty, resulting inevitably in a detrimental impact on access to care and clinical outcomes for patients who experience this debilitating complication.

The lowest reported rate of infection for total hip replacement is 0.4 % and for the total knee is up to 0.6 %. The question is then whether it is only difficult or impossible to reduce the infection rate. Dedicated joint replacement surgical teams help in decreasing the infection rates which have been higher in community-based hospitals [41 – 43]. If "lowest rates" had been reached by all hospitals there would have been huge cost savings and much less suffering. Following the process of clean room technology in the operative theatre environment is also of paramount importance whereas continuum and random evaluation should also be the basic priority of each surveillance committee.

Focusing on the three specific health care strategies including the prevention, diagnosis and effective treatment of infection, the wise use of antimicrobials and the prevention of transmission, the industry, the technology and especially biomedical engineering should proceed with priority on the manufacturing of implants which are less vulnerable to bacterial attachment.

The importance of economic analysis in the allocation of critical resources and evaluation of treatment options in orthopaedics is demonstrated by the growing number of papers that have been published on the subject [6, 15, 18 – 21, 24, 26, 28, 30, 32, 36, 40, 44, 46 – 53, 55, 57 – 60, 62, 63, 67, 70 – 72, 74, 79]. Unfortunately, very few of these studies adhered to the principles of sound economic analysis. In a review of forty economic evaluations of total knee arthroplasty published between 1966 and 1996, Saleh et al. found that none met the established criteria for a comprehensive economic evaluation [67]. In fact, many studies that are claimed to be so-called cost-effectiveness analyses are actually retrospective cost-identification analyses [15, 49]. The vast majority of the orthopaedic economic evaluations published over the past decade have been cost-identification or cost-minimization analyses. Many have focused on the costs associated with total joint arthroplasty [6, 22, 32, 49, 50, 57, 63, 79].

As far as septic joint arthroplasties are concerned, none of the published studies calculated total costs and especially direct medical costs and non- medical or indirect costs to the patient and to society associated with lost wages and productivity. So, limited data are available to payers who comprise increasingly demanding evidence of real costs and cost-effectiveness analyses. Also, limiting the analysis to data from a single institution potentially limits the generalizability of the results.

It is concluded from many economic studies that control of variable costs and basically implant's cost plays an important role in cost containment programmes. Research efforts should focus on the recycling of used or unused implants through biomechanics departments. Standardization and rationing of implants through competitive bidding systems should be an integral part of health care system and hospital-based strategies. Each hospital should promote a utilization control for reduction of services and unnecessary supplies. Early transfer to rehabilitation centres is a cost-shifting method by reducing the hospital cost. Control quality of practices and construction specialized in infectious diseases centres should be promoted by each national health care system.

Physicians, society members and politicians need to adopt a global view point of the musculoskeletal infections not only from the medical but also from the financial and the social–functional one. There is an urgent need for identification of the burden through further studying of the natural history of each separate group of orthopaedic infections, estimation of epidemiologic indices and selection of the best estimates, so that better practices are established to reduce the Burden.

References

1. Economic analysis of health care technology. A report on principles. Task Force on Principles for Economic Analysis of Health Care Technology (1995). Ann Intern Med 123(1):61–70
2. How to read clinical journals: VII. To understand an economic evaluation (part A) (1984) Can Med Assoc J 130(11):1428–1434
3. How to read clinical journals: VII. To understand an economic evaluation (part B) (1984). Can Med Assoc J 130(12):1542–1549
4. Ahnfelt L, Herberts P, Malchau H et al (1990) Prognosis of total hip replacement. A Swedish multicenter study of 4,664 revisions. Acta Orthop Scand Suppl (238):1–26
5. Baldwin DC Jr, Adamson TE, Self DJ et al (1996) Moral reasoning and malpractice. A pilot study of orthopedic surgeons. Am J Orthop 25(7):481–484
6. Barber TC, Healy WL (1993) The hospital cost of total hip arthroplasty. A comparison between 1981 and 1990. J Bone Joint Surg (Am) 75(3):321–325
7. Barrack RL (1995) Economics of revision total hip arthroplasty. Clin Orthop Relat Res (319):209–214
8. Barrack RL (1996) Implant matching has no clinical or scientific basis. J Arthroplasty 11(8):969–971
9. Barrack RL (1999) The evolving cost spectrum of revision hip arthroplasty. Orthopedics 22(9):865–866
10. Barrack RL, Engh G, Rorabeck C et al (2000) Patient satisfaction and outcome after septic versus aseptic revision total knee arthroplasty. J Arthroplasty 15(8):990–993
11. Barrack RL, Hoffman GJ, Tejeiro WV et al (1995) Surgeon work input and risk in primary versus revision total joint arthroplasty. J Arthroplasty 10(3):281–286
12. Barrack RL, Sawhney J, Hsu J et al (1999) Cost analysis of revision total hip arthroplasty. A 5-year followup study. Clin Orthop Relat Res (369):175–178
13. Behrens C, Henke K (1988) Cost of illness studies: no aid to decision making: Reply to Shiell et al. (Health Policy, 8 (1987) 317–323). Health Policy 10(2):137–141
14. Blumenthal D (2001) Unhealthy hospitals: addressing the trauma in academic medicine. Harvard Magazine, (ed.). www.harvardmagazine.com/on-line/0301138.html 103, 29–31. (GENERIC)
15. Boettcher WG (1992) Total hip arthroplasties in the elderly. Morbidity, mortality, and cost effectiveness. Clin Orthop Relat Res (274):30–34
16. Bozic KJ, Ries MD (2005) The impact of infection after total hip arthroplasty on hospital and surgeon resource utilization. J Bone Joint Surg (Am) 87(8):1746–1751
17. Brandt CM, Sistrunk WW, Duffy MC et al (1997) Staphylococcus aureus prosthetic joint infection treated with debridement and prosthesis retention. Clin Infect Dis 24(5):914–919
18. Burstein AH (1989) Cost-effectiveness of orthopaedic research. J Bone Joint Surg (Am) 71(7):1094–1097
19. Chan CL, Villar RN (1996) Obesity and quality of life after primary hip arthroplasty. J Bone Joint Surg (Br) 78(1):78–81
20. Chang RW, Pellisier JM, Hazen GB (1996) A cost-effectiveness analysis of total hip arthroplasty for osteoarthritis of the hip. JAMA 275(11):858–865
21. Clark CR (1994) Cost containment: total joint implants. J Bone Joint Surg (Am) 76(6): 799–800
22. Clark R, Anderson MB, Johnson BH et al (1996) Clinical value of radiologists' interpretations of perioperative radiographs of orthopedic patients. Orthopedics 19(12):1003–1007

23. Crockarell JR, Hanssen AD, Osmon DR et al (1998) Treatment of infection with debridement and retention of the components following hip arthroplasty. J Bone Joint Surg (Am) 80(9):1306–1313

24. Daellenbach HG, Gillespie WJ, Crosbie P et al (1990) Economic appraisal of new technology in the absence of survival data--the case of total hip replacement. Soc Sci Med 31(12):1287–1293

25. Drummond MF, Richardson WS, O'Brien BJ et al (1997) Users' guides to the medical literature. XIII. How to use an article on economic analysis of clinical practice. A. Are the results of the study valid? Evidence-Based Medicine Working Group. JAMA 27719):1552–1557

26. Faulkner A, Kennedy LG, Baxter K et al (1998) Effectiveness of hip prostheses in primary total hip replacement: a critical review of evidence and an economic model. Health Technol Assess 2(6):1–133

27. Fisman DN, Reilly DT, Karchmer AW et al (2001) Clinical effectiveness and cost-effectiveness of 2 management strategies for infected total hip arthroplasty in the elderly. Clin Infect Dis 32(3):419–430

28. Fitzpatrick R, Shortall E, Sculpher M et al (1998) Primary total hip replacement surgery: a systematic review of outcomes and modelling of cost-effectiveness associated with different prostheses. Health Technol Assess 2(20):1–64

29. Giar AH (1998) Orthopedic malpractice; prosecuting a case of failure to diagnose compartment syndrome. Medical Malpractice Law and Strategy 15:1

30. Gillespie WJ, Pekarsky B, O'Connell DL (1995) Evaluation of new technologies for total hip replacement. Economic modelling and clinical trials. J Bone Joint Surg (Br) 77(4):528–533

31. Hamblen DL (1993) Diagnosis of infection and the role of permanent excision arthroplasty. Orthop Clin North Am 24(4):743–749. Review

32. Healy WL, Finn D (1994) The hospital cost and the cost of the implant for total knee arthroplasty. A comparison between 1983 and 1991 for one hospital. J Bone Joint Surg (Am) 76(6):801–806

33. Hebert CK, Williams RE, Levy RS et al (1996) Cost of treating an infected total knee replacement. Clin Orthop Relat Res (331):140–145

34. Hodgson TA (1983) The state of the art of cost-of-illness estimates. Adv Health Econ Health Serv Res (4):129–164

35. Hodgson TA (1989) Cost of illness studies: no aid to decision making? Comments on the second opinion by Shiell et al (Health Policy, 8(1987):317–23). Health Policy 11:57–60

36. Hollingworth W, Mackenzie R, Todd CJ et al (1995) Measuring changes in quality of life following magnetic resonance imaging of the knee: SF-36, EuroQol or Rosser index? Qual Life Res 4(4):325–334

37. Hope PG, Kristinsson KG, Norman P et al (1989) Deep infection of cemented total hip arthroplasties caused by coagulase-negative staphylococci. J Bone Joint Surg (Br) 71(5):851–855

38. Hsiao WC, Braun P, Dunn D et al (1988) Resource-based relative values. An overview. JAMA 260(16):2347–2353

39. Jackson WO, Schmalzried TP (2000) Limited role of direct exchange arthroplasty in the treatment of infected total hip replacements. Clin. Orthop Relat Res (381):101–105

40. Jobanputra P, Parry D, Fry-Smith A et al (2001) Effectiveness of autologous chondrocyte transplantation for hyaline cartilage defects in knees: a rapid and systematic review. Health Technol Assess 5(11):1–57

41. Katz JN, Barrett J, Mahomed NN et al (2004) Association between hospital and surgeon procedure volume and the outcomes of total knee replacement. J Bone Joint Surg (Am) 86(9):1909–1916

42. Katz JN, Losina E, Barrett J et al (2001) Association between hospital and surgeon procedure volume and outcomes of total hip replacement in the United States medicare population. J Bone Joint Surg (Am) 83(11):1622–1629

43. Katz JN, Phillips CB, Baron JA et al (2003) Association of hospital and surgeon volume of total hip replacement with functional status and satisfaction three years following surgery. Arthritis Rheum. 48(2):560–568

44. Kocher MS, Erens G, Thornhill TS et al (2000) Cost and effectiveness of routine pathological examination of operative specimens obtained during primary total hip and knee replacement in patients with osteoarthritis. J Bone Joint Surg (Am) 82(11):1531–1535

45. L.Liaropoulos (2004) Hellenic Representative. Organization of Economic Cooperation and Development (OECD). Personal Communication
46. Launois R, Henry B, Marty JR et al. (1994) Chemonucleolysis versus surgical discectomy for sciatica secondary to lumbar disc herniation. A cost and quality-of-life evaluation. Pharmacoeconomics 6(5):453–463
47. Laupacis A, Bourne R, Rorabeck C et al (1994) Costs of elective total hip arthroplasty during the first year. Cemented versus noncemented. J Arthroplasty 9(5):481–487
48. Laupacis A, Feeny D, Detsky S et al (1992) How attractive does a new technology have to be to warrant adoption and utilization? Tentative guidelines for using clinical and economic evaluations. CMAJ 146(4):473–481
49. Lavernia CJ (1998) Cost-effectiveness of early surgical intervention in silent osteolysis. J Arthroplasty 13(3):277–279
50. Lavernia CJ, Drakeford MK, Tsao AK et al (1995) Revision and primary hip and knee arthroplasty. A cost analysis. Clin Orthop Relat Res (311):136–141
51. Liang MH, Cullen KE, Larson MG et al:(1986) Cost-effectiveness of total joint arthroplasty in osteoarthritis. Arthritis Rheum 29(8):937–943
52. Liang MH, Wade J, Hartley RM et al (1987) Social and health policy issues in total joint replacement surgery. Int J Technol Assess Health Care 3(3):387–395
53. Lord J, Victor C, Littlejohns P et al (1999) Economic evaluation of a primary care-based education programme for patients with osteoarthritis of the knee. Health Technol Assess 3(23):1–55
54. Mandell DB (2006) Malpractice trap can be sneaky. Am Acad Orthop Surg Bull Anonymous. 26, 1–3. (GENERIC)
55. Maniadakis N, Gray A (2000) Health economics and orthopaedics. J Bone Joint Surg (Br) 82(1):2–8. Review
56. Mendenhall S (2002) 2002 Hip and knee implant review. Orthop Network News 13(3):1–16
57. Meyers SJ, Reuben JD, Cox DD et al (1996) Inpatient cost of primary total joint arthroplasty. J Arthroplasty 11(3):281–285
58. Nakai,T, Masuhara K, Matsui M et al (2000) Therapeutic effect of transtrochanteric rotational osteotomy and hip arthroplasty on quality of life of patients with osteonecrosis. Arch Orthop Trauma Surg 120(5–6):252–254
59. Norman-Taylor FH, Palmer CR, Villar RN (1996) Quality-of-life improvement compared after hip and knee replacement. J Bone Joint Surg (Br) 78(1):74–77
60. Norman-Taylor FH, Villar RN (1997) Hybrid hip arthroplasty in the younger patient. Quality of life. J Arthroplasty 12(6):646–650
61. O'Donoghue MA, Allen KD (1992) Costs of an outbreak of wound infections in an orthopaedic ward. J Hosp Infect 22(1):73–79
62. Parker MJ, Myles JW, Anand JK et al (1992) Cost-benefit analysis of hip fracture treatment. J Bone Joint Surg (Br) 74(2):261–264
63. Reuben JD, Meyers SJ, Cox DD et al (1998) Cost comparison between bilateral simultaneous, staged, and unilateral total joint arthroplasty. J Arthroplasty 13(2):172–179
64. Ries MD, Bertino JS Jr, Nafziger AN (1997) Distribution of orthopaedic surgeons, lawyers, and malpractice claims in New York. Clin Orthop Relat Res (337):256–260
65. Rorabeck CH, Bourne RB, Laupacis A et al (1994) A double-blind study of 250 cases comparing cemented with cementless total hip arthroplasty. Cost-effectiveness and its impact on health-related quality of life. Clin Orthop Relat Res (298):156–164
66. Rothfuss J, Mau W, Zeidler H et al (1997) Socioeconomic evaluation of rheumatoid arthritis and osteoarthritis: a literature review. Semin Arthritis Rheum 26(5):771–779
67. Saleh KJ, Gafni A, Macaulay WB et al (1999) Understanding economic evaluations: a review of the knee arthroplasty literature. Am J Knee Surg 12(3):155–160
68. Salvati EA (2003) The infected total hip arthroplasty. Instr Course Lect (52):223–245
69. Sharkey PF, Shastri S, Teloken MA et al (2004) Relationship between surgical volume and early outcomes of total hip arthroplasty: do results continue to get better? J Arthroplasty 19(6):694–699
70. Shvartzman L, Weingarten E, Sherry H et al (1992) Cost-effectiveness analysis of extended conservative therapy versus surgical intervention in the management of herniated lumbar intervertebral disc. Spine 17(2):176–182

71. Sommers LS, Schurman DJ, Jamison JQ et al (1990) Clinician-directed hospital cost management for total hip arthroplasty patients. Clin Orthop Relat Res (258):168–175

72. Swiontkowski MF, Chapman JR (1995) Cost and effectiveness issues in care of injured patients. Clin Orthop Relat Res (318):17–24

73. Ure KJ, Amstutz HC, Nasser S et al (1998) Direct-exchange arthroplasty for the treatment of infection after total hip replacement. An average ten-year follow-up. J Bone Joint Surg (Am) 80(7):961–968

74. Wang C, Ghalambor N, Zarins B et al (2005) Arthroscopic versus open Bankart repair: analysis of patient subjective outcome and cost. Arthroscopy 21(10):1219–1222

75. Washington, DUSGPO (2001) The Council of Economic Advisors. Economic Report of the President. Anonymous. 107–58. 2001 (GENERIC)

76. Weycker DA, Jensen GA (2000) Medical malpractice among physicians: who will be sued and who will pay? Health Care Manag Sci 3(4):269–277

77. Whitehouse JD, Friedman ND, Kirkland KB et al (2002) The impact of surgical-site infections following orthopedic surgery at a community hospital and a university hospital: adverse quality of life, excess length of stay, and extra cost. Infect Control Hosp Epidemiol 23(4):183–189

78. Wiklund I, Romanus B (1991) A comparison of quality of life before and after arthroplasty in patients who had arthrosis of the hip joint. J Bone Joint Surg (Am) 73(5):765–769

79. Zuckerman JD, Kummer FJ, Frankel VH (1994) The effectiveness of a hospital-based strategy to reduce the cost of total joint implants. J Bone Joint Surg (Am) 76(6):807–811

Orthopaedic Device-related Infections

Epidemiology and Classification of Septic Total Hip Replacement

G. SESSA, V. PAVONE, L. COSTARELLA

Deparment of Surgical Medical Sciences, Section of Orthopaedics and Traumatology
University of Catania, Italy

Introduction

The list of potential complications following total hip arthroplasty is extensive. Aside from the life threatening complications of total hip replacement, no post-operative complication can be more devastating than infection.

Deep post-operative wound infection complicating total hip replacement were relatively uncommon since the new era of joint replacement began with Sir John Charnley in the early sixties [3]. The infection rate in those years ranged from 7 % to 10 % and has been relatively stable since the introduction of prophylactic antibiotics with gradual improvement (Table 1).

The actual rate of infection ranged from 0.5 % to 3.0 % for primary total hip replacement and 3 – 6 % after revision hip surgery. These values were achieved by the access to laminar flow, body exhaust suite, high airflow, ultraviolet lights, improvements in room discipline (limiting the number of personnel, decreasing traffic, improved barrier draping, use of sterile suction systems), and better surgical approaches and techniques [7]. Antibiotic prophylaxis together with a more careful preoperative evaluation of patients has also been effective in decreasing the infection rate. *Staphylococcus aureus* is the most common cause of acute infection after surgery, *Staphylococcus epidermidis* and *Staphylococcus albus* are common causes of late infection [16] (Table 2). The awareness of the emergence of resistant bacterial flora

Table 1. Incidence of septic primary total hip arthroplasty

Authors	Years	Incidence
Charnley, Eftekhar [3]	1969	6.80
Wilson et al [18]	1972	11.00
Patterson, Brown [11]	1972	8.20
Brady et al [1]	1975	1.30
Hill et al [8]	1981	1.50
Salvati et al [13]	1982	2.00
Lidwell et al [10]	1982	1.50
Schutzer, Harris [15]	1988	1.20
Fitzgerald [7]	1995	0.50
Di Giovanni et al [5]	2000	1.00
Joseph et al [9]	2003	0.30–2.00
Phillips et al [12]	2003	0.50–2.00
Sessa et al [16]	2006	2.2

Micro-Organism	Incidence
Staphylococcus epidermidis	36%
Staphylococcus aureus	29%
Enterococcus faecalis	4%
Escherichia coli	3%
Pseudomonas spp.	2%
Polymicrobial agents	16%
Anaerobes	5%
Others	5%

Table 2. Infecting agents in primary total hip arthroplasty

and the capacity of micro-organism to form the glycocalyx, a polysaccharide biofilm that permits increased adherence and survival of bacteria on biosynthetic surfaces, thereby conferring resistance to the hosts' humoral and cellular defences has been helpful in treating delayed infections.

Coventry classified infected total hip in 1975 into three categories: acute postoperative infections (infection is caused by contamination at the time of the operation), delayed infections (usually at least eight weeks after operation in the form of an indolent, chronic, low grade infection) and late hematogenous infections (it can happen at any time with a presentation similar to that of acute infection [4]. This classification was revised by Fitzgerald on the basis of when the symptoms begin and the cause of the infection. Stage I (Acute postoperative infections) include the classic fulminant postoperative infection, the infected hematoma and the superficial infection that progresses to a deep infection [7]. In this stage purulent materials draining from a red and swollen postoperative wound in a febrile patient can be seen and the major challenge consists in differentiating a superficial from a deep infection. Stage II (Delayed deep infections) is characterized by a painful total hip replacement with a patient that has a well healed wound. Usually the patient has had pain from the time of surgery without history of fever, chills or postoperative wound drainage. Clinical signs and radiographic findings can simulate aseptic mechanical loosening of one or both components of the implant. Laboratory findings such as serum C-reactive protein level, ESR, haemoglobin level, peripheral leukocyte count, may or may not be elevated. Aspiration of the hip permits recovery of the causative agent in more than two thirds of cases of infected total hip arthroplasty. Scintigraphy, especially the new modern modalities, is gradually becoming more specific and accurate and could be helpful in distinguishing aseptic from septic loosening of painful arthroplasties [7]. Stage III (Late hematogenous infections) diagnosis poses little difficulty. Patients typically complain of an acute onset of pain, with laboratory tests usually revealing elevation in sedimentation rate, C-reactive protein, and white blood cell count [7].

Other classifications are described in literature. To better characterize the cause of deep periprosthetic infection, Schmalzried et al described four modes of infections: Mode 1 characterized by surgical contaminations, Mode 2 by haematogenous spread, Mode 3 by a recurrence of sepsis in a previously infected hip and Mode 4 by contiguous spread of infection from local source [14].

Tsukayama et al proposed another four category classification: positive intraoperative cultures only (need of revision); early postoperative infections (occurring less than one month postoperatively); late chronic infections (occurring more than one month postoperatively with an insidious onset); and acute haematogenous infections [17].

Estrada et al refined the classification of periprosthetic infection proposed by Coventry in 1975, with the addition of a category to add the patient who had positive intraoperative cultures without other features of obvious infection [6]. Those authors described postoperative infections as occurring either early (within one month after the operation) or late (more than one month after the operation). In addition, acute haematogenous infection may present at any stage in a hip joint that has been asymptomatic.

Although classifications are important, diagnosis of infected total hip replacement is not easy. In our opinion it is imperative to perform an integrated assessment utilizing all data available through a precise, in depth history, careful physical examination, laboratory parameters, imaging procedures and microbiological analysis in order to identify the micro organism responsible for the infection. Often pathogen identification can be reached only with aspiration of joint fluid or with intraoperative histological examination of pathologic specimen. With a correct diagnosis it is possible to establish the best operative treatment with different options that include debridement with retention of the prosthesis, immediate one stage exchange arthroplasty, excision arthroplasty either as a definitive, permanent procedure or as the first of a two or even three stage reconstructive procedure. The choice of a particular treatment is influenced by many factors including the acuteness or chronicity of the infection, the causative micro organism, its sensitivity profile to antibiotics, its ability to manufacture glycocalyx, the overall health of the patient, the fixation of the implant, the quality and availability of bone stock, and the experience of the surgeon.

Case Series

At the Orthopaedic and Traumatologic Clinic of Catania University, between January 1995 and February 2005, 1422 total hip replacement were performed in 1380 patients with a mean age of 70 years (range 55 – 87 years). In 557 cases the implant was cemented in both acetabular and femoral component in 865 we utilized biological prosthesis. The implant was necessary for both degenerative (58 % of cases) and traumatic disorders (42 %). We had 31 deep infected prosthesis (2.2 %) in 20 females and 11 males with a mean age of 69 years (range 64 – 78 years). According to the classification proposed by Coventry [4] the infection were acute (3), chronic (23), haematogenous (5). There were 13 cemented and 18 biological prosthesis that failed after a mean time of 2 years. One or more co morbidities were present in all of our patients (Table 3). 67 % of our group of study comprised actual or former smoker for more than 35 years. *S. epidermidis* and *S. aureus* were the most frequently isolated causal organism making up 65% of all cases.

The group of study was treated with one stage revision procedure in two cases, with definitive Girdlestone in 3 cases and with two stage procedure for 26 patients (Fig. 1). We utilized an antibiotic loaded spacer in 63 % of cases, systemic antibiotic therapy was performed for 35 days, reconstructive procedure was carried out after a mean time of 8 months when all the laboratory parameter, imaging procedures and aspiration were negative.

Factor	Incidence
Inflammatory arthritis	8%
Chronic renal insufficiency	17%
Malignacy	13%
Metabolic diseases	11%
Immunodeficency	7%
Obesity	11%
Skin disorders	6%
Diabetes mellitus	20%
Other conditions	7%

Table 3. Co-morbidity in septic primary total hip arthroplasty

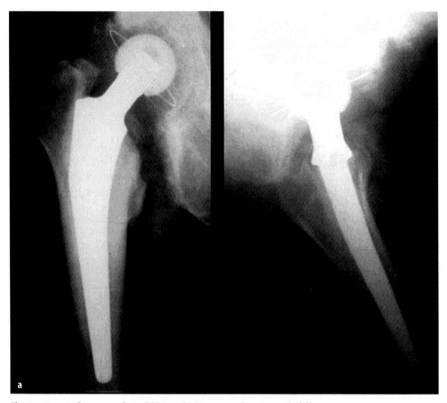

Fig. 1a. X-ray of cemented total hip replacement at the 6-month follow-up

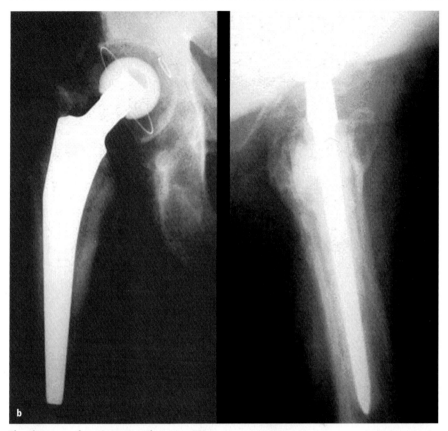

Fig. 1b. X-ray of septic THR at the 1-year FU

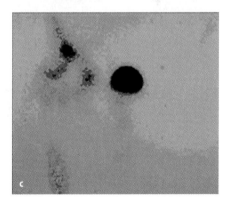

Fig. 1c. Bone scintigraphy positive at the 15-months FU. Joint aspiration identified *S. aureus.*

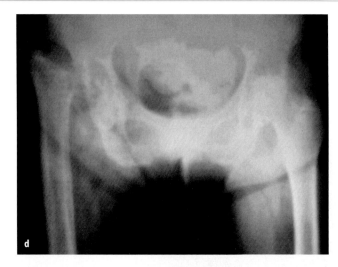

Fig. 1d. X-ray with excision arthroplasty after 1 year of prosthesis removal

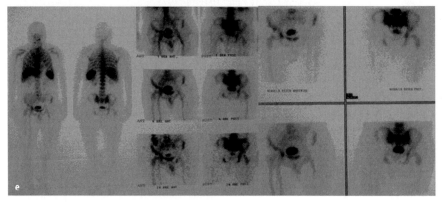

Fig. 1e. Bone scintigraphy negative after 1 year of prosthesis removal. Preoperative joint aspiration negative

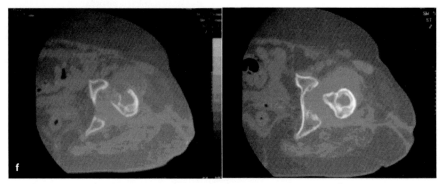

Fig. 1f. CT-scan performed for preoperative planning to evaluate residual bone stock

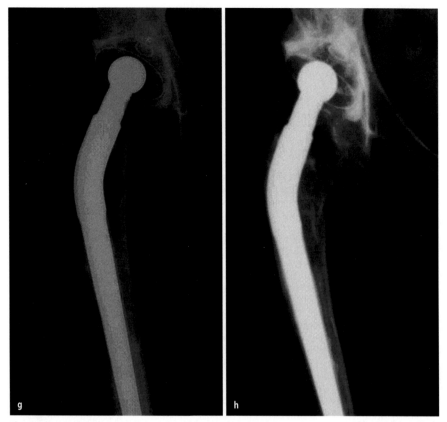

Fig. 1g. X-ray showing revision arthroplasty with antibiotic cemented cup and biological long stem at the 6-months FU; **h** follow-up at 3,5 years from revision arthroplasty

At a mean follow up of 43 months, 30 on 31 patients had no evidence of recurrent infection with only one patient presented with a definitive wound infection treated with a resection arthroplasty. We had two postoperative dislocation treated conservatively and the modified Harris hip score improved from 39 pre operatively to 71 (range 51–92). Radiographically we had two cases of heterotopic ossification (Brooker 2) [2], one acetabular component migration that was revised and one peri-prosthetic fracture.

Conclusion

In conclusion the incidence of deep infection after total hip replacement has decreased significantly with improvements in operating room discipline and surgical technique, better preoperative assessment of the patient and the prophylactic administration of antibacterial agents. Classification is important but the diagnosis of deep sepsis is not always easy. It can be made on the basis of clinical history, physical examination, laboratory and imaging studies. It is mandatory to detect the micro organism in order to establish the best treatment.

References

1. Brady LP, Enneking WF, Franco JA (1975) The effect of operating room environment on the infection rate after Charnley low-friction total hip replacement. J Bone Joint Surg (Am) 57(1):80–83.
2. Brooker AF, Bowerman JW, Robinson RA et al (1973) Ectopic ossification following total hip replacement. Incidence and a method of classification. J Bone Joint Surg (Am) 55(8): 1629–1632.
3. Charnley J, Eftekhar N (1969) Postoperative infection in total prosthetic replacement arthroplasty of the hip-joint: with special reference to the bacterial content of the air of the operating room. Br J Surg 56(9):641–649.
4. Coventry MB (1975) Treatment of infections occurring in total hip surgery. Orthop Clin North Am 6(4):991–1003.
5. Di Giovanni CW, Saleh KJ, Salvati EA et al (2000) Deep Infection Complicating Total Hip Arthroplasty. In Orthopaedic Knowledge Update (2000) AAOS, 137–149.
6. Estrada R, Tsukayama D, Gustilo R (1994) Management of THA infections. A prospective study of 108 cases. Orthop Trans (17):1114–1115.
7. Fitzgerald MD, Robert H (1995) Infected total hip arthroplasty: diagnosis and treatment. J Am Acad Orthop Surg (3):249–262.
8. Hill C, Mazas F, Flamant R et al (1981) Prophylactic cefazolin versus placebo in total hip replacement: report of a multicentre double-blind randomised trial Lancet 1(8224):795–796.
9. Joseph TN, Chen AL, Di Cesare P (2003) Use of antibiotic impregnated cement in total joint arthroplasty. J Am Acad Orthop Surg 11(1):38–47.
10. Lidwell OM, Lowbury EJL, Whyte W et al (1982) Effect of ultraclean air in operating rooms on deep sepsis in the joint after total hip or knee replacement: a randomised study, Br Med J 285(6334):10–14.
11. Patterson FP, Brown CS (1972) The McKee-Farrar total hip replacement: preliminary results and complication of 368 operation performed in five general hospitals, J Bone Joint Surg (Am) 54(2):257–275.
12. Phillips CB, Barrett JA, Losina E et al (2003) Incidence rate of dislocation pulmonary embolism, and deep infection during the first six months after elective total hip replacement. J Bone Joint Surg (Am) 85(1):20–26.
13. Salvati EA, Robinson RP, Zeno SM et al (1982) Infection rates after 3175 total hip and total knee replacements performed with and without a horizontal unidirectional filter air-flow system, J Bone Joint Surg (Am) 64(4):525–535.
14. Schamalzried TP, Amstutz HC, Au MK (1992) Etiology of deep deep sepsis in total hip arthroplasty: the significance of hematogenous and recurrent infections. Clin Orthop Relat Res (280):200–207.
15. Schutzer SF, Harris WH (1988) Deep-wound infection after total hip replacement under contemporaney aseptic condition J Bone Joint Surg (Am) 70(5):724–727.
16. Sessa G, Costarella L, Pavone V et al (2006) Diagnostic protocol for septic total hip replacement: our experience. In XXV Annual Meeting of European Bone and Joint Infection Society.
17. Tsukayama DT, Estrada R, Gustilo RB (1996) Infection after total hip arthroplasty: a study of the treatment of one hundred and six infections. J Bone Joint Surg (Am) 78(4):512–523
18. Wilson PD, Amstutz HC, Czerniecki A et al (1972) Total hip replacement with fixation by acrylic cement: a preliminary study of 100 consecutive Mckee-Farrar prosthetic replacements. J Bone Joint Surg (Am) 54(2):207–236.

Early Radiological Diagnosis and Differential Diagnosis of Infection in Orthopaedic Surgery

M.B. Gallazzi, R. Chiapparino, P.G. Garbagna

Department of Radiology, "G. Pini" Orthopaedic Institute, Milan, Italy

Introduction

Today, peri-prosthetic septic complications are considered rare (between 1–2% of joint arthroplasties) due to the improvement of prophylactic measures and techniques developed in orthopaedic surgery in the recent years, which have enabled to control infections. However, these are particularly negative in terms of the patients' outcome due to the high morbidity and the considerable medical costs related to their management. In the event of infection, two operations are often required after the original one to try to eradicate it and in many cases the treatment is not successful, having to sacrifice the prosthesis itself and leaving the patient heavily disabled in his movements. In the United States it was estimated that a minimum cost of 50,000 $ would be required for the treatment of each single patient, with an annual cost of 250 million $ [11, 18].

Moreover, if in the past identifying a patient carrying an infection around the prosthetic hardware was considered an uncommon event outside the major hospitals where this type of surgery is a routine practice, nowadays this problem can be frequently found even in Radiology Departments of small hospitals, according to the diffusion of prosthetic surgery.

Due to the high diagnostic and the therapeutic management costs spent on septic patients, as well as the infection's pronounced tendency to become chronic and to relapse with time, it is very important to define specific guidelines aimed at reaching an early and accurate diagnosis of the infection and/or monitoring relapses, thus avoiding a dangerous waste of economic and instrumental resources through a correct use of the various diagnostic techniques.

Radiological Techniques

About 60 % of peri-prosthetic infections depend on direct implant of bacteria during the operation. In the other cases, contamination takes place through the blood, originating from endogenous centres of chronical infection. During the period straight after the surgery, traumatized ischemic soft tissues are an ideal ground for the implant of bacteria. Furthermore, the barrier effect assured by the fasciae is missing due to their surgical incision. The deep peri-prosthetic tissues are thus exposed to septic contamination [8, 15, 16].

Once implanted, the prosthesis is progressively coated by a glycoprotein layer, which favours the superficial adhesion of bacteria. These are, themselves, coated with a biofilm composed of polysaccharides (glycocalyx) which protects them from the host's immunity system and from antibiotics [3, 7, 24].

This physiopathological background is essential to understand the different ways in which infections develop, according to the time of onset after the surgical traumatism. Early infections (1–2 months after the operation) are normally only limited to peri-prosthetic soft tissues, without affecting the bone-prosthesis interface.

Delayed or late infections (from 6 months to many years after the operation) have as main target the peri-prosthetic bone. Soft tissues around the prosthesis may or may not be involved in a subordinate way according to the aggressiveness of the process and its extension in the tissues [1, 17].

In the diagnosis of peri-prosthetic infections, the role and the diagnostic power of the various radiological techniques strongly depend on these critical aspects.

The radiological work-up that can be used in the diagnosis of peri-prosthetic infections is varied and complicated. This implies that the doctor who prescribes the radiological tests has a good knowledge of their characteristics as well as their strong and weak points. This is the only way in which specific diagnostic protocols can be created, which enable an accurate but even a cost-effective approach to the infection at the same time.

Radiography

In order to maximize the diagnostic power of plain radiography (PR), it is essential to have a correct executive technique. In particular, it is important to carry out at least 2 projections (AP and axial for hip prostheses, AP and LL for knee prostheses), since this is the only way of evaluating the whole bone-prosthesis interface, thus avoiding "blind areas" that can interfere with the analysis of the radiologist and that can possibly delay the diagnosis. Furthermore, the correct exposure of the radiogram must be carefully verified. In fact, underexposures can hide initial signs of infection, while overexposures are often the cause of false positive results. In this context, digital radiology is certainly better than the conventional technique, since it has wider exposure latitude and reduces the frequency of exposure errors. Finally, in order to allow a better evaluation of the details, it is always recommended to have post-operation radiograms which show the bone-prosthesis situation at "time zero" making it possible to identify even minimal changes during follow-up studies, which would not be otherwise identifiable.

Despite the development of more sophisticated radiological techniques, PR still remains the mainstay in evaluating arthroplasties. This is both because X-ray films are easily available at a low cost (no matter how specialized the hospital is) and because it is essential for a correct interpretation of the information that can be collected from other diagnostic techniques to be eventually applied. In particular, PR is important for the exclusion of non-septic causes that can cause a painful prosthesis (sprain, mechanical movement, stress shielding with a tip effect, peri-prosthetic calcification, etc.). PR is specific: if typical signs of a septic process are identified on X-ray films (peri-prosthetic osteoporosis, periosteal reaction, erosions of the endosteal profile, peri-prosthetic osteolysis) the diagnosis is already carried out (Fig. 1). In

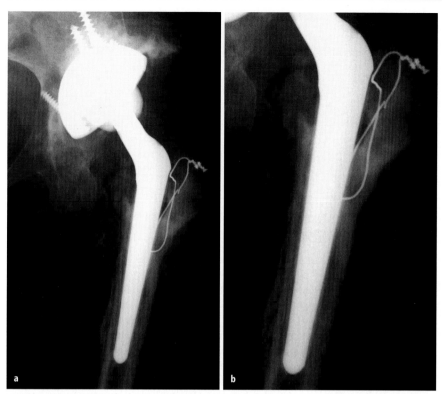

Fig. 1. Radiological signs of femoral peri-prosthetic infection (**a**) osteolysis of the trochanters, multi-laminated periosteal reaction on the internal diaphyseal cortical profile; (**b**) the same radiographic findings are better seen in the expanded view of the meta-diaphyseal region

this case all other radiological techniques only have a complementary role: they are only needed to evaluate the extension of the infection.

Unfortunately, PR has poor sensitivity. Between 3–6 months may be required from the clinical onset of the infection to have the radiological evidence of the process. There is also no correlation between the presence of the infection and the mobilization degree [6, 9, 17, 22, 23].

As a result, the test only has a predictive value if it is positive, but it has a limited predictive value if it is negative. For painful prostheses, PR must therefore be recommended as a screening procedure in addition to blood inflammation tests [9]. If it has a negative result, the diagnosis procedure must continue, since the infection cannot be totally ruled out only on the basis of negative X-ray films.

Finally, it is worth underlining that PR gives informations only on the bone-prosthesis interface, while it does not provide significant evidence on what is going on in the soft tissues around the prosthesis which, as we have reminded, are the main target of early infections and can be also involved in delayed and late infections.

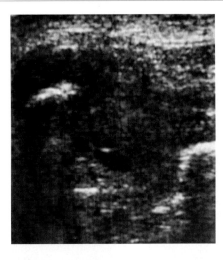

Fig. 2. US picture of bulky corpuscolated inflammatory collection between pseudo-capsule and prosthesis

Ultrasonography

In the last few years, ultrasonography (US) has acquired a growing importance in the diagnostic identification and in the follow-up of peri-prosthetic infections. Thanks to its high spatial resolution, US can easily identify abscesses in soft tissues (Fig. 2) defining their morphological characters and dimensions, their spatial relations with local and regional vascular bundles, the existence of fistulous tracts (joined or not to the skin surface). US is also the most common guiding technique for biopsies, aspirations and for placing drain tubes into abscesses. It is therefore a fundamental diagnostic technique. However, US also has some limitations: it is operator dependent, and, moreover, it is unable to evaluate bony involvement by infectious processes. It is therefore a cause of false negative results of peri-prosthetic infections that are limited to the bone. Finally, US has a limited specificity in the differential diagnosis between abscess and haematoma.

Aspiration/Biopsy of Peri-prosthetic Collections

This is a main step of the diagnostic procedure for peri-prosthetic infections. In fact, withdrawing peri-prosthetic specimens, not only enables to confirm or exclude the infection, but it also allows the identification of the bacterial agent. This goal is considered important for at least two reasons.

The first one is that the bacterial strain determines the biological behaviour of the infection. For example, *Staphylococcus aureus* can cause acute and extremely aggressive infections. Instead if the pathogenous are coagulase-negative *Staphylococcus* or Gram-negative bacteria, the infectious processes can be more subtle and have a slower clinical evolution but it has a high tendency to become chronic. In this way the isolation of the organism in infected prosthesis gives one forecast of the aggressiveness the infection.

The second reason is that the identification of the bacteria enables to test their sensitivity towards various antibiotics. It is therefore possible to order a specific and therefore more effective antibiotic therapy.

In fact data from literature indicate that antibiotic sensitivity is extremely variable in bacterial strains that most frequently cause peri-prosthetic infections. *S. aureus* sensitivity to methicillin and cephalosporins ranges between 53 % and 95 %. *S. epidermidis* sensitivity to methicillin is 70 %. The resistance of peri-prosthetic *Enterococcus* to vancomycin reaches 23 % [5]. These data emphasizes the need of identifying the pathogen before starting with the antibiotic therapy.

Clinical studies dealing with the role of peri-prosthetic aspiration in the diagnosis of infections have also been shown variable sensitivity (ranging from 50 to 92 %) and specificity (ranging from 88 to 97 %) [4, 10, 20]. The technique used to perform the aspiration is a critical factor [23]. The patient should not have been treated for at least two weeks before the procedure. US or CT must be the imaging modalities of choice for guiding the aspiration or at least it has to take place under fluoroscopy, in order to obtain a precise withdrawal. It is also important to collect as much material as possible (fluid and tissue specimens from the abscess). If direct aspiration is insufficient, wash-out by means of peri-prosthetic injection of physiological solution is recommended. Part of the material obtained must be submitted to histological evaluation because if a significative number of neutrophils is found in the sampled tissue, this can contribute to carry out the diagnosis.

CT and MR

CT and MR are not routinely used in the diagnostic work-up of peri-prosthetic infections, since the metallic implants heavily degrade the quality of the studies to the point that they loose most of their clinical significance [25]. Modified acquisition techniques to the MR have recently been introduced. They reduce the weight of the metal artefacts and seem to improve the ability of MR in evaluating the location and extension of peri-prosthetic osteolysis. If these preliminary data will be confirmed by further studies, in future MR may have a role in the diagnosis of peri-prosthetic infections [14]. Finally, CT suffers from the same diagnostic limitations of MR due to metal artefacts, but, anyway, it can be used to guide peri-prosthetic aspiration procedures, as an alternative technique to fluoroscopy or US (Fig. 3).

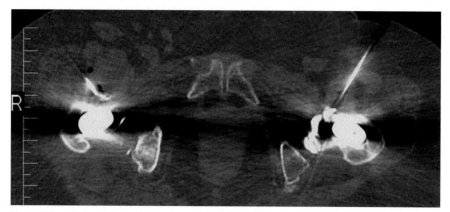

Fig. 3. CT-guided needle-aspiration in peri-prosthetic bilateral inflammatory collection

Radionuclide Imaging

Radionuclide imaging gives an important contribution to the diagnosis of patients suspected of having infection. Particular reference must be made to three-phase bone scan (BS) and labelled autologous leukocyte scintigraphy (WBS), while the role of the FDG-PET in distinguishing aseptically loosened prosthesis and infected one is still uncertain and it is currently under investigation.

BS with Tc99m methylendiphosphonate (MDP) is the most common nuclear medicine procedure used. MDP tends to spread into the tissues, having a bimodal distribution. At an early stage (from the moment of injection up to a few minutes later) it diffuses in soft tissues and bone, according to the local blood flow. At a later stage (2–4 hours after the injection) its main target is the bone, where it concentrates in an amount depending on the rate of new bone formation.

BS is a highly sensitive technique but it is not very specific for infections, since even only small alterations in the local bone metabolism, despite their matrix, can produce a positive bone scan. Furthermore, BS shows an increase local uptake for many months after the prosthesis implant, even if it is well tolerated, which greatly limits its diagnostic use during the period straight after the operation (normally up to 6 months). A cautious use even for longer periods after surgery is also recommended [1].

However, an important consideration needs to be made. A completely negative BS (in all its phases) virtually excludes the infection. A positive BS (hyperaemia of the peri-prosthetic tissues in the early stages, late increase of the uptake in the bone), even if this scintigraphic pattern is not limited to the infection, makes the presence of an infection suspected and therefore justifies further diagnostic procedures addressed to rule out this complication [13, 19].

Tc99m-hexamethylprophyleneamine oxime (HMPAO) WBS is the currently radionuclide gold standard in the diagnosis of peri-prosthetic infections in immunocompetent patients. Since most of the labelled cells are neutrophils, this procedure is useful especially in imaging inflammations which have neutrophils as cellular effectors. To this purpose, it should be underlined that aseptic mobilization is in many cases caused by an aseptic immune reaction towards the prosthesis, but in these cases the peri-prosthetic inflammatory infiltrate is mainly composed of hystiocytes, macrophages and lymphocytes while neutrophils (the principal cellular line in the infection) are virtually absent. This explains why WBS is negative in case of aseptic mobilization, while it is positive in case of septic one, with a diagnostic accuracy higher than 90 % [12].

Unfortunately WBS has same practical limitations. It is a technique based on a complicated procedure of "*in vitro*" cell labelling, which requires specialized equipment and staff. It is, therefore, expensive both in terms of time and of economic resources employed. It is not indicated as a screening technique for peri-prosthetic infections, but only for those patients that, on the basis of a preliminary diagnostic work-up, are suspected to harbour a peri-prosthetic infection. In other words, WBS cannot be performed on patients having a negative BS, since the pre-test probability of infection is extremely low and therefore the WBS does not give a significant diagnostic contribution. Similarly, its use is questionable for those patients whose infection diagnosis is already sure, on the basis of tests that have already been carried out. Even in this case, it does not provide any additional information.

Finally, WBS can give both false positive results (especially if carried out during the first 2–3 months after surgery, when reactive/reparatory phenomena related to the surgical trauma are still in course) and false negative results (in chronical peri-prosthetic infections which have a low activity or if performed without an adequate break in the antibiotic therapy). Late acquisitions (usually after 24 hours) have shown to improve the specificity of WBS in these conditions.

As stated before the role of FDG-PET in the diagnosis of peri-prosthetic infections is still under debate. Initial investigations were encouraging, reporting sensitivity and specificity higher than 90 % [2, 26]. More recent studies highlight aspecific uptake of 18F-FDG even in non-infected prosthesis, thus questioning the ability of FDG-PET to provide a clear diagnosis [21].

Diagnostic Purposes in Infections

Once the features of the available radiological techniques have been defined, their position with respect to clinical problems needs to be clarified.

In general, the aims of the diagnosis in infections are:

- Differential diagnosis: in the event of a painful prosthesis it is important to distinguish if the pain is generated by a mechanical intolerance/mobilization or by an infection. Moreover, it should be noted that an accurate diagnosis of the infection is not sufficient. It must be carried out as quickly as possible because the process can be controlled with minimally invasive medical or surgical therapies only if it has a limited extension in the tissues. Otherwise, if it is extensive, radical intervention is required which causes serious limitations to the patient's *"quoad valetudinem"* prognosis. It is also more difficult in this case to eradicate the infection completely.
- Staging: once the infection has been identified, in order to plan a proper surgery it is important to give to the surgeon clear information on the local extension of the infection, on its distance from local and regional vascular bundles and on its eventual spreading to adjacent anatomical districts (a typical example is the spreading of infections from hip prosthesis to the pelvic area). In fact, in case of limited processes focal surgical "toilette" may be effective, thus sparing the prosthesis. Otherwise, the implant needs to be removed and a two-stage surgery should be planned.
- Identification of the bacterial strain that causes the infection on the basis of the above described considerations.
- Monitoring of the relapses: since therapies in many cases do not allow a complete healing of the septic process but they obtain only its transformation into a chronic form with a low biological activity, which may develop one or more other acute relapses during the rest of the patient's life, it is critical to establish a follow-up programme based on few but significant tests in order to improve the diagnostic yield, while minimizing management costs.

Radiological Diagnostic Protocols

Considering the forementioned diagnostic purposes, the various types of imaging techniques need to be carefully used in order to get a specific diagnosis, but taking into account that since time is a critical factor for the success of therapies, an over-use of diagnostic procedures is often harmful. This imaging over-use, usually, not only fails to provide further contributions in the management of the patient's infections, but it lengthens the time interval between the clinical onset of the sickness and its diagnostic identification.

The differential diagnosis obviously represents the nodal and also the most critical point. First of all, the radiologist needs to know the patient's clinical background (existence of local and/or general risk factors, general symptoms and local signs suggesting infection) as well as laboratory data (white blood cells count, erythrocyte sedimentation rate, C-reactive protein). As indicated above, in order to decide the best instrumental approach, it is also important to distinguish infections on the basis of the time that elapsed between their onset and surgery, because their biological behaviour is different and each type has particular properties that influence the diagnostic and therapeutic options. According to this criterion, infections can be classified in:

- Early: they occur within the first-second month after the prosthetic implant. These infections are related to bacteria that are implanted during the operation and they are normally located in the soft peri-prosthetic tissues, since surgical trauma (producing ischemia, tissue necrosis and haematomas) creates the ideal conditions in the muscles and connectives that favour the implant and development of bacteria, thus causing abscesses. Usually, the bone-prosthesis interface is not involved and this explains why these infections have a good prognosis and tend to heal and spare the prosthesis if they are rapidly identified. Considering these characters, if an early infection is clinically suspected, the first diagnostic technique of choice is US. If US is negative, it virtually rules out the infection. On the contrary, if it highlights the existence of deep and/or superficial hypo-anechoic collections, it supports the clinical suspicion, even if the picture is not specific. In fact, as noted above, it is not always possible to distinguish a simple post-surgical haematoma from an abscess only on the basis of sonographic elements. Unfortunately in the case of early infections, both BS and WBS share with US the same limits of specificity. PR does not normally provide any particular contribution both because the bone usually is not involved in early infections and because PR, anyway, has a long latency in manifesting the bony signs of the infection. An effective diagnosis of infection is performed by means of US or CT guided needle aspiration/biopsy of the collections, withdrawing tissue samples that are submitted to microbiological and histological evaluations. In particular, counting white blood cells in the aspirated peri-prosthetic fluid is very useful. Indeed, if the number of white cells is higher than $400/mm^3$ this strongly suggests an infection around the prosthesis. It is also highly probable when the number of neutrophils (per high power field at a magnification of x 400) detected in peri-prosthetic frozen tissue is more than five. In our institutional experience, peri-prosthetic aspiration/biopsy has revealed to be a simple method that has a low cost and allows a reliable diagnosis and monitoring of infections. Once the real nature of the process has been established, US provides the surgeon with precious information on the process's extension in the soft tissues, so that he can correctly plan a surgical "toilette" to support the antibiotic therapy.
- Delayed and late: these types of infection occur between a few months and 10 – 15 years after the prosthesis has been implanted. It should be considered that if the

infection risk reduces with time, it never falls to zero. Delayed and late infections are caused by a haematogenous spreading of bacteria localized in remote areas (lungs, intestine, urinary system, teeth, etc.). But the possibility of a local reactivation of bacteria that reached the bone-prosthesis interface during surgery and harboured there in a latent way cannot be totally excluded. Unlike early infections, they originate in the bone and only later can colonize the peri-prosthetic soft tissues. PR can show signs of the infection (porosis and/or osteolysis of the peri-prosthetic bone, periostal reactions, etc.) but due to its well-known sensitivity limits, it can be falsely negative even if a peri-prosthetic infection is going on. In any case, US must follow PR. Indeed, if the diagnosis has already been established on radiographic elements, US completes the evaluation of the extension of the process, identifying a possible involvement of soft tissues. If PR is negative and US highlights some collections in the peri-prosthetic soft tissues, the diagnosis of infection is almost certain. This is because a relatively long period of time has passed after surgery and its effects have been completely reabsorbed by the tissues. To complete the diagnostic process, a needle aspiration/biopsy should be carried out, with the aim of identifying bacterial strain and its specific antibiogram. However, as remembered above, false negative results are also possible not only with PR, but also with US, when infections are still limited to the bone-prosthesis interface. In this case, a significant role is played by nuclear medicine procedures, and in particular by WBS which, if positive, can give a decisive diagnostic contribution, if associated to the clinical elements and laboratory data, identifying a peri-prosthetic infection, that would not have otherwise been detected (Fig. 4).

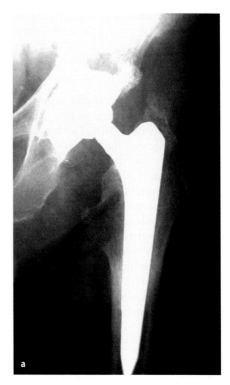

Fig. 4. Painful hip arthroplasty: PR negative for infection (**a**), BS picture suggesting infection: early peri-prosthetic hyperperfusion and late increased peri-prosthetic uptake (**b**), WBS acquired at 24 hours showing peri-prosthetic pathological concentration of labelled white blood cells, more evident in the paratrochanteric soft tissues confirming the septic complication (**c**)

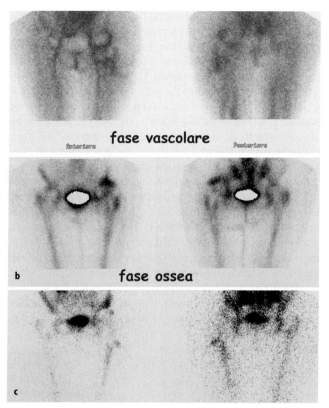

Fig. 4 (*Cont.*)

The patient's follow-up is primarily based on clinical and laboratory data. If these elements are negative there is practically no need to carry out any radiological test. Eventually in case of painful arthroplasty, plain radiographs can be prescribed, which give indications on the bone's conditions, identifying any local complications different from infection (pathological fractures, calcifications, mobilization of the implant etc.). Instead, if laboratory data and clinical background suggest a relapse of the infection, scintigraphic techniques have a major role in monitoring the process. In fact, the structural changes of peri-prosthetic tissues (related to the complicated overlapping of lesions connected to the infection, to surgical traumatisms and to the post-therapy restructuring processes) make the PR and US pictures not completely reliable. In this context, finding a positive WBS (especially if it is interpreted taking into account radiographs and sonography and making an integrated analysis of the different elements) increases the diagnostic specificity in a decisive way, confirming the clinical and laboratory suspicion of a relapse of the infection. Even in this case, needle aspiration/biopsy completes the diagnostic work-up.

Conclusions

Peri-prosthetic infections are currently considered a rare complication owing to the improvement of prophylactic measures and surgical techniques. However, when infections occur, they are characterised by high morbidity, and high costs for therapy and patient management. Time is often a critical factor in deciding the patient's outcome. Any delay in the proper diagnosis, often involves the risk to sacrifice the implanted prosthesis, with obvious consequences on the patient's *"quoad valetudinem"* prognosis. These considerations highlight the critical need to give an accurate and early diagnosis of the infection. Radiology, with its various diagnostic techniques, has a major role in the diagnostic process. Plain radiography still remains the first diagnostic aid. However, due to its limited sensitivity, a negative X-ray study does not exclude the diagnosis. Sonography and Radionuclide imaging, particularly scintigraphy with labelled autologous leucocytes, give a fundamental contribution in the specific identification of the process. Needle aspiration/biopsy guided by the mean of US or CT is a critical step in the diagnostic process, both to confirm the nature of the complication and to identify the bacterial strain that causes it, in order to prepare targeted antibiotic therapies.

References

1. Barberan J (2006) Management of infections of osteoarticular prosthesis. Clin Microbiol Infect 12(Suppl 3):93–101.
2. Chacko TK, Zhuang H, Stevenson K et al. (2002) The importance of the location of fluordeoxyglucose uptake in periprosthetic infection in painful prostheses. Nucl Med Commun 23(9):852–855.
3. Donlom RM (1991) Biofilm formation: a clinically relevant process. Clin Infect Dis 33(8): 1387–1392. Review.
4. Fehring TK, Cohen B (1996) Aspiration as a guide to sepsis in revision total hip arthroplasty. J Arthroplasty 11(5):543–547.
5. Garvin KL, Hinrinhs, Urban JA (1999) Emerging antibiotic-resistant bacteria: their treatment in total joint arthroplasty. Clin Orthop Relat Res (369):110–123.
6. Goergen TG, Dalinka MK et al. (2000) Evaluation of the patient with painful hip or knee arthroplasty. American College of Radiology. ACR Appropriateness Criteria. Radiol 215 (Suppl):295–298.
7. Gristina AG (1987) Biomaterial-centered infections: microbial adhesion versus tissue integration. Science 237(4822):1588–1595.
8. Hanssen AD, Rand JA (1998) Evaluation and treatment of infection at the site of a total hip arthroplasty. Instr Course Lect J Bone Joint Surg (Am) 80(6):910–922.
9. Itasaka T, Kawai A, Sato T et al. (2001) Diagnosis of infection after total hip arthroplasty. J Orthop Sci 6(4):320–326.
10. Lachiewictz PF, Rogers GD Thomason HC (1996) Aspiration of the joint before revision total hip arthroplasty: clinical and laboratory factors influencing attainment of a positive culture. J Bone Joint Surg (Am) 78(5):749–754.
11. Masterson EL, Masri BA, Duncan CP (1997) Treatment of infection at the site of total hip replacement. Instr Course Lect J Bone Joint Surg (Am) 79(11):1740–1749.
12. Palestro CJ, Kim CK, Swyer AJ et al (1990) Total hip arthroplasty: periprosthetic indium 111leukocyte activity and complementary technetium 99m-sulfur colloid imaging in suspected infection. J Nucl Med 31(12):1950–1955.
13. Palestro CJ, Torres MA (1997) Radionuclide imaging in orthopaedic infections. Semin Nucl Med 27(4): 334–345. Review.

14. Potter HG, Nestor BJ, Sofka CM et al (2004) Magnetic resonance imaging after total hip arthroplasty: evaluation of periprosthetic soft tissues. J Bone Joint Surg (Am) 86(9): 1947–1954.
15. Petty W (1978) The effect of methylmethacrylate on bacterial phagocitosis and killing by human polymorphonuclear leukocytes. J Bone Joint Surg (Am) 60(6):752–757.
16. Pretty W, Spaniers S, Shuster JJ et al. (1985) The influence of skeletal implants on incidence of infections. J Bone Joint Surg (Am) 67(8):1236–1244.
17. Saccente M (1998) Periprosthetic joint infections: a review for clinicians. Infect Dis Clin Pract 7:431–441.
18. Sculco TP (1995) The economic impact of infected joint arthroplasty. Orthopedics 18(9): 871–873.
19. Smith SL, Wastie ML, Forster I (2001) Radionuclide bone scintigraphy in the detection of significant complications after total knee joint replacement. Clin Radiol 56(3):221–224.
20. Spangehl MJ, Masri BA, O'Connell JX et al. (1999) Prospective analysis of preoperative and intraoperative investigations for diagnosis of infection at the sites of two hundred and two revision total hip arthroplasty. J Bone Joint Surg (Am) 81(5):672–683.
21. Stumpe KD, Noztli HP, Zanetti M et al. (2004) FDG PET for differentiation of infection and aseptic loosening in total hip replacements: comparison with conventional radiography and three-phase bone scintigraphy. Radiology 231(2):333–341.
22. Tigges S, Stiles RG, Roberson JR (1994) Appearance of septic hip prosthesis on plain radiographs. Am J Roentgenol 163(2):377–380.
23. Toms TA, Davidson D, Masri BA et al ((2006) The management of periprosthetic infection in total joint arthroplasty. J Bone Joint Surg (Br) 88(2):149–155.
24. Vuong C, Gerke C, Somerville GA et al (2003) Quorum-sensing control biofilm factors in the Staphylococcus epidermidis. J Infect Dis 188(5):706–718.
25. White LM, Kim JK Mehta M et al (2000) Complication of total hip arthroplasty: MR imaging initial experience. Radiology 215(1):254–262.
26. Zhuang H, Chacko TK, Hickeson M et al (2002) Persistent non specific FDG uptake on PET imaging following hip. Eur J Nucl Med Mol Imaging 29(10):1328–1333.

Bacterial Strategies of Implant Colonization and Resistance

C. von Eiff, C. Heilmann, G. Peters

Institute of Medical Microbiology, University Hospital of Münster, Münster, Germany

Introduction

Staphylococcus aureus remains a frequent cause of infections in both the community and the hospital. This pathogen accounts for about 13 % of all nosocomial blood infections, and is the second most common cause of these infections. *S. aureus* has been implicated in a multitude of diseases, ranging from minor wound infections to more serious diseases, including endocarditis, pneumonia, osteomyelitis, and septic shock. Worldwide, the increasing resistance of *S. aureus* to various antibiotics complicates treatment of infections due to this microorganism. In contrast, coagulase-negative staphylococci (CoNS), such as *Staphylococcus epidermidis*, have long been dismissed as culture contaminants since they are commonly seen among the normal flora of human skin and mucous membranes. Bacteraemia caused by CoNS is rarely life-threatening, especially, if treated promptly and adequately. However, frank sepsis syndrome and fatal outcome may occur, especially in immunocompromised patients and/or if one of the more virulent species, such as *Staphylococcus lugdunensis*, is involved.

Staphylococci produce a large number of factors that enable them to adhere specifically to host substrates, evade host defenses, and resist antibiotic therapy. The versatility of these pathogens, in particular their ability to adhere to and to accumulate on surfaces, and thus to form a biofilm, but also their ability to hide within host cells and to form a sub-population which may persist intracellularly, enables staphylococci to resist treatment with antimicrobial agents and host immune defense. Among others, these strategies which may be responsible for persistent and recurrent infections due to this pathogen are discussed in this short overview.

Discussion

S. aureus can be considered as a facultative intracellular microorganism. Both, adherence and cellular invasion appear to be involved in complicated *S. aureus* infections. While some of the basic molecular mechanisms have been elucidated in detail in the past years, there are still many aspects to be clarified.

Several lines of evidence suggest a central role of fibrinogen-binding proteins (FnBPs) as *S. aureus* invasins for the establishment of endovascular infections, and inducing the full-fledged disease *in vivo*. This is based on a cooperative binding of fibrinogen and fibronectin, but only the latter confers the ability to invade and settle in the endothelial lining.

Recently identified modulators of invasion, such as *pls*/Pls have been shown to strongly reduce cellular invasion. In particular, the pathogenesis of endovascular infections by *S. aureus*, such as infective endocarditis appears to be a complex process, involving several host and pathogen systems. In addition, cellular invasion may also play a role in the pathogenesis of invasive and metastatic infection upon hematogenous dissemination, such as osteomyelitis and abscess formation. Of particular interest, the fibrinolytic capacity appears not to be substantially affected by staphylococci *in vitro*, as observed in mesothelial cells.

The pathogenesis of foreign-body-associated infections due to staphylococci is characterised by the ability of these pathogens to colonise the surface of an inserted or implanted device by the formation of a thick, multi-layered biofilm. Small numbers of bacteria from the patient's skin or mucous membranes probably contaminate the foreign body during the surgical implantation of the device. Biofilm formation is a two-step process: first, the bacteria rapidly adhere to the polymer material. During the following accumulation phase, the bacteria proliferate to form multi-layered cell clusters on the polymer surface, which are embedded in extracellular material. The presence of such large adherent biofilms on the surfaces of foreign bodies has been shown by scanning electron microscopy. In the past ten years, significant progress has been made in the definition of molecular mechanisms involved in staphylococcal biofilm formation.

Transposon mutagenesis of a biofilm-positive *S. epidermidis* strain demonstrated that different genetic loci are involved in the adherence phase and accumulation phase of biofilm formation. Cloning and characterization of the genes that were inactivated by transposon insertion revealed that adherence to a polymeric surface is mediated by an autolysin – the autolysin/adhesin AtlE. Generally, autolysins are bacteriolytic enzymes involved in cell separation and cell division, but they also mediate adherence, invasion, virulence, and antibiotic-induced cell lysis. Shortly after insertion of a medical device, its surface becomes coated with host factors, such as the plasma and extracellular matrix proteins fibrinogen, fibronectin, vitronectin, thrombospondin, elastin, and collagen. Moreover, platelets may be immobilised on surfaces and thus can mediate the staphylococcal colonization of medical devices or host tissues, such as a damaged endocardium. The autolysin/adhesin AtlE also binds to vitronectin suggesting that it not only mediates adherence to the naked polymer surface, but also to host factor coated medical devices or host tissues. Besides AtlE, another autolysin/adhesin, Aae from *S. epidermidis* and the homologous protein Aaa from *S. aureus*, are bacteriolytic enzymes that also bind to fibrinogen, fibronectin, and vitronectin with high affinity and thus may be involved in colonization. Aae and Aaa are surface-associated proteins probably bound to the surface by hydrophobic and/or hydrophilic interactions, because they do not contain the LPXTG motif typical for Gram-positive cell wall-anchored proteins. Phage display revealed *S. aureus* factors that mediate adherence to platelets, such as the extracellular fibrinogen-binding proteins coagulase and Efb and the fibronectin-binding cell wall proteins FnBPA and FnBPB. Furthermore, FnBPA, but not FnBPB is able to induce platelet aggregation, which may lead to an enlargement of the vegetation on a medical device or on a damaged heart valve involved in the pathogenesis of infective endocarditis, and further recruitment of bacteria. Adherence to fibronectin deposited on a polymeric surface or on host tissue may also be mediated by teichoic acid or the extracellular adherence protein Eap. Once adhered to a surface, bacteria proliferate and accumulate to form the multi-layered biofilms. Multiple factors are also involved in the accumulation phase of S. epidermidis, i.e. the polysaccharide intercellular adhesin (PIA), which is also produced by S. aureus. Synthesis of PIA, which is a ß-1,6 linked N-acetylglucosaminoglycan, is mediated by the icaADBC (intercellular adhesion) gene cluster. IcaA together with IcaD leads to the synthesis of short chains of the N-acetylglucosaminpolymer, while IcaC seems to be involved in their transport across the cytoplasmic membrane, where finally the polymer consisting of more than 130 N-acetylglucosamin-units is built up. PIA not only mediates intercellular adhesion and accumulation, but also adherence to glass and hemagglutination. Moreover, epidemiological studies demonstrated a pathogenetic role for the icaADBC gene cluster: more than 85 % of strains that were associated with septicemia contained the icaADBC operon and were able to form a biofilm, while the icaADBC operon and biofilm formation only rarely were detectable with harmless skin isolates. Furthermore, the importance of the autolysin/adhesin AtlE and PIA in pathogenesis was suggested in an experimental rat model of intravascular catheter-associated infection. Besides PIA, a protein, the accumulation-associated protein AAP is involved in the biofilm accumulation. Recent results demonstrated that proteolytic processing of AAP by either staphylococcal or host proteases is involved in the induction of AAP-mediated biofilm formation.

In addition, there is growing evidence that other, more chronic, polymer-associated clinical syndromes may also at least partly be associated with CoNS, particularly with S. epidermidis. These syndromes include the aseptic loosening of hip or other joint prostheses, fibrous capsular contracture syndrome after mammary augmentation with silicone prostheses, and late-onset endophthalmitis after implantation of artificial intraocular lenses after cataract surgery. In these studies, identical clones were isolated at different times and/or at various multiple sites, indicating the significance of the isolated bacteria.

Beside formation of a biofilm, persistent and relapsing infections may also be related to live S. aureus bacteria actively residing inside epithelial cells. Internalization of S. aureus by epithelial cells was found to be time and dose dependent. Transmission electron microscopy revealed that internalized bacteria resided within endocytic vacuoles without any evidence of lysosomal fusion in a 24-h period. The results of internalization experiments and time-lapse fluorescence microscopy of epithelial cells infected with green fluorescent S. aureus indicated that, after an initial lag period, intracellular bacteria began to replicate, with three to five divisions in a 24-h period, leading to apoptosis of infected cells. Induction of apoptosis required bacterial internalization and was associated with intracellular replication. The slow and gradual replication of S. aureus inside epithelial cells hints at the role of host factors or signals in bacterial growth and further suggests possible cross talk between host cells and S. aureus.

Since the past decade, many reports and prospective studies have supported a pathogenic role for so-called "Small-Colony Variants" (SCVs), a sub-population of S. aureus or CoNS in patients with antibiotic-refractory, recurrent, and/or persistent staphylococcal infections. In particular, patients with chronic osteomyelitis or cystic fibrosis patients were found to be infected with these variants. Phenotypically, SCVs display a slow rate of growth and atypical colony morphology, thereby exhibiting a high rate of reversion into the normal morphotype. Furthermore, SCVs cultivated from clinical specimens are often auxotrophic for hemin, menadione and/or thymidine and have further unusual biochemical features making them a challenge for clinical microbiologists to identify. Several studies revealed that *S. aureus* SCVs are able to persist within non-professional phagocytes such as endothelial cells due to decreased alpha-toxin production. It was assumed that the intracellular location of these variants might shield SCVs from host defences and antibiotics, thus providing one explanation for the difficulty in removing this subpopulation from host tissues. To study the physiological characteristics of *S. aureus* SCVs, stable mutants in electron transport were generated by interrupting hemin (*hemB*) or menadione (*menD*) biosynthetic genes in *S. aureus*. In various approaches comprising genomic, transcriptomic, proteomic, and metabolomic investigations, the SCV concept, in particular their significance in chronic and persistent infections, was studied.

To compare the transcriptome of a clinical *S. aureus* isolate with normal morphotype to its *hemB* mutant mimicking the SCV phenotype, a full-genome DNA microarray was applied. With the standard statistical analysis of the acquired genome-wide transcription data, pooling values from different growth phases, 170 genes were found to be significantly changed when comparing the parent strain and the *hemB*-disrupted strain. Compared to its parental strain with normal phenotype, 48 of these genes were significantly down-regulated and 122 genes were significantly up-regulated in the *hemB* mutant. Furthermore, systems biology advances were used to identify reporter metabolites and to achieve a more detailed survey of genome-wide expression differences between both morphotypes. Of particular interest, genes encoding enzymes involved in glycolytic and fermentative pathways were found to be up-regulated in the mutant. Among others, profound differences were identified in the purine biosynthesis as well as in the arginine and proline metabolism. A hypothetical gene of the Crp/Fnr family being part of the arginine-deiminase pathway, whose homologue in *Streptococcus suis* is assumed to be involved in intracellular persistence, revealed a significantly increased transcription in the mutant. The *hemB* mutant potentially uses the up-regulated arginine-deiminase pathway to produce ATP or (through ammonia production) to counteract the acidic environment that prevails intracellularly.

In a proteomic approach, proteins whose levels were changed by the mutation in *hemB* were identified. Proteins involved in the glycolytic pathway and related pathways as well as in fermentation pathways were found to be induced in exponentially growing cells of the *hemB* mutant. These observations indicated that the *hemB* mutant generates ATP from glucose or fructose only by substrate phosphorylation. In addition, the arginine deiminase pathway was induced providing ATP as well. With regards to the extracellular protein patterns of the parent strain and its *hemB* mutant in the stationary growth phase, the comparative proteomic analysis revealed very strong differences: Most of the known virulence factors expressed during the late exponential phase were not found in the mutant or were present at low levels.

Both, the *menD* and the *hemB* mutant were also studied in a metabolomic approach. Using Phenotype MicroArrays (PM), the *hemB* mutant was shown to be defective in utilizing a variety of carbon sources including Krebs cycle intermediates and compounds that ultimately generate ATP via electron transport. The features of the *menD* mutant were similar to those of the *hemB* mutant, but the defects in carbon metabolism were more pronounced than seen with the *hemB* mutant. Hexose phosphates and other carbohydrates that provide ATP in the absence of electron transport stimulated growth of both mutants.

Conclusion

Taken together, this overview shows the enormous versatility of the genus *Staphylococcus*. Pathogenic members of this genus are able to resist antimicrobial agents by classical mechanisms, but also able to change the phenotype to survive intracellulary, and/or to form a biofilm, and thus, to resist the host immune defense or the action of antibiotics.

References

1. Fey PD, Ulphani JS, Götz F et al (1999) Characterization of the relationship between polysaccharide intercellular adhesin and hemagglutination in Staphylococcus epidermidis. J Infect Dis 179(6):1561–1564
2. Grundmann H, Aires-de-Sousa M, Boyce J et al (2006) Emergence and resurgence of meticillin-resistant Staphylococcus aureus as a public-health threat. Lancet 368(9538):874–885
3. Grundmeier M, Hussain M, Becker P et al (2004) Truncation of fibronectin-binding proteins in Staphylococcus aureus strain Newman leads to deficient adherence and host cell invasion due to loss of the cell wall anchor function. Infect Immun 72(12):7155–7163
4. Haslinger-Löffler B, Wagner B, Bruck M et al (2006) Staphylococcus aureus induces caspase-independent cell death in human peritoneal mesothelial cells. Kidney Int 70(6):1089–1098
5. Heilmann C, Gerke C, Perdreau-Remington F et al (1996) Characterization of Tn917 insertion mutants of Staphylococcus epidermidis affected in biofilm formation. Infect Immun 64(1):277–282
6. Heilmann C, Hartleib J, Hussain MS et al (2005) The multifunctional Staphylococcus aureus autolysin aaa mediates adherence to immobilized fibrinogen and fibronectin. Infect Immun 73(8):4793–4802
7. Heilmann C, Herrmann M, Kehrel BE et al (2002) Platelet-binding domains in 2 fibrinogen-binding proteins of Staphylococcus aureus identified by phage display. J Infect Dis 186(1):32–39
8. Heilmann C, Hussain M, Peters G et al (1997) Evidence for autolysin-mediated primary attachment of Staphylococcus epidermidis to a polystyrene surface. Mol Microbiol 24(5):1013–1024
9. Heilmann C, Niemann S, Sinha B et al (2004) Staphylococcus aureus fibronectin-binding protein (FnBP)-mediated adherence to platelets, and aggregation of platelets induced by FnBPA but not by FnBPB. J Infect Dis 190(2):321–329
10. Heilmann C, Schweitzer O, Gerke C et al (1996) Molecular basis of intercellular adhesion in the biofilm-forming Staphylococcus epidermidis. Mol Microbiol 20(5):1083–1091
11. Heilmann C, Thumm G, Chhatwal GS et al (2003) Identification and characterization of a novel autolysin (Aae) with adhesive properties from Staphylococcus epidermidis. Microbiology 149(Pt 10):2769–2778
12. Hussain M, Haggar A, Heilmann C et al (2002) Insertional inactivation of Eap in Staphylococcus aureus strain Newman confers reduced staphylococcal binding to fibroblasts. Infect Immun 70(6):2933–2940
13. Hussain M, Heilmann C, Peters G et al (2001) Teichoic acid enhances adhesion of Staphylococcus epidermidis to immobilized fibronectin. Microb Pathog 31(6):261–270

14. Hussain M, Herrmann M, von Eiff C et al (1997) A 140-kilodalton extracellular protein is essential for the accumulation of Staphylococcus epidermidis strains on surfaces. Infect Immun 65(2):519–524

15. Juuti KM, Sinha B, Werbick C et al (2004) Reduced adherence and host cell invasion by methicillin-resistant Staphylococcus aureus expressing the surface protein Pls. J Infect Dis 189(9):1574–1584

16. Kahl BC, Goulian M, van WW et al (2000) Staphylococcus aureus RN6390 replicates and induces apoptosis in a pulmonary epithelial cell line. Infect Immun 68(9):5385–5392

17. Kipp F, Becker K, Peters G et al (2004) Evaluation of different methods to detect methicillin resistance in small-colony variants of Staphylococcus aureus. J Clin Microbiol 42(3):1277–1279

18. Kipp F, Kahl BC, Becker K et al (2005) Evaluation of two chromogenic agar media for recovery and identification of Staphylococcus aureus small-colony variants. J Clin Microbiol 43(4):1956–1959

19. Kohler C, von Eiff C, Peters G et al (2003) Physiological characterization of a heme-deficient mutant of Staphylococcus aureus by a proteomic approach. J Bacteriol 185(23):6928–6937

20. Proctor RA, von Eiff C, Kahl BC et al (2006) Small colony variants: a pathogenic form of bacteria that facilitates persistent and recurrent infections. Nat Rev Microbiol 4(4):295–305

21. Rohde H, Burdelski C, Bartscht K et al (2005) Induction of Staphylococcus epidermidis biofilm formation via proteolytic processing of the accumulation-associated protein by staphylococcal and host proteases. Mol Microbiol 55(6):1883–1895

22. Rupp ME, Fey PD, Heilmann C et al (2001) Characterization of the importance of Staphylococcus epidermidis autolysin and polysaccharide intercellular adhesin in the pathogenesis of intravascular catheter-associated infection in a rat model. J Infect Dis 183(7):1038–1042

23. Seggewiß J, Becker K, Kotte O et al (2006) Reporter metabolite analysis of transcriptional profiles of a Staphylococcus aureus strain with normal phenotype and its isogenic hemB mutant displaying the small colony variant phenotype. J Bacteriol 15(in press)

24. Seifert H, Oltmanns D, Becker K et al (2005) Staphylococcus lugdunensis pacemaker-related infection. Emerg Infect Dis 11(8):1283–1286

25. Seifert H, von Eiff C, and Fatkenheuer G (1999) Fatal case due to methicillin-resistant Staphylococcus aureus small colony variants in an AIDS patient. Emerg Infect Dis 5(3):450–453

26. Seifert H, Wisplinghoff H, Schnabel P et al (2003) Small colony variants of Staphylococcus aureus and pacemaker-related infection. Emerg Infect Dis 9(10):1316–1318

27. Sinha B and Herrmann M. (2005) Mechanism and consequences of invasion of endothelial cells by Staphylococcus aureus. Thromb Haemost 94(2):266–277

28. von Eiff C, Becker K, Metze D et al (2001) Intracellular persistence of Staphylococcus aureus small-colony variants within keratinocytes: a cause for antibiotic treatment failure in a patient with darier's disease. Clin Infect Dis 32(11):1643–1647

29. von Eiff C, Bettin D, Proctor RA et al (1997) Recovery of small colony variants of Staphylococcus aureus following gentamicin bead placement for osteomyelitis. Clin Infect Dis 25(5):1250–1251

30. von Eiff C, McNamara P, Becker K et al. (2006) Phenotype microarray profiling of Staphylococcus aureus menD and hemB mutants with the small-colony-variant phenotype. J Bacteriol 188(2):687–693

31. von Eiff C, Peters G, and Heilmann C (2002) Pathogenesis of infections due to coagulase-negative staphylococci. Lancet Infect Dis 2(11):677–685

32. Ziebuhr W, Heilmann C, Götz F et al (1997) Detection of the intercellular adhesion gene cluster (ica) and phase variation in Staphylococcus epidermidis blood culture strains and mucosal isolates. Infect Immun 65(3):890–896

Pathological Findings of Septic Loosening

G. Gasparini, S. Cerciello, M. Vasso, C. Fabbriciani

Orthopaedic department, Catholic University, Rome, Italy

Introduction

Bone loss secondary to an infectious process in total joint replacement progresses in different stages. The first stage is primary osteolysis which is the direct action of the infecting bacteria and by the host's immune response to these bacteria. Implant removal causes additional damage to the bone if not performed carefully. If a two-stage revision is planned a temporary antibiotic loaded spacer that is not stable can also cause further bone loss. The soft tissues are involved with a progressive thickening of the joint capsule, and with an iperplasia of the synovial membrane (Fig. 1). In the active phase of the infectous process, synovial membrane exudate can be found in the joint space. In the chronic phase this exudate evolves into a scar tissue.

Primary Osteolysis

Invading bacteria produce enzymes and exotoxins that induce enzymatic degradation, activation of the fibrinolytic pathway, loss of vasculature, and cell death leading

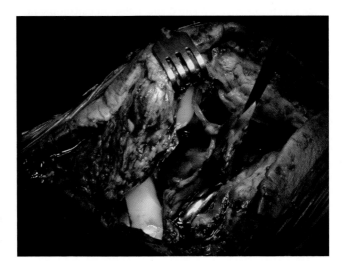

Fig. 1. Soft tissue removal is an essential step in revision surgery for septic loosening.

to bone necrosis. In addition to this pathway, another set of events that leads to host-cell activation rather than cell death, occurs. During infection, the series of events that are induced may be initiated by bacterial endotoxin (lipopolysaccharide). It is well recognised that lipopolysaccharides exert potent effects on a variety of target cells associated with both nonspecific inflammatory and specific immune responses, including macrophages, neutrophils, and B-lymphocytes. Bone macrophages and osteoblasts are activated by lipopolysaccharides, as evidenced by cell proliferation, cytokine secretion, and increased bone resorption. Because cells of both hematopoietic and stromal cell lineage respond to bacterial endotoxin, exposure of marrow cells to lipopolysaccharides from invading organisms results in the activation of cells from many different systems [7]. As part of this activation, host cells secrete a genetically predetermined (and therefore specific) set of cytokines: interleukin-1, granulocyte-macrophage colony stimulating factor, tumor necrosis factor, and interleukin-6 [9]. Some cytokines are involved in the induction of osteoclastic bone resorption; others are involved in bone cell maturation, which results in increased number of osteoclasts and possibly macrophages. This is the common pathway of osteomyelitis; when these phenomena develop at the bone-implant interface, the endpoint of the process, i.e. osteolysis, causes bone resorption along the interface with cement or metal which makes the prosthesis unstable. In fact the main pathogenic mechanism in biomaterial-associated infections is microbial colonization of biomaterials. Microbial adhesion is basically a chemical bonding of bacterial extracapsular structures to the surface of an implant, where they adhere, grow and proliferate forming a biofilm. The biofilm mode of growth offers enhanced protection for the infecting organism against natural host defences and antibiotics allowing infection and bone damage progression along the interface.

First Stage Procedure

The surgical procedure to remove an infected implant can cause significant bone loss. If the prosthesis is uncemented and stable an osteotomy must be performed to prevent devastating bone loss. If unstable the prosthesis usually can be easily removed but a wider debridement of infected bone may be required. In cemented prosthesis, implant removal is easier if debonding occurs at the cement-implant interface. If the cement is stable, its removal can be difficult and special equipment required to prevent excessive bone loss. Aggressive debridement is an important step in the success of reimplantation after septic loosening. Soft tissue (synovial membrane, scar tissue and fibrous or pyogenic membranes) and all infected bone must be resected.

Cement Spacer

Most of the authors suggest the use of antibiotic loaded cement spacers to prevent recolonization in the surgical field after septic loosening in joint replacement. Custom made and commercial spacers are available for the hip and knee. Static spacers in the knee have the disadvantage of creating a fix articulation with extensor mechanism shortening, stiffness and more difficult exposure at the time of reoperation.

Conversely articulating spacers in the knee permit postoperative passive and active motion with lower risk of stiffness and extensor mechanism shortening. Unfortunately these articulating spacers spread cement micro-particles into the articulation stimulating a synovial membrane inflammation which may be a source of further bone and soft tissue damage. Moreover shear forces at the bone cement interface during knee joint movement produces micromotion, which may lead to further bone destruction.

In case of infected hip arthroplasties the choice between commercial and custom made spacers has less impact. Commercial spacers have a stem with a large head diameter which articulates with the acetabular cavity. The smooth surface of the head may avoid acetabular erosion and minimize bone loss. Custom made spacers follow the same philosophy but are less expensive and the surface is rougher, which may lead to some bone erosion of the acetabulum.

Second Stage Procedure

At the time of revision surgery, in addition to the osteolysis caused by micromovements at the bone spacer interface, further bone damage may be caused by spacer removal. Careful debridement of the articular surfaces and of the medullary canals is necessary. With re-implantation bone loss must be accounted for to gain stability. Modular implants may be required to fill in defects.

Classfication of Bone Defects in Joint Replacement

The Anderson Orthopaedic Research Institute (AORI) bone defect classification was proposed by Engh [3] to define the severity of bone loss on the femoral side (F1, F2, F3) and the tibial side (T1, T2, T3) in total knee replacements. Type 1 defects (F1 and T1), have almost intact metaphyseal segments with only small defects in the cancellous portions of the bone with no component subsidence or osteolysis (Fig. 2). Type 2 defects involve metaphyseal bone in one (F2A and T2A) or both (F2B and T2B) femoral or tibial condyles; on the femoral side we have a component subsidence or osteolysis distal to epicondyles, on the tibial side a component subsidence or osteolysis up to or below tip of fibula head (Fig. 3). Type 3 defects (F3 and T3) include major deficiencies of metaphyseal segments, occasionally incorporating loss of ligamentous structures. On the femoral side we have a component subsidence or osteolysis at or beyond level of epicondyles (Fig. 4), on the tibial side a component subsidence or osteolysis at or beyond level of tubercle (Fig. 5). The AORI classification can be helpful and simple to use but it does not distinguish between contained and uncontained defects [5]. The contained or cavitary defects have an intact cortical ring which surrounds the area of bone loss, while the uncontained or segmental defects are more peripheral and they have not a surrounding intact cortical ring.

Rand has classified these defects according to symmetry, location, and extent [6]. A symmetric deficiency would exist with subsidence of a tibial implant into the centre of the tibia from an undersized prosthesis. An asymmetric defect would follow angular subsidence of an implant into the tibia resulting in bone loss on one side alone.

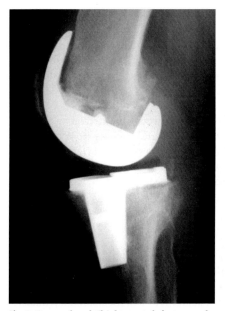 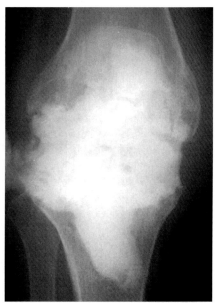

Fig. 2. Femoral and tibial type 1 defect according to the AORI classification

Fig. 3. Femoral and tibial type 2B defect; bone loss involves both femoral and tibial condyles

The location of the deficiency may be considered either central or peripheral on the tibial plateau. A central defect frequently exists from loosening of an older resurfacing implant, leaving an intact peripheral rim of bone. A peripheral defect occurs in association with angular deformities in primary arthroplasty and it is usually located posteromedially in varus knee. On the femoral side, bone loss associated with revision procedures is located distally, posteriorly, or combined. The extent of the deficiency can be subdivided into minimal (Type I), moderate (Type II), extensive (Type III), and massive cavitary (Type IV) types. The extent of bone loss is estimated after the initial tibial and femoral bone cuts have been made. A minimal defect would comprise less than 50 % of a single condyle with a depth of less than 5 mm. A moderate defect would comprise an area 50 % – 70 % of a single condyle to a depth of 5 – 10 mm. An extensive bone defect would comprise greater than 70 % of a condyle to a depth of greater than or equal to 10 mm. A massive cavitary defect can be considered as two types: with an intact peripheral rim (a), and with a deficient peripheral rim (b).

The American Academy of Orthopaedic Surgeons (AAOS) Committee on the Hip introduced a comprehensive classification system of femoral abnormalities in total hip replacements [2]. This classification system has two basic categories: segmental and cavitary. A segmental defect is defined as any bone loss in the supporting cortical shell of the femur. A cavitary defect is a contained lesion and represents an excavation of the cancellous or endosteal cortical bone with no violation of the outer cortical shell of the femur. Levels of bone loss involvement are given. Level I is defined as bone proximal to the inferior border of the lesser trochanter, Level II is from the inferior lesser trochanter to 10 cm distal, Level III involves bone distal to Level II. Segmental

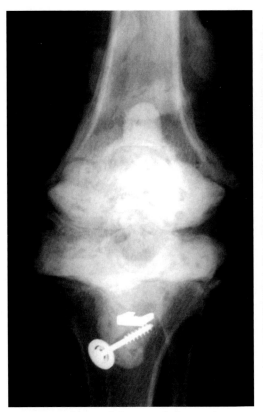 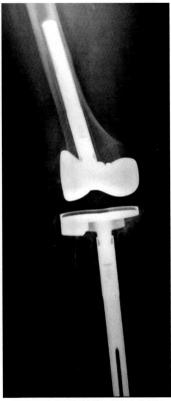

Fig. 4. Femoral type 3 defect: osteolysis extends beyond the level of the epicondyles. A tibial type 2B defect cohexists

Fig. 5. Tibial type 3 defect: bone loss extends distally to the tibial tuberosity. A femoral type 3 defect cohexists

proximal deficiencies can be further subdivided into partial or complete. Partial segmental bone loss can be located anteriorly, medialy, or posteriorly and can exist from proximal though any distal level of the femur. An intercalary defect is segmental cortical bone loss with intact bone above and below such as a cortical window. The greater trochanter fracture is listed as a separate segmental defect because of the unique and difficult problems that it can present in femoral reconstruction. Cavitary defects are classified according to the degree of bone loss within the femur. Cancellous cavitary defects involve only the medullary bone. Cortical cavitary defects suggest a more severe type of erosion where, in addition to cancellous loss, the femoral cortex is eroded from within. Finally, ectasia is an enlargement of the femoral medullary canal often associated with thinning of the diaphyseal cortex. A separate category of combined defects designates the situation where segmental and cavitary abnormalities co-exist. This may result from osteolysis, stem movement, or iatrogenic circumstances. Next, the classification system addresses malalignment abnormalities and femoral stenosis. Finally, femoral discontinuity describes the lack of bony integrity that exists with fractures of the femur.

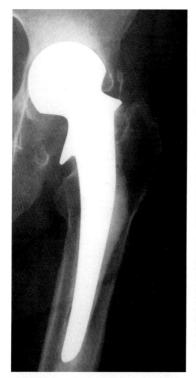

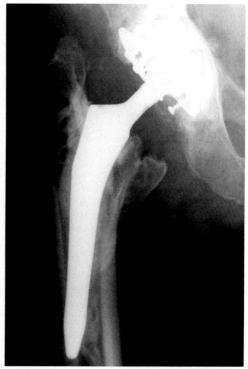

Fig. 6. Femoral type I defect according to Paprosky classification: minimal damage of the proximal metaphysis

Fig. 7. Femoral type II defect: metaphyseal damage with minimal diaphyseal damage

The Paprosky femoral defects classification has the advantage to be more indicative for surgical strategies [8]. Type I defects present minimal damage of the proximal metaphysic (Fig. 6). Type II defects present metaphyseal damage with minimal diaphyseal damage (Fig. 7). Type IIIA defects represent a metadiaphyseal bone loss where 4 cm scratch-fit can be obtained at isthmus (Fig. 8). Type IIIB defects represent a metadiaphyseal bone loss where scratch-fit cannot be obtained at isthmus but more distally (Fig. 9). Finally, Type IV defects represent an extensive metadiaphyseal damage with thin cortices and widened femoral canal (Fig. 10).

The American Academy of Orthopaedic Surgeons (AAOS) Committee on the Hip devised a classification system for acetabular deficiencies too [1]. This classification is simple, is applicable to both primary and revision cases, and facilitates an approach to both preoperative planning and treatment. This classification system has two basic categories: segmental and cavitary. A segmental deficiency is any complete loss of bone in the supporting hemisphere of the acetabulum (including the medial wall). Cavitary defects represent a volumetric loss in bony substance of the acetabular cavity (including the medial wall), but the acetabular rim remains intact. Segmental deficiencies (Fig. 11) can be classified as peripheral (superior, posterior, or anterior) or central (medial). These deficiencies may be isolated or may exist in combination.

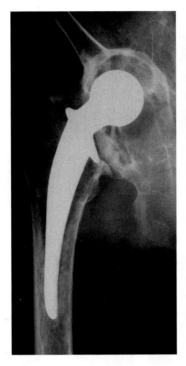
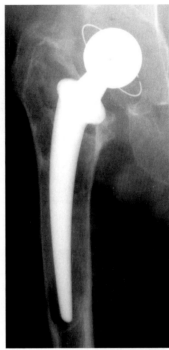

Fig. 8. (*left*) Femoral type IIIA defect: metadiaphyseal bone loss; 4 cm scratch-fit can be obtained at isthmus

Fig. 9. (*right*) emoral type IIIB defect: metadiaphyseal bone loss; scratch-fit can be obtained distally to the isthmus

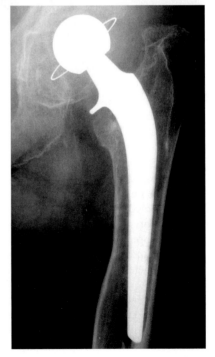

Fig. 10. Femoral type IV defect: extensive metadiaphyseal damage with thin cortices and widened femoral canal

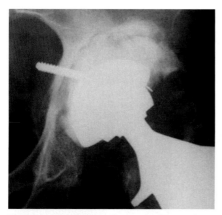

Fig. 11. Segmental bone loss according to the AAOS acetabular defect classification

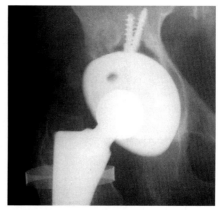

Fig. 12. Superior cavitary acetabular defect

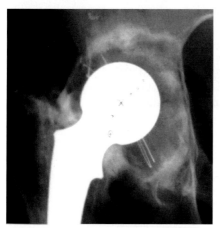

Fig. 13. Combined segmental and cavitary defect

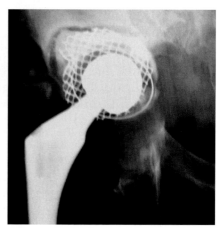

Fig. 14. Pelvic discontinuity

Cavitary deficiencies (Fig. 12), likewise, are peripheral (superior, posterior, or anterior) or central (medial wall intact). Similarly, they may be isolated or exist in combination. It is important to underline that a medial cavitary deficiency implies excavation of the medial wall without violation of the medial rim, even in the case of protrusio. Therefore, it must be distinguished from a medial segmental defect where the complete absence of a portion of the inner medial wall or rim is present. Combined segmental and cavitary deficiencies may coexist (Fig. 13). For example, a superior segmental defect and a posterior cavitary defect are frequently present in congenital hip dysplasia, or with proximal migration of an endoprosthesis. It is not uncommon to experience superior and posterior segmental deficiencies with coexistent posterior and superior cavitary deficiencies when socket pelvic migration have occurred. Pelvic discontinuity is a defect across the anterior and posterior columns with total separation of the superior from the inferior acetabulum (Fig. 14). Arthrodesis is not associated with acetabular bone loss; nevertheless it is included in this classification because it represents a technical problem.

The Paprosky acetabular defects classification system [4] is based upon the presence or absence of an intact acetabular rim and its ability to provide initial rigid support for an implanted acetabular component. Defects are classified by type, indicating whether the remaining acetabular structures are completely supportive (type 1), partially supportive (type 2), or not supportive (type 3) of the revision component. Type 1 acetabular defects present minimal deformity. Cancellous bone is often retained while lytic defects are present. On the preoperative radiograph the component displays no migration, suggesting that the dome is intact. The teardrop is present indicating that the medial wall is uninvolved, and ischial bone lysis is absent suggesting that the posterior wall is intact. Type 2 acetabular defects represent a distortion of the acetabular hemisphere with distruction of the dome and/or medial wall but retention of the anterior and posterior columns. Cancellous bone is often sparse and replaced with sclerotic bone. Type 2A defects are a generalized oval enlargement of the acetabulum. Superior bone lysis is present but the superior rim remains intact. Type 2B defects are similar to type 2A but the dome is more distorted and the superior rim is absent. Type 2C defects involve destruction of the medial wall. Type 2A and type 2B defects present less than 2 cm of component migration. In type 2A the cup migrates superiorly because of the cavitation of the dome, while In type 2B the cup migrates superolaterally because the superior rim is absent. Both type 2A and 2B defects show no lysis of the teardrop or the ischium. In type 2C the teardrop is obliterated. The cup may migrates because the medial wall is absent. Type 3 acetabular defects demonstrate severe bone loss resulting in maior destruction of the acetabular rim and supporting structures. Type 3A bone loss pattern usually extends from the ten o'clock to the two o'clock position around the acetabular rim. In type 3B defects the acetabular rim is absent from the nine o'clock to the five o'clock position. In both 3A and 3B defects the component usually migrates more than 2 cm superiorly. Type 3A defects present moderate but not complete destruction of the teardrop and moderate lysis of the ischium. Because the medial wall is present, the component usually migrates superolaterally. Type 3C defects show complete obliteration of the teardrop and severe lysis of the ischium, usually resulting in superomedial cup migration.

These classifications generally refer to the periprosthetic bone loss with no specific reference to the aetiology of the loosening. In case of infection the process evolves with some peculiarities. At the beginning the progression of the infection along the bone-implant interface determines a linear bone loss. Later several osteolysis areas occur as the consequence of bone abscesses; their confluence lead to cavitary defects with instability of the implant that is cause of further bone loss on mechanical basis. The process can evolve to segmental defects even because of the additional iatrogenic bone damage.

References

1. D'Antonio JA, Capello WN, Borden LS et al (1989) Classification and management of acetabular abnormalities in total hip arthroplasty. Clin Orthop Relat Res (243):126–137
2. D'Antonio J, McCarthy JC, Bargar WL et al (1993) Classification of femoral abnormalities in total hip arthroplasty. Clin Orthop Relat Res (296):133–139

3. Engh GA, Bone loss classification. In: Engh GA, Rorabeck CH (1997) Revision total knee arthroplasty. Williams and Wilkins, Baltimore
4. Paprosky WG, Perona PG, Lawrence JM (1994) Acetabular defect classification and surgical reconstruction in revision arthroplasty. A 6-year follow-up evaluation. J Arthroplasty 9(1): 33 – 44
5. Patel JV, Masonis JL, Guerin J et al (2004) The fate of augments to treat type-2 bone defects in revision knee arthroplasty. J Bone Joint Surg (Br) 86(2):195 – 199
6. Rand JA (1991) Bone deficiency in total knee arthroplasty. Use of metal wedge augmentation. Clin Orthop Relat Res (271):63 – 71
7. Rennick D, Yang G, Gemmell L et al (1987) Control of hemopoiesis by a bone marrow stromal cell clone: Lipopolysaccharide and interleukin-1-inducible production of colony-stimulating factors. Blood 69(2):682 – 681
8. Sporer SM, Paprosky WG (2003) Revision total hip arthroplasty. The limits of fully coated stems. Clin Orthop Relat Res (417):203 – 209
9. Thorens B, Mermod JJ, Vassalli P (1987) Phagocytosis and inflammatory stimuli induce GM-CSF mRNA in macrophages through posttranscriptional regulation. Cell 48(4):671 – 679

Antimicrobial Prophylaxis in Orthopaedic Surgery 5

A. Soriano[1], S. García-Ramiro[2], J. Mensa[1]

[1] Department of Infectious Diseases; Hospital Clínic, Barcelona, Spain
[2] Department of Orthopaedic Surgery, Hospital Clínic, Barcelona, Spain

General Concepts in Antimicrobial Prophylaxis

Research in antimicrobial prophylaxis started in the 70's when Miles and Burke [23] established that the efficacy of antibiotics in reducing the wound size after subcutaneous bacterial inoculation in a guinea pig model was associated with its administration during surgery or few hours after wound closing. By delaying the administration of antibiotics by only 3 or 4 hours, the resulting lesions were identical in size to those of animals not receiving antibiotic prophylaxis. Afterwards, this concept was confirmed in a large study including surgical procedures performed in 2847 patients [6]. Patients receiving antibiotics between 24 h and 2 h before surgery or 3 h after finishing surgery had an infection rate over 3 %. The lower infection rate (0.6 %) was observed among those patients who received the antibiotic just prior to the intervention. Once the precise moment for the administration was established, many other studies were conducted to identify the best antibiotic for different types of surgery and its optimal duration. The information from these studies could be summarized as follows: 1) the antibiotic chosen should cover the main contaminant flora present in the skin or mucosa disrupted by incision, 2) it is necessary to achieve high antibiotic concentrations during surgery, therefore, the best moment for antibiotic infusion is 15–30 minutes by intravenous route before starting surgery and 3) the administration of one preoperative dose of antibiotic is probably sufficient. The third point is still controversial and many international guidelines maintain an antibiotic prophylaxis during 24 h after surgery. Since contamination occurs in the majority of cases while the wound is open, it is reasonable to conclude that a preoperative dose is the most effective which is supported by a large clinical trial [6].

Risk Factors and Scores to Predict the Risk for Surgical Site Infection

Several factors have been associated to a high risk of surgical site infection (SSI). The most important are those related to the level of bacterial contamination and the host capacity to eradicate these microorganisms (Fig. 1). The level of bacterial contamination basically depends on the type of surgery following the traditional wound classification which stratifies wounds into: clean, clean-contaminated, contaminated and dirty. Quantitatively, it has been shown that if a surgical site is contaminated with $> 10^5$ microorganisms per gram of tissue, the risk of SSI is markedly increased [19].

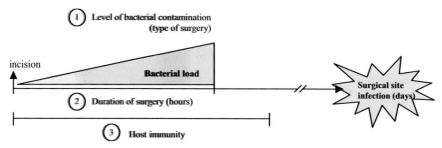

Fig. 1. Predicting factors of surgical site infection (type of surgery is classified according to the level of bacterial contamination in clean, clean-contaminated, contaminated and dirty).

For clean surgery (i.e. arthroplasty), the bacterial load into the wound depends on: 1) the correct application of barrier measures to avoid the contamination from the skin of patients and surgeons (skin decontamination, gloves or masks), the environment (laminar airflow, reducing the number of persons in the operating theatre) and the surgical material (sterilization), 2) the duration of surgery, and 3) the virulence of the microorganism. On the other hand, the bacterial load is balanced by the general and local host immune system. Chronic systemic illnesses, such as diabetes mellitus have been clearly associated with high SSI rates. However, the precise mechanisms for explaining these observations are still being investigated. For example, glucose level [21], subcutaneous oxygen tension [14] or low body temperature [20] during and after surgery have been implicated as a risk factors for SSI. All these factors have demonstrated, in vitro, a deleterious effect on the activity of polymorphonuclear leucocytes essential for killing contaminating bacteria. But probably many other factors previously associated to SSI such as pain, poor nutritional status, obesity or old age, also impair the local immune system. In order to control all these parameters the collaboration from all staff members involved in surgery and post-surgery is necessary.

The Centre for Disease Control developed a risk index that helps the surgeons to predict the risk of SSI [22]. This includes three variables: 1) the classification of oper-

Table 1. The American Society of Anaesthesiologists physical status classification

Class	Physical status	Example
I	A completely healthy patient	A fit patient with an inguinal hernia
II	A patient with mild systemic disease	Essential hypertension, mild diabetes without end organ damage
III	A patient with severe systemic disease that is not incapacitating	Angina, moderate to severe COPD
IV	A patient with incapacitating disease that is a constant threat to life	Advanced COPD, cardiac failure
V	A moribund patient who is not expected to live 24 hours with or without surgery	Ruptured aortic aneurysm, massive pulmonary embolism
E	Emergency case	

Table 2. NNIS (National Nosocomial Infection Surveillance system) risk index

ASA score of 3, 4, or 5	1 point
Contaminated or dirty procedure	1 point
Length of procedure > T hours*	1 point
Use of laparoscope	Minus 1 point

* T hours = 75th percentile duration of specific procedure.

Table 3. Surgical site infections in hip and knee arthroplasty by NNIS risk index category.

Type of arthroplasty	Duration (75th percentile)	Infection rates for NNIS risk index		
		0	1	2
Hip	2	0.89	1.53	2.38
Knee	2	0.85	1.28	2.21

Table 4. Major pathogens in deep surgical wound infections after arthroplasty.

Pathogen	Infection percent*
Gram positive cocci	
S. aureus	50
Coagulase-negative staphylococci	14
E. faecalis	3
Gram negative rods	
E. coli	15
Other Enterobacteriaceae sp	8
P. aeruginosa	8
Negative cultures	2

* from Hospital Clínic of Barcelona

ative wounds by level of bacterial contamination (clean, clean-contaminated, contaminated or dirty) 2) the duration of surgery and 3) the American Society of Anaesthesiologists physical status classification as a marker of the immune status of the patient (Table 1). The index to assess the individual risk of developing surgical wound infection is shown in Table 2 and the surgical site infection rate reported by NNIS for hip and knee arthroplasty in Table 3.

In orthopaedic surgery *Staphylococcus aureus* is the most common pathogen (Table 4) and the most difficult to treat [4]. The available data on the role of being a nasal carrier is summarized in the next section.

Role of Nasal Carriage of *S. aureus* in the Development of Surgical Site Infection

S. aureus colonizes the anterior nares of humans and cross-sectional studies yield a prevalence of approximately 30 % of nasal carriers in the general population, who some of them are persistent and some intermittent carriers [18]. Carriage of *S. aureus* has been identified as a risk factor for the development of infections in surgical patients (general, orthopaedic and thoracic surgery). Kalmeijer et al [17] found that persons who did not have nasal carriage compared to those carriers who underwent orthopaedic surgery, had a relative risk of 8.9 for developing a SSI in the univariate analysis (95 % CI, 1.7–45.5) and in the multivariate analysis it was an independent risk factor associated with SSI due to *S. aureus*. These findings led to the hypothesis that nasal decolonisation before surgery could reduce the incidence of infection rate by *S. aureus*. Kalmeijer et al [16] randomized 614 patients to receive mupirocin or a placebo the day before surgery. In this study, mupirocin nasal ointment did not significantly reduce the global SSI rate (3.8 % in the mupirocin group and 4.7 % in the placebo group) or SSI by *S. aureus* (mupirocin group, 1.6 % versus placebo, 2.7 %). However, molecular typing of *S. aureus* from nasal mucosa and wound infection demonstrated that endogenous *S. aureus* infection (when nasal and wound strains were identical) was 5 times less likely in the mupirocin group than in the placebo (RR 0.19, 95 % CI 0.02 – 1.62, p> 0.05), suggesting that mupirocin could prevent endogenous infections. In another clinical trial involving general surgery [26] and with a similar design (randomized and doble-blind), the authors observed a significant decrease in nosocomial infections due to *S. aureus*, however the SSI rate was similar in the mupirocin group and the placebo probably due to the unexpected low number of SSI caused by endogenous *S. aureus* in both arms. In conclusion, the information available demonstrates that nasal colonization with *S. aureus* is an important risk factor for developing a SSI due to this microorganism and probably decolonisation of selected patients would be an effective preventing measure. In the future it would be necessary to define the candidates and to investigate new regimens for decolonisation since the resistance to mupirocin is increasing.

Particular Concepts on Antimicrobial Prophylaxis in Orthopaedic Surgery

Generally, orthopaedic and trauma surgery consists in the implantation of foreign materials such as prosthesis, plates or nails. It is well recognized from animal models, that the bacterial load necessary to cause infections, when an implant is present, could be reduced 10,000-fold in comparison to those without foreign bodies (i.e., 100 staphylococci per gram of tissue introduced on silk sutures) [9]. This fact is associated with the impairment of fagocyte function on the inert surfaces and the ability of microorganisms to grow forming complex community embedded in a polysaccharide matrix called biofilm which is characterized by a high resistance to fagocytosis and antibiotics. As a consequence, the infection on an orthopaedic implant is particularly harmful since it requires several interventions, prolonged hospitalisation and antibiotic treatment for weeks or months [30].

Another characteristic of orthopaedic surgery with foreign body implantation is that the infections may be diagnosed months or even years after the surgery. Although the pathogenesis of early infections (those diagnosed during the first 3 months after surgery) is well understood, this is not the case of delayed infections (after the first 3 months). In early infections the contamination takes place, in the majority of cases, while the wound is open and the most frequent source of the microorganisms is the patient's endogenous flora. However, other factors like contaminated surgical instruments, skin, mucous or clothing from operating room staff have all been implicated as potential sources. Hours or days after surgery the wound is immersed in the complex process of healing and during this period, the blood flow could be in contact with the wound and foreign material implanted, for this reason it could be possible that bacteremia due to any microorganism seeding in this place;

however, the hematogenous source has rarely been documented [2]. It is not well defined for how long the orthopaedic implant is exposed to blood flow and therefore at a high risk to be colonized during an episode of bacteremia. This is an important question in order to better understand the pathogenesis of delayed infections and to advise antimicrobial prophylaxis prior to dental, genitourinary or gastrointestinal invasive procedures. The American Academy of Orthopaedic Surgeons and the American Dental Association analysed the frequency of prosthetic joint infections related to a previous dental procedure and found an increased risk among patients with coexisting immuno compromised status (such as diabetes mellitus) and during the first 2 years after surgery. As a result, they recommend antibiotic prophylaxis only for these patients [7].

The pathogenesis of delayed infections is still unclear. It is difficult to establish if these infections result from intraoperative bacterial seeding on the prosthetic device followed by a prolonged dormancy or from a true postoperative bacteremia. Carlsson et al [5] in a randomized, prospective, controlled study of antibiotic prophylaxis in hip arthroplasty, demonstrated that deep wound infections that developed over 2.5 years after surgery, were more likely to have occurred among placebo versus cloxacillin recipients (13.7 % versus 3.3 % respectively, $p < 0.05$). In addition, other authors observed a decrease in the incidence rate of late infections when prostheses were cemented with an antibiotic [9]. These data strongly suggest that bacteria inoculated into the wound at the time of surgery may lie dormant (forming biofilms on the inert surface of foreign material) for years being responsible for late infections. The fact that the most frequent microorganism isolated in delayed infections is coagulase-negative staphylococci also supports this hypothesis. This data confers even more importance to the investigation on pathophysiology, prevention and surveillance of surgical wound infection. In the next section the experience in our hospital during the 1980's and early 90's about prophylaxis in orthopaedic surgery will be discussed.

Previous Experience in Prevention of Infection in Orthopaedic Surgery

Several randomized and double blind studies were conducted in our hospital from 1982 to 1990. The patients included in the consecutive studies were patients who needed an internal fixation due to a femoral neck fracture. In the first study [13], prophylaxis with cefamandol 1 g every 8 h (a second generation cephalosporin with 0.8 h of half-life) was compared to a placebo. The infection rate was statistically significantly lower in the cefamandol group ($p < 0.05$). The second study [12], compared cefamandol 2 g preoperatively, 2 g at 2 h postoperative and 1 g at 8 h, 14 h and 20 h postoperative to only one dose of 2 g preoperatively. None of the patients assigned to the first regimen and 6.6 % of those in the mono-dose regimen had an infection ($p = 0.03$). Since in the multiple doses arm the second dose of cefamandol was administered 2 h after the initiation of surgery and the half-life of this antibiotic is only 0.8 h, our results suggest that the maintenance of high plasmatic levels during surgery is associated to a better efficacy. In order to demonstrate this hypothesis, we compared the efficacy of one preoperative dose of 2 g of cefonicid, a second-generation cephalosporin with a half-life of 4 h, with multiple doses of cefamandol [11]. In this case there were also no differences in the infection rate between groups were found. Since the most frequently recommended antibiotic in orthopaedic surgery is cefazolin (half-life of 1.7 h), 2 doses of cefazolin 30' preoperative and 2 h postoperative were compared with multiple doses of cefamandol and no differences were observed between both regimens (Lozano ML, García S, Gatell JM et al. Prophylaxis in clean orthopaedic surgery requiring implantable devices, New Orleans: 36th ICAAC 1996). Our studies support the importance of maintaining a high antibiotic concentration during surgery. This objective is achievable by administrating: 1) two doses of a first or second-generation cephalosporin with short half-life at intervals no longer than 2-fold the half-life of the antibiotic or 2) one dose when the half-life of the antibiotic is over 4 h.

During the last years, the incidence of methicillin-resistant staphylococci in wound infections is on the increase. This raises the question about the need of modifying the prophylaxis from cephalosporins to glycopeptides. The following section deals with a recently study conducted in our hospital on this subject.

Prevention of Methicillin-resistant *S. aureus* (MRSA) Infection

During the last 15 years the prevalence of methicillin-resistant *S. aureus* (MRSA) infections in orthopaedic surgery has increased [28]. One important factor that may explain this finding in the developed world is the increasing number of patients admitted to the hospitals colonized or infected by MRSA. In fact, since 2002 the number of patients colonized by MRSA admitted from the community has increased and now they represent about 40 % of the total MRSA isolates in our hospital. Since nasal colonization with *S. aureus* is a well-recognized independent risk factor for developing a surgical-site infection (SSI), the increase of SSI by MRSA among patients operated for femoral neck fracture is not surprising because this population has a high risk to be colonized by MRSA (most of them are living in a nursing home or had been previously hospitalized). In order to control these endogenous infections, one of the preventive measures is the use of a glycopeptide in prophylaxis. Periti et al [24], reviewed the articles published comparing teicoplanin versus cephalosporins as prophylaxis in orthopaedic surgery and they showed that both regimens were equally effective. However, the prevalence of MRSA in the studied populations was low. The objective of our study was to evaluate the impact of adding 600 mg of teicoplanin to cefuroxim during induction of anaesthesia on the prevalence of MRSA infections in a population with a previously documented high prevalence of infections due to MRSA [29].

The global and MRSA infection rates in internal fixation for femoral fracture in our hospital during 2002 were 5.07 % and 2.73 %, respectively, using cefuroxim as antibiotic prophylaxis. Pulse-field gel electrophoresis demonstrated that there was no clonal relationship among MRSA strains and no nasal carriers of MRSA were detected among health workers. During the following year, 600 mg of teicoplanin were added to cefuroxim and infused at anaesthetic induction. The global and MRSA infection rates were significantly lower during the second period than those in the first period, 2.36 % (p = 0.04) and 0.19 % (p = 0.002), respectively. The selection of high dose teicoplanin was based on a previous experience in cardiac surgery where 400 mg of teicoplanin showed lower efficacy than cloxacillin plus tobramycin in prevention of Gram-positive infections. The explanation for these findings could be related to the high protein binding showed by teicoplanin (> 90 %) since only the free fraction of an antibiotic is microbiologically active and it could be surpassed using high doses. On the other hand, we consider that it is necessary to maintain cephalosporin in order to prevent infections due to Gram-negative bacilli (GNB). In fact, reviewing the microbiological aetiology in those clinical trials, those patients receiving teicoplanin had a higher percentage of GNB infections than those receiving cephalosporins. In conclusion, our study suggests that teicoplanin and cefuroxim is an effective prophylactic regimen for those patients who undergo surgical treatment of a femoral neck fracture and who may be at high risk of developing a post-operative MRSA wound infection.

The Impact of a Tourniquet in the Efficacy of Antimicrobial Prophylaxis in Orthopaedic Surgery

Since the major bacterial contamination occurs while the wound is open, the most important factor associated with the efficacy of antimicrobial prophylaxis is the presence of a high antibiotic concentration in the tissues and blood bathing the wound during the whole surgery period (Fig. 1). As mentioned earlier, it is possible to achieve this objective infusing an antibiotic with a short half-life during the induction of anaesthesia if the duration of surgery is less than 2 hours. This is the case of the majority of orthopaedic procedures and it explains the well-documented efficacy of cefazolin or cefuroxim [25]. However, when the surgery is performed under ischemia (i.e. total knee arthroplasty) the antibiotic is administered before inflating the tourniquet. The precise timing for infusing the antibiotic was established by several authors [10, 15] that measured the antibiotic concentration in bone and fat during total knee arthroplasty after administering the antibiotic at different intervals before inflating the tourniquet. The conclusion was that infusing the antibiotic 10 minutes before inflating the tourniquet the concentration in bone and fat was over the minimal inhibitory concentration of cephalosporins for the main pathogens. However, in spite of applying these precautions some authors have observed a higher infection rate in knee arthroplasty than in hip arthroplasty. Furthermore, two pilot studies that compared the outcome of knee arthroplasty performed with or without tourniquet or early release of tourniquet, observed a lower rate of infectious complications in the arm operated without tourniquet or with early release of it [1, 3]. A possible explanation is that the haematoma formed around the prosthesis should contain a high antibiotic concentration to kill the contaminant microorganisms. In the case of knee arthroplasty, the blood reaches the wound and form haematomas after the tourniquet release. This means a delay of about 60 to 80 minutes from the infusion of the antibiotic to the moment of tourniquet release (10–30 minutes before tourniquet plus approximately 50 minutes of ischemia, data from personal experience in 900 knee arthroplasties performed in our hospital). Therefore, if we use an antibiotic with a half-life of 1h at the moment of tourniquet release the blood bathing the wound will have a low antibiotic concentration. Richardson et al [27], measured the concentration of cephamandole (a cephalosporin with 0.8 h of half-life) in serum and drain fluid to determine the benefit of an intravenous dose of antibiotic at the time of tourniquet deflation in 32 knee replacement operations. The most important findings were: 1) the concentration of cephamandole in drain fluid was directly proportional to the serum concentration at the time of tourniquet release and 2) the addition of a 'tourniquet-release' dose of antibiotic increased concentration of drain fluid three-fold. Therefore, in the future it is necessary to design clinical trials to investigate the best moment for antibiotic administration in knee arthroplasty.

References

1. Abdel-Salam A, Eyres KS (1995) Effects of tourniquet during total knee arthroplasty. A prospective randomised study. J Bone Joint Surg (Br) 77(2):250–253
2. Ainscow DA, Denham RA (1984) The risk of haematogenous infection in total joint replacements. J Bone Joint Surg (Br) 66(4):580–582
3. Barwell J, Anderson G, Hassan A et al (1997) The effects of early tourniquet release during total knee arthroplasty: a prospective randomized double-blind study. J Bone Joint Surg (Br) 79(2):265–268
4. Brandt CM, Sistrunk WW, Duffy MC et al (1997) Staphylococcus aureus prosthetic joint infection treated with debridement and prosthesis retention. Clin Infect Dis 24(5):914–919
5. Carlsson AK, Lidgren L, Lindberg L (1977) Prophylactic antibiotics against early and late deep infections after total hip replacements. Acta Orthop Scand 48(4):405–410
6. Classen DC, Evans RS, Pestotnik SL et al (1992) The timing of prophylactic administration of antibiotics and the risk of surgical-wound infection. N Engl J Med 326(5):281–286
7. Curry S, Phillips H (2002) Joint arthroplasty, dental treatment, and antibiotics: a review. J Arthroplasty 17(1):111–113
8. Engesaeter LB, Lie SA, Espehaug B et al (2003) Antibiotic prophylaxis in total hip arthroplasty: effects of antibiotic prophylaxis systemically and in bone cement on the revision rate of 22,170 primary hip replacements followed 0–14 years in the Norwegian Arthroplasty Register. Acta Orthop Scand 74(6):644–651
9. Falcieri E, Vaudaux P, Huggler E et al (1984) Role of bacterial exopolymers and host factors on adherence and phagocytosis of Staphylococcus aureus in foreign body infection. J Infect Dis 155(3):524–531
10. Friedman RJ, Friedrich LV, White RL et al (1990) Antibiotic prophylaxis and tourniquet inflation in total knee arthroplasty. Clin Orthop Relat Res (260):17–23
11. Garcia S, Lozano ML, Gatell JM et al (1991) Prophylaxis against infection. Single-dose cefonicid compared with multiple-dose cefamandole. J Bone Joint Surg (Am) 73(7):1044–1048
12. Gatell JM, Garcia S, Lozano L et al (1987) Perioperative cefamandole prophylaxis against infections. J Bone Joint Surg (Am) 69(8):1189–1193
13. Gatell JM, Riba J, Lozano ML et al (1984) Prophylactic cefamandole in orthopaedic surgery. J Bone Joint Surg (Am) 66(8):1219–1222
14. Greif R, Akca O, Horn EP et al (2000) Supplemental perioperative oxygen to reduce the incidence of surgical-wound infection. Outcomes Research Group. N Engl J Med 342(3):161–167
15. Johnson DP (1987) Antibiotic prophylaxis with cefuroxime in arthroplasty of the knee. J Bone Joint Surg (Br) 69(5):787–789
16. Kalmeijer MD, Coertjens H, Nieuwland-Bollen PM et al (2002) Surgical site infections in orthopedic surgery: the effect of mupirocin nasal ointment in a double-blind, randomized, placebo-controlled study. Clin Infect Dis 35(4):353–358
17. Kalmeijer MD, Nieuwland-Bollen E, Bogaers-Hofman D et al (2000) Nasal carriage of Staphylococcus aureus is a major risk factor for surgical-site infections in orthopedic surgery. Infect Control Hosp Epidemiol 21(5):319–323
18. Kluytmans JA, Wertheim HF (2005) Nasal carriage of Staphylococcus aureus and prevention of nosocomial infections. Infection 33(1):3–8
19. Krizek TJ, Robson MC (1975) Evolution of quantitative bacteriology in wound management. Am J Surg 130(5):579–584
20. Kurz A, Sessler DI, Lenhardt R (1996) Perioperative normothermia to reduce the incidence of surgical-wound infection and shorten hospitalization. Study of Wound Infection and Temperature Group. N Engl J Med 334(19):1209–1215

21. Latham R, Lancaster AD, Covington JF et al (2001) The association of diabetes and glucose control with surgical-site infections among cardiothoracic surgery patients. Infect Control Hosp Epidemiol 22(10):607–612

22. Mangram AJ, Horan TC, Pearson ML et al (1999) Guideline for Prevention of Surgical Site Infection, 1999. Centers for Disease Control and Prevention (CDC) Hospital Infection Control Practices Advisory Committee. Am J Infect Control 27(2):97–132

23. Miles AA, MIiles EM, Burke J (1957) The value and duration of defence reactions of the skin to the primary lodgement of bacteria. Br J Exp Pathol 38(1):79–96

24. Mini E, Nobili S, Periti P (1997) Methicillin-resistant staphylococci in clean surgery. Is there a role for prophylaxis? Drugs 54(Suppl 6):39–52

25. Oishi CS, Carrion WV, Hoaglund FT (1993) Use of parenteral prophylactic antibiotics in clean orthopaedic surgery. A review of the literature. Clin Orthop Relat Res (296):249–255

26. Perl TM, Cullen JJ, Wenzel RP et al (2002). Intranasal mupirocin to prevent postoperative Staphylococcus aureus infections. N Engl J Med 346(24):1871–1877

27. Richardson JB, Roberts A, Robertson JF et al (1993) Timing of antibiotic administration in knee replacement under tourniquet. J Bone Joint Surg (Br) 75(1):32–35

28. Ridgeway S, Wilson J, Charlet A et al (2005) Infection of the surgical site after arthroplasty of the hip. J Bone Joint Surg (Br) 87(6):844–850

29. Soriano A, Popescu D, Garcia S et al (2006) Usefulness of teicoplanin for preventing methicillin-resistant Staphylococcus aureus infections in orthopedic surgery. Eur J Clin Microbiol Infect Dis 25(1):35–38

30. Zimmerli W, Trampuz A, Ochsner PE (2004) Prosthetic-joint infections. N Engl J Med 351(16):1645–1654

The Limits of Systemic Antibiotics in Device-related Infections

P. Baiocchi[1], P. Martino[2]

[1] Department of Clinical Medicine, University "La Sapienza", Rome, Italy
[2] Department of Human Biopathology University "La Sapienza", Rome, Italy

Introduction

Infection rate following implatation of an orthopedic device has continuously decreased during the last 50 years [4] but, since the numbers of trauma and aged patients requiring joint replacement is steadily increasing, the absolute number of patients with device-associated infection is raising [10]. The infection rate should not exceed 1% in patients with primary hip replacement and 2% in those with knee replacement [6, 7, 14]. However, the real overall risk per patient-life is unknown, since in most case series only the first 2 years after implantation are considered.

Main

During the past decade considerable progress has been made in the treatment of orthopaedic implant-associated infections [11, 19]. The goal of treating infection associated to a prosthetized joint is a pain-free, functional joint. This can best be achieved by infection eradication. Various therapies have been used, including surgical removal of all infected tissue and the implant, and a combination of debridement with implant retention and long-term antimicrobial therapy that is active against biofilm microrganisms. In North America, debridement with device retention and one-stage exchange (in which the infected prosthesis is removed and a new one implanted in the same procedure) is performed less frequently than in Europe, and the interval between resection and reimplantation of the prosthesis, two-stage exchange, is generally longer (typically six weeks) [8, 18].

In addition, long-term therapy with suppressive oral antimicrobial agents is commonly used in North America; in Europe, this treatment is reserved mainly for patients in whom surgery is contraindicated [17].

The proposed standard procedure is a two-stage exchange with meticulous removal of all foreign material (device and bone cement) combined with a finite course of antimicrobial treatment. Alternatively, lifelong suppressive oral antimicrobial treatment without surgical intervention is suggested. The traditional two-stage exchange is fastidious, time-consuming and the functional result may be suboptimal due to delayed re-implantation of the prosthesis. Alternatively, long-term suppressive antimicrobial therapy without exchange usually controls clinical manifestation of the infection, but does not eradicate infection [15]. The ultimate goal of a successful therapy, namely the eradication of infection associated with a pain-free functional joint, can only be accomplished with a combination of both surgical and antimicrobial treatment.

In prosthesis-associated infection, standard antimicrobial-susceptibility tests cannot used to reliably predict the outcome [2, 20, 22]. Ideally, the antimicrobial agent should have bactericidal activity against surface-adhering, slow-growing, and biofilm-producing microrganism [20, 22]. Really, the optimal antimicrobial therapy is well defined in staphylococcal orthopaedic implant-associated infections. This therapy includes rifampicin in susceptible pathogens [23]. Rifampin has excellent activity in slow-growing and adherent staphylococci but it must always be combined with a drug of a different class to prevent emergence of resistance in staphylococci. Quinolones are excellent combination drugs because of their good bioavailability, activity and safety. Newer quinolones such as moxifloxacin and levofloxacin have better *in vitro* activity against quinolone-susceptible staphylococci compared to ciprofloxacin or ofloxacin. However, when administered alone levofloxacin was shown to be unable to eliminate adherent staphylococci "*in vitro*" or "*in vivo*" [12]. In contrast to older quinolones, no controlled clinical trials of quinolones in implant-associated infection with a sufficient follow-up period have been conducted. Moreover, possible interaction of newer quinolones with rifampicin have not yet been systematically assessed. In addition, safety data for long-term therapy with moxifloxacin are not available. For levofloxacin long-term experience is only available by extrapolating from the ofloxacin experience and from studies in patients with mycobacterial infection [5, 21]. Because of increasing resistance to quinolones, other anti-staphylococcal drugs have been combined with rifampicin. Rifampin combinations with minocycline or cotrimoxazole may have higher success rates, but sufficient clinical data are lacking. High-dose oral cotrimoxazole was used in the treatment of infected implants in 39 patients with an overall success rate of 67 %, though removal of unstable components was conducted within 3 to 9 months of treatment [16]. Increasing antimicrobial resistance of staphylococci prompted the search for new antibiotics or novel combinations.

Recently, in a retrospective study of linezolid in 20 patients with prosthetic joint infections (MRSA 14 strains, methicillin-resistant coagulase-negative, 5 strains and *Enterococcus* spp., 1 strain) who either refused further surgical intervention or in

Table 1. Treatment of staphylococcal infection of orthopaedic devices in animal models: role of rifampin +/– quinolone +/– glycopeptide

Therapy	% Failure	Comment
Rifampin	> 80	development of resistance
Quinolone	> 80	development of resistance
Quinolone + Rifampicin	0 – 60	idem !!!
Glycopeptide + Quinolone + Rifampicin	< 10	no resistance ?

From
1. Tobin EH (1999) Prosthetic joint infections: controversies and clues. Lancet 353(9155): 770 – 771.
2. Widmer AF, Frei R, Rajacic Z et al (1990) Correlation between in vivo and in vitro efficacy of antimicrobial agents against foreign body infections. J Infect Dis 162(1):96 – 102.
3. Rissing JP (1997) Antimicrobial therapy for chronic osteomyelitis in adults: role of the quinolones. Clin Infect Dis 25(6):1327 – 1333.

whom surgical removal was not feasible, reported a cure rate of 80 % [1]. The overall duration of treatment was 7.2 +/- 2 weeks (range 6 – 10 weeks), linezolid was well tolerated and no drug-related event leading to discontinuation of treatment were recorded [1]. There are no data on cotrimoxazole and linezolid in combination with rifampicin.

Penicillin-susceptible streptococcal prosthetic joint infections have been successfully treated, with prosthetic retention, using intravenous penicillin or ceftriaxone, followed by oral amoxicillin- rifampin [9].

Few data are available on the treatment of gram-negative bacilli. *In vitro* studies and in animal model showed that ciprofloxacin had better efficacy against gram negative bacilli than did beta-lactam [22]. For *P. aeruginosa* infected prostheses, two-stage exchange remains the treatment of choice, altought in a recent study using a combination of ceftazidime and ciprofloxacin, reported a cure in four of five patients without implant removal [15].

Antibiotic therapy alone for long-term suppression is a reasonable option for patients in whom surgery is contraindicated for different reasons or who refuse further procedures. Its goal is to reduce the clinical manifestations rather than eradicating the infection, and preserving joint function. The prerequisites for long term suppressive antimicrobial therapy are: stability of the prosthesis, relatively avirulent pathogen sensitivity to an orally well absorbed antibiotic, absence of systemic infection, good tolerability of oral antibiotic therapy and compliance of the patient. There are no guidelines regarding the duration of this approach [13]. The suppressive approach is not without risk, the main being the emergence of secondary resistance, the extension of the localised septic process to adjacent tissue possibly heading to systemic infection, and the potential side-effects of long term antibiotic therapy.

Conclusion

Antibiotic therapy has a important role in the treatment of device related infection but there are some considerations regarding its limits. These including emergence of resistence, possible toxicity and infection due to *Clostridium difficile*. Other limits may be due to patient and the socio-economic condition compliance to tratment.

There is no single approach that is the best. Stability of the prosthesis, duration of the symptoms, pathogen detection and its antibiotic susceptibility to oral antimicrobial agents with activity against surface-adhering microorganisms, condition of soft tissues, patient preference and health status need to be considered in selecting the approach to therapy.

Large-scale multicentre trials are still necessary to determine the influence of the multiple variables involved in arthroplasty infections.

References

1. Bassetti M, Vitale F, Melica G (2005) Linezolid in the treatment of Gram positive prosthetic joint infections. J Antimicrob Agents 55(3):387 – 390
2. Brandt CM, Sistrunk WW, Duffy MC (1997) Staphylococcus aureus prosthetic joint infection treated with debridement and prosthesis retention. Clin Infect Dis 24(5):914 – 919

3. Brouqui P, Raousseau MC, Stein A e al (1995) Treatment of Pseudomonas aeruginosa infected orthopedic prostheses with ceftazidime-ciprofloxacin antibiotic combination. Antimicrob Agents Chemother 39(11):2423–2425

4. Carvin K, Hanssen AD (1995) Infection after total hip arthroplasty. Past, present and future. J Bone Joint Surg (Am) 77(10):1576–1588

5. Drancourt M, Stein A, Argenson JN et al (1990) Oral rifampin plus ofloxacin for treatment of Staphylococcus infected orthopedic implants. Antimicr Agents Chemother 37(6):1214–1218

6. Harris WH, Sledge CB (1990) Total hip and total knee replacement (1). N Engl J Med 323(11):725–731. Review

7. Harris WH, Sledge CB (1990) Total hip and total knee replacement (2) N Engl J Med 323(12):801–807. Review

8. Langlais F (2003) Can we improve the results of revision arthroplasty for infected total hip replacement? J Bone Joint Surg (Br) 85(5):637–640

9. Meehan AM, Osmon DR, Duffy MC et al (2003) Outcome of penicillin-susceptible streptococcal prosthetic infections treated with debridement and retention of the prosthesis. Clin Infect Dis 36(7):845–849

10. NIH consensus conference: Total hip replacement. NIH Consensus Development Panel on Total Hip Replacement (1995) JAMA 273(24):1950–1956

11. Sanderson PJ (1999) Orthopaedic implant infections. Opin Infect Dis 12(4):347–350

12. Schwank S, Rajack Z, Zimmerly W et al (1998) Impact of bacterial biofilm formation on in vitro and in vivo activities of antibiotics. Antimicrob Agents Chemother 42(4):895–898

13. Segreti J, Nelson JA, Trenholme GM (1998) Prolonged suppressive antibiotic therapy for infected orthopaedic prostheses. Clin Infect Dis 27(4):711–713

14. Spangehl MI, Younger AS, Masri BA et al (1998) Diagnosis of infection following total hip arthroplasty. Instr Course Lect (47):285–295

15. SteckelbergJM, Osmon DR (2000) Prosthetic joint infection, In Infections associated with indwelling medical devices. Bisno AL, Vladogel FA eds. American Society for Microbiology. Washington DC USA 173–209

16. Stein A, Batails JF, Drancourt M et al (1998) Ambulatory treatment of multidrug-resistant Staphylococcus- infected orthopedi implants with high-dose oral co-trimoxazole (trimethoprim- sulfamethoxazole) Antimicrob Agents Chemother 42(12):3086–3091

17. Tsukayama DT, Wicklund B, Gustilo RB (1991) Suppressive antibiotic therapy in chronic prosthesis joint infections. Orthopedics 14(8):841–844

18. Westrich GH, Salvati EA, Brause B (1999) in: Bono JV, Mc Carty JC, Thornhill TS, Bierbaum BE, Turner RH, eds. Revision total hip arthroplasty. NY: Springer-Verlag 371–390

19. Widmer AF (2001) New developments in diagnosis and treatment of infection in orthopedic implants. Clin Infect Dis 33(Suppl 2):S94–106. Review

20. Widner AF, Frei R, Rajacic Z et al (1990) Correlation between in vivo and in vitro efficacy of antimicrobial agents against foreign body infection. J Infect Dis 162(1):96–102

21. Yew WW, Chan CK, Laung CC et al (2003) Comparative roles of levofloxacin and ofloxacin in the treatment of multidrug-resistant tuberculosis. Preliminary results of a retrospective study from Hong Kong. Chest 124(4):1476–1481

22. Zimmerli W, Frei R , Widner AF et al (1994) Microbiological tests to predict treatment outcome in experimental device-related infections due to Staphylococcus aureus. J Antimicrob Chemother 33(5):959–967

23. Zimmerli W, Witner AF, Blatter F et al (1996) Role of rifampin for treatment of orthopedic implant related staphylococcal infections: a rondomized controlled trial. Foreign Body Infection (FBI) Study Group J Am Med Assoc 279(19):1537–1541

7 Antibiotic Bone Cement as a Prophylactic Means in Joint Replacement Surgery

A. Lundberg, H. Hedlund

Department of Orthopaedics, Karolinska University Hospital, Stockholm, Sweden

Introduction

The use of some form of cement as an alternative to direct mechanical fixation (press-fit, screws etc) dates back to the earliest period of joint replacement surgery. The first void-filling agent to be tried by Gluck in 1890 was a combination of plaster, pumice and resin. At this time there were no antibiotics, and the experiments failed for this and other obvious reasons [13]. When methyl methacrylate as a bone cement was made popular in the field of implant fixation in the 1960's, antibiotics were available and the first documented use of antibiotic loaded bone cement occurred within this decade [4].

From the start of the joint replacement era, gentamicin and other agents belonging to the aminoglycoside group, which has heat resistance as a major characteristic, dominated the market. However, many other agents have been used, and in recent years there has been an upsurge in the attention given to several of the many heat resistant antibiotics avaiable, mainly as a result of increased presence of gentamycin resistant bacteria [17].

Over the years, many combinations of cement and antibiotic have also been used in the treatment of manifest infection. however, this review only covers prophylactic use of bone cement/antibiotic.

In this field, the main points of controversy have been:

- The efficacy of antibiotic loaded cement in preventing implant infection
- The risk of allergic reaction to the antibiotic agent
- The risk of alterations in the mechanical properties of bone cement caused by the antibiotic additive
- The risk of toxic reaction to the antibiotic agent
- The risk of altered resistance patterns of different bacteria caused by extensive use of antibiotic additives in routine joint replacement surgery, and
- The risk of the presence of antibiotics influencing assessment of infection in the patient.

Available Documentation

Experimental

There are large volumes of documentation available, relating to the antibiotic release properties, the influence (or lack of influence) of antibiotic agents on the mechanical properties of different bone cements as well as the in vitro antimicrobial effects of different combinations of bone cement and antibiotic agent.

Antibiotic Release Properties

These properties vary between different combinations of cement and antibiotic agent. The period of described elution of significant amounts of antibiotics has usually been in the range from 7 to 14 days, but considerably higher values have also been suggested [2, 4, 9, 16, 18, 21]

Mechanical Properties

The results generally support the view that the mechanical properties of bone cement are not significantly altered by up to 4–5 % by volume of an antibiotic additive. This corresponds to the range where antibiotic additives for prophylactic use are normally kept, and there seems to be relative consensus that influence on mechanical properties is not a problem with these amounts of antibiotic [7, 14].

Antimicrobial Efficacy

In vitro studies have shown inhibition of bacterial growth by antibiotic loaded cement [3, 17], but also increased presence of strains resistant to the used antibiotic [20].

Clinical

Efficacy

1. RCT evidence
   Few RCT studies have been performed where different cements and/or antibiotic prophylaxis regimens have been compared. Chiu et al have shown in two studies, one on otherwise healthy patients, the other on diabetic patients, that there was a significant reduction in the incidence of infection when an antibiotic was added to the cement [5, 6]. In another study antibiotic loaded cement was also found to be efficient in reducing the risk of infection in the early postoperative period [12].

2. Epidemiological evidence
   Most of the national registers of implant surgery have addressed the issues of prophylactic antibiotics. The most commonly quoted publication today comes from the Norwegian national register [8] and shows that antibiotics administered systemically and locally as an additive to the cement have cumulative effect on the risk of revision for septic loosening. Data from the Swedish national hip register have also shown a decreased incidence of septic loosening of hip implants with the use of antibiotic loaded cement [15].

Excluding the few studies that have shown no difference in joint infection incidence, the difference in the rate of deep infection between cement containing antibiotic and not containing antibiotic has varied between 1:2 and 1:4 [5, 6, 8, 12, 15]. A very rough estimate of the corresponding cost difference at the time of primary surgery (assuming a cost of USD 30,000 for a two-stage procedure and not including other costs) would yield USD 200–400. The cost for the antibiotic additive is approximately USD 40.

Safety

1. Influence on mechanical properties of the bone cement
   There are few clinical studies of the influence of antibiotics on the mechanical properties of cement. Studies using radiostereometric analysis have supported the experimental finding that the addition of antibiotics in prophylactic amounts does not significantly alter the mechanical properties of bone cement [1]

2. Toxic effects
   The most commonly used agent, gentamicin, was known at the time that it was first used as an adjunct in bone cement to show a large variation in uptake when administered systemically. The amounts used in bone cement are large, but clinical studies have not shown risks of toxic reactions even in the presence of renal impairment [10].

3. Hypersensitivity
   Hypersensitivity is much less common for aminoglycosides than for β-lactam antibiotics, which are less commonly used in cement. As with the metals contained in joint implants, final proof that there is no risk of hypersensitivity at all is lacking.

4. Influence on bacterial resistance patterns and clinical decision making
   Influence of antibiotic additives on bacterial resistance patterns can mainly be expected in situations where the release rate of the antibiotic gives lower concentrations than the MIC value. This has been seen as related to the increased incidence of gentamicin resistance in particularly coagulase-negative staphylococci (CNS) [11].

5. Clinical decision making
   A further possible problem relates to clinical decision making. It has been shown that the antibiotic contained in old cement mantles may influence the reliability of cultures taken from the joint by aspiration [9] as well as during revision surgery [19].

Discussion

There is wide consensus that the addition of antibiotics to bone cement reduces the risk of septic loosening, although there is a possibility that this correlation is much stronger in patients with an increased risk of infection due to risk factors such as diabetes. Toxicity is according to most investigators not a problem. There are now several studies conclusively showing that the quality of the cement mantle is not significantly impaired by the addition of antibiotic in the amounts used for prophylactic purposes.

The main concerns voiced against the routine use of prophylactic antibiotic additives in bone cement relate to the risk of hypersensitivity and the risk of adverse influence on bacterial patterns of resistance to antibiotics. While the latter is a real and important concern, it seems unlikely that the use of antibiotics as additives to bone cement should constitute a more serious risk for future multi-resistance patterns in bacteria. Hypersensitivity to antibiotics may be a more serious concern, particularly as the spectrum of agents used widens. A single case of serious allergic reaction to an antibiotic agent may overthrow the gains from a decade of persistent use of all means available to reduce the infection rate after total joint reaction. It is also important to consider the presence of antibiotics in the cement mantle of patients with joint implants when evaluating aspirate and tissue cultures.

References

1. Adalberth G, Nilsson KG, Karrholm J et al (2002) Fixation of the tibial component using CMW-1 or Palacos bone cement with gentamicin: similar outcome in a randomized radiosteReometric study of 51 total knee arthroplasties. Acta Orthop Scand 73(5):531–538
2. Armstrong M, Spencer RF, Lovering AM et al (2002) Antibiotic elution from bone cement: A study of common cement-antibiotic combinations. Hip International (12):23–27
3. van de Belt H, Neut D, Schenk W et al (2000) Gentamicin release from polymethylmethylacrylate bone cement and staphylococcus aureus biofilm formation. Acta Orthop Scand 71(6):625–629
4. Buchholz HW, Elson RA, Engelbrecht E et al (1981) Management of deep infection of total hip replacement. J Bone Joint Surg (Br) 63(3):342–353
5. Chiu FY, Lin C-FJ, Chen CM et al (2001) Cefuroxime-impregnated cement at primary total knee arthroplasty in diabetes mellitus. A prospective, randomized study. J Bone Joint Surg (Br) 83(5):691–695
6. Chiu FY, Chen CM, Lin C-FJ et al (2002). Cefuroxime-impregnated cement in primary total knee arthroplasty: a prospective, randomized study of three hundred and forty knees. J Bone Joint Surg (Am) 84(5):759–762
7. Davies J, O'Connor DO, Harris WH (1984). Comparison of the mechanical properties of Palacos, Palacos-gentamicin and Simplex P. Orthop Trans (8):400–401
8. Espehaug B, Engesaeter LB, Vollset SE et al (1997). Antibiotic prophylaxis in total hip arthroplasty. Review of 10,905 primary cemented total hip replacements reported to the Norwegian arthroplasty register, 1987 to 1995. J Bone Joint Surg (Br) 79(4):590–595
9. Fletcher MDA, Spencer RF, LangkamerVG et al (2004). Gentamicin concentrations in diagnostic aspirates from 25 patients with hip and knee arthroplasties. Acta Orthop Scand 75(2):173–176
10. Forsythe ME, Crawford S, Sterling GJ et al (2006). Safeness of Simplex-tobramycin bone cement in patients with renal dysfunction undergoing total hip replacement. J Orthop Surg 14(1):38–42
11. Hansen AD (2004). Prophylactic use of antibiotic bone cement: an emerging standard – in opposition. J Arthroplasty 19(suppl 1):73–77
12. Josefsson G, Kolmert L (1993). Prophylaxis with systematic antibiotics versus gentamicin bone cement in total hip arthroplasty: A ten-year survey of 1,688 hips. Clin Orthop Relat Res (292):210–214
13. LeVay D (1990). The history of orthopaedics. Parthenon, Carnforth
14. Lewis G, Bhattaram A (2006). Influence of a pre-blended antibiotic (gentamicin sulfate powder) on various mechanical, thermal and physical properties of three acrylic bone cements. J Biomater Appl 20(4):377–408

15. Malchau H, Herberts P, Ahnfelt L (1993). Prognosis of total hip replacement in Sweden. Follow-up of 92,675 operations performed 1978–1990. Acta Orthop Scand 64(5):497–506
16. Masri BA, Duncan CP, Beauchamp CP (1998). Long-term elution of antibiotics from bone cement: an in vivo study using the prosthesis of antibiotic-loaded acrylic cement (PROSTA-LAC) system. J Arthroplasty 13(3):331–338
17. Neut D, Hendriks JGE, van Horn JR et al (2006). Antimicrobial efficacy of gentamicin-loaded acrylic bone cements with fusidic acid or clindamycin added. J Orthop Res 24(2):291–299
18. Penner MJ, Duncan CP, Masri BA (1999). The in vitro elution characteristics of antibiotic-loaded CMW and Palacos-R bone cements. J Arthroplasty 14(2):209–214
19. Powles JW, Spencer RF, Lovering AM (1998). Gentamicin release from old cement during revision hip arthroplasty. J Bone Joint Surg (Br) 80(4):607–610
20. Thornes B, Murray P, Bouchier-Hayes D (2002) Development of resistant strains of staphylococcus epidermidis on gentamicin loaded bone cement in vivo. J Bone Joint Surg (Br) 84(5):758–760
21. Trippel SB (1986) Antibiotic impregnated cement in total joint arthroplasty. J Bone Joint Surg (Am) 68(8):1297–1302

The Limits of the Local Antibiotic Therapy

E. Witsø

Department of Orthopaedic Surgery, St. Olavs University Hospital; Norwegian University of Science and Technology; Trondheim, Norway

Introduction

This presentation will focus on two subjects: a) does the slow release of antibiotics from bone cement have a particular antibiotic resistant promoting effect, and b) does the use of local antibiotics in orthopaedic surgery have any allergic or toxic side effects.

The Emergence of Resistant Bacterial Strains and Biofilm Formation

The amount of antibiotics eluted from antibiotic-impregnated bone cement shows a high early release with exponential decay, both *in vitro* and *in vivo* [2, 17, 18, 22, 24, 31]. Studies of antibiotic release from different combinations of bone cement and antibiotics have reported on antibiotic concentration in drainage fluid from the hip joint, with peak values (mean) ranging from 25 – 118 mg/L of gentamicin and 9 – 43 mg/L of tobramycin [4 – 6, 9, 20, 23, 37, 38, 49, 50]. After the initial phase of exponential decay, bone cement elutes small amounts of antibiotic for many years *in vitro* and *in vivo* [44, 49], and gentamicin has been recovered in urine two years postoperatively [44].

There is an increasing concern regarding the decreasing effectiveness of antibiotics [19]. Bacterial genes coding for resistance against most antibiotics occur naturally [8, 41], and the widespread use and misuse of antibiotics have selected antibiotic resistant bacterial strains. *In vitro* studies have demonstrated the development of aminoglycoside-resistant strains of *Staphylococcus aureus* and *Staphylococcus epidermidis* on the surface of different types of bone cement containing gentamicin, tobramycin and vancomycin [16, 28, 45, 46]. *In vivo*, resistant strains of *S. epidermidis* developed both on cement containing gentamicin and on cement with no antibiotics, but at a significantly higher rate in the gentamicin group. The author of the study concluded that *"Antibiotic-impregnated cement provides an excellent environment for the development of resistant strains of Staphylococcus epidermidis"* [40]. The emergence of gentamicin-resistant Small Colony Variant form of bacteria has also been associated with the use of antibiotic-containing bone cement [27, 47].

Probably as a result of billions of years of adaptation, and as a strategy for bacterial survival, more than 90 % of all bacteria adhere, colonize and form biofilm on all types of surfaces. It is a thousand times more difficult for the body's natural defense or antimicrobial therapy to eradicate bacteria that have established themselves in a biofilm.

Fig. 1. A picture of live bacteria (green stain), embedded in a biofilm on gentamicin containing bone cement (Copyright: Daniëlle Neut)

The use of biomaterials, including orthopaedic implants in general and bone cement in particular, entails the risk of biofilm formation on their surfaces [25, 43]. *In vitro*, bone cement containing gentamicin does not inhibit biofilm formation [27, 46] (Fig. 1).

The slow release of antibiotics from bone cement has been considered as a potential risk for the emergence of antibiotic resistant bacterial strains. Previously, *in vitro* studies have shown reduced adherence of bacteria to surfaces when exposed to sub-inhibitory concentrations of different antibiotics [21, 36]. However, there is increasing evidence for a specific effect of antibiotics used in low concentrations, and that this effect is distinct from their inhibitory effect [11]. Beta-lactams in sub-inhibitory concentrations stimulate the expression of virulence-associated genes in *S. aureus* [29], and sub-inhibitory concentrations of aminoglycosides, ciprofloxacin, tetracycline and erythromycin promote bacterial adherence and biofilm formation, *in vitro* [3, 13, 34]. In an *in vitro* model simulating the clinical situation with high gentamicin concentration in the interfacial gap, sensitive strains of *S. aureus*, *S. epidermidis* and *Pseudomonas aeruginosa* did not adhere to the cement [12]. The same result was observed when antibiotic-containing bone cement eluted for three weeks in saline was employed. To my knowledge, there are no *in vivo* studies that have properly addressed the possible emergence of resistant bacterial strains as resulting from prolonged slow release of antibiotics from bone cement.

Very few clinical studies have focused on the clinical relevance of the above mentioned *in vitro* and *in vivo* studies. Hope [15] reviewed 91 patients with an infected cemented prosthesis. A preliminary biopsy confirmed the diagnosis of deep infection in all cases. Joint fluid and peri-prosthetic tissue samples were obtained using a cannula. The number of biopsies taken is not mentioned in the paper. The biopsies and joint fluid were inoculated immediately in broth and incubated for 12 days. Peri-operative biopsies were also taken and cultured. The result of these cultures is not mentioned in the report. In 52 patients infected with gentamicin-sensitive *S. epidermidis*, four of them had previously been operated with the use of gentamicin-containing bone cement. In contrast, of the 39 patients infected with gentamicin-resistant *S. epidermidis*, 30 of them had previously received bone cement containing gentamicin. In another report the antibiotic susceptibility of 49 bacterial isolates recovered from revised hip prosthesis was studied [42]. A high number of gentamicin-resistant bacteria were isolated. Although the exact number is not mentioned, the authors state that virtually all the removed implants had been fixed with gentamicin-impregnated bone cement. There was no control group in this study. Furthermore, 19 of 28 isolates recovered from the surface of gentamicin-loaded PMMA beads were considered gentamicin-resistant [26]. In 12 out of 18 patients, bacterial growth occurred only after extensive laboratory procedure including aerobically and anaerobically incubation for seven days. Finally, in a study on staphylococcal isolates recovered from patients with hip and knee prosthetic infection, 41 (66 %) of 93 isolates (93 patients) were resistant to gentamicin and tobramycin [1]. Previous exposure to aminoglycoside-impregnated bone cement did not correlate with resistance to gentamicin or tobramycin. However, in only 40 (43 %) of the patients, the previous use of either plain or antibiotic-containing bone cement was ascertainable.

In conclusion, molecular mechanism coding for increased antibiotic resistance and biofilm formation due to sub-inhibitory antibiotic concentrations are becoming more evident. To what extent this is a problem related to the use of local antibiotics in orthopaedic surgery has to be proven, by preference in an experimental *in vivo* model. Every department of orthopaedic surgery should survey the resistance profile of different bacterial strains cultured from infected orthopaedic implants in general, and infected prosthesis in particular.

Hypersensitivity and Toxic Side Effects

Due to the risk of hypersensitivity, the beta-lactams have been avoided as local antibiotic agents in orthopaedic surgery [51]. To my knowledge there are no reports on allergic reaction when using bone cement containing gentamicin. *In vitro* studies have shown that methylmethacrylate impairs several immune functions [30, 32, 33]. The clinical implication of this observation is not documented.

All aminoglycosides share the potential for renal and oto-vestibular toxicity [35]. The toxixity of aminoglycosides has been associated with persistent exposure to elevated serum levels of the drug, i.e., high and prolonged trough serum values (Fig. 2). Aminoglycosides have been administered as a once-daily dose with high peak serum values and with no recordable toxic effects [10, 14]. There are two reports on toxic serum levels of gentamicin when using gentamicin containing PMMA spacers and beads or gentamicin-containing sponges [39, 48]. 12 patients with postoperatively infected total hip arthroplasty were operated with soft tissue debridement and implantation of gentamicin-containing sponges (520–780 mg gentamicin). Toxic serum gentamicin levels were registered in seven patients, one to ten days after surgery and a decrease in creatinine clearance observed in 10 patients [39].

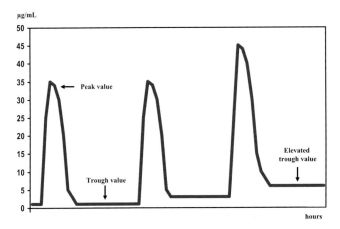

Fig. 2. In clinical trials, peak serum levels ranging from 20 to 40 µg/mL of aminoglycosides have been recorded without changes in auditory, vestibular or renal function. However, elevated minimum (trough) serum values for prolonged time is associated with toxicity

In revision prosthetic surgery impaction of cancellous bone impregnated in aminoglycoside solution results in very high local antibiotic concentration. When 50 gram of cancellous bone were impregnated with netilmicin, 100 mg/mL, the highest netilmicin concentration recorded in serum was 4.0 mg/L. Neither renal nor otovestibular toxicity was reported [52]. Furthermore, in another clinical study no nephrotoxicity was reported when an average of three morcellized femoral heads mixed with three grams of vancomycin was impacted in the femur and/or the acetabulum [7]. At our institution, the current protocol for antibiotic impregnation of cancellous bone is as follows:

Vancomycin: 1000 mg per femoral head (max 1500 mg); gentamicin: 800 mg per femoral head (max 1200 mg); clindamycin: 1200 mg per femoral head (max 1800 mg).

To conclude, there is a limit concerning the amount of antibiotics that can be used safely locally. Caution should be taken when using aminoglycoside-containing vehicles with an elution profile of very high early release, such as collagen sponge and cancellous bone. A particular precaution should be taken in patients with impaired renal function.

Acknowledgments

I would thank Daniëlle Neut for giving me the permission to use her picture shown in Figure 1.

References

1. Anguita-Alonso P, Hanssen AD, Osmon DR et al (2005) High rate of aminoglycoside resistance among staphylococci causing prosthetic joint infection. Clin Orthop Relat Res (439):43–47
2. Becker PL, Smith RA, Williams RS et al (1994) Comparison of antibiotic release from polymethylmethacrylate beads and sponge collagen. J Orthop Res 12(5):737–741
3. Bisognano C, Vaudaux PE, Lew DP et al (1997) Increased expression of fibronectin-binding protein by fluoroquinolone-resistant Staphylococcus aureus exposed to subinhibitory levels of ciprofloxacin. Antimicrob Agents Chemother 41(5):906–913

4. Brien WW, Salvati EA, Klein R et al (1993) Antibiotic impregnated bone cement in total hip arthroplasty. Clin Orthop Relat Res (296):242–248
5. Bunetel L, Segui A, Cormier M et al (1989) Release of gentamicin from acrylic bone cement. Clin Pharmacokinet 17(4):291–297
6. Bunetel L, Segui A, Cormier M et al (1990) Comparative study of gentamicin release from normal and low viscosity acrylic bone cement. Clin Pharmacokinet 19(4):333–340
7. Buttaro M, Gimenez MI, Greco G et al (2005) High local levels of vancomycin without nephrotoxicity released from impacted bone allograft in 20 revision hip arthroplasties. Acta Orthopaedica 76 (3):336–340
8. D'Costa VM, McGrann KM, Hughes DW et al (2006) Sampling the antibiotic resistome. Science 311(5759):374–377
9. Della Valle AG, Bostrom M, Brause B et al (2001) Effective bactericidal activity of tobramycin and vancomycin eluted from acrylic bone cement. Acta Orthop Scand 72(3):237–240
10. Gilbert DN (1991) Once-daily aminoglycoside therapy. Antimicrob Agents Chemother 35(3):399–405
11. Goh E-B, Yim G, Tsui W et al (2002) Transcriptional modulation of bacterial gene expression by subinhibitory concentrations of antibiotics. Proc Natl Acad Sci USA 99(26):17025–17030
12. Hendriks JGE, Neut D, van Horn JR et al (2005) Bacterial survival in the interfacial gap in gentamicin-loaded acrylic bone cements. J Bone Joint Surg (Br) 87(2):272–276
13. Hoffman LR, Dárgenio DA, MacCross MJ et al (2005) Aminoglycoside antibiotics induce bacterial biofilm formation. Nature 436(7054):1171–1175
14. Hollender LF, Bahnini J, De Manzini N et al (1989) A multicentric study of netilmicin once daily versus thrice daily in patients with appendicitis and other intra-abdominal infections. J Antimicrob Chemother 23(5):773–783
15. Hope PG, Kristinsson KG, Norman P et al (1989) Deep infection of cemented total hip arthroplasties caused by coagulase-negative staphylococci. J Bone Joint Surg (Br) 71(5):851–855
16. Kendall RW, Duncan CP, Smith JA et al (1996) Persistence of bacteria on antibiotic loaded acrylic depots: A reason for caution. Clin Orthop Relat Res (329):273–280
17. Klekamp J, Dawson JM, Haas DW et al (1999) The use of vancomycin and tobramycin in acrylic bone cement. Biomechanical effects and elution kinetics for use in joint arthroplasty. J Arthroplasty 14(3):339–346
18. Lawson KJ, Marks KE, Brems J et al (1990) Vancomycin vs tobramycin elution from polymethylmethacrylate: An in vitro study. Orthopedics 13(5):521–524
19. Levy SB (1992) The antibiotic paradox. How miracle drugs are destroying the miracle. Plenum Publishing Corporation, New York, USA
20. Lindberg L, Önnerfält R, Dingeldein E et al (1991) The release of gentamicin after total hip replacement using low or high viscosity bone cement. Int Orthop15(4):305–309
21. Lorian V (1993). Medical relevance of low concentrations of antibiotics. J Antimicrob Chemother 31(Suppl. D):137–148
22. Mader JT, Calhoun J, Cobos J (1997). In vitro evaluation of antibiotic diffusion from antibiotic-impregnated biodegradable beads and polymethylmethacrylate beads. Antimicrob Agents Chemother 41(2):415–418
23. Masri BA, Duncan CP, Beauchamp CP (1998) Long-term elution of antibiotics from bonecement. J Arthroplasty 13(3):331–338
24. Miclau T, Dahners LE, Lindsey RW (1993) In vitro pharmacokinetics of antibiotic release from locally implantable materials. J Orthop Res 11(5):627–632
25. Naylor PT, Myrvik QN, Gristina A (1990) Antibiotic resistance of biomaterial-adherent coagulase-negative and coagulase-positiv staphylococci. Clin Orthop Relat Res (261):126–133
26. Neut D, van de Belt H, Stokroos I et al (2001) Biomaterial-associated infection of gentamicin-loaded PMMA beads in orthopaedic revision surgery. J Antimicrob Chemother 47(6):885–891
27. Neut D, Hendriks JGE, van Horn JR et al (2005) Pseudomonas aeruginosa biofilm formation and slime excretion on antibiotic-loaded bone cement. Acta Orthopaedica 76 (1):109–114
28. Oga M, Arizono T, Sugioka Y (1992) Inhibition of bacterial adhesion by tobramycin-impregnated PMMA bone cement. Acta Orthop Scand 63(3):301–304
29. Ohlsen K, Ziebuhr W, Koller K-P et al (1998) Effects of subinhibitory concentrations of antibiotics on alpha-toxin (hla) gene expression of methicillin-sensitive and methicillin-resistant Staphylococcus aureus isolates. Antimicrob Agents Chemother 42(11):2817–2863

30. Panush RS, Petty RW (1978) Inhibition of human lymphocyte responses by methylmethacrylate. Clin Orthop Relat Res (134):356–363
31. Penner MJ, Duncan CP, Masri BA (1999) The in vitro elution characteristics of antibiotic-loaded CMW and Palacos-R bone cements. J Arhroplasty 14(2):209–214
32. Petty W (1978) The effect of methylmethacrylate on bacterial phagocytosis and killing by human polymorphonuclear leukocytes. J Bone Joint Surg (Am) 60(6):752–757
33. Petty W, Caldwell JR (1977) The effect of methylmethacrylate on complement activity. Clin Orthop Relat Res (128):354–359
34. Rachid S, Ohlsen K, Witte W et al (2000) Effect of subinhibitory antibiotic concentrations on polysaccharide intercellular adhesin expression in biofilm-forming Staphylococcus epidermidis. Antimicrob Agents Chemother 44(12):3357–3363
35. Ristuccia AM (1984). Aminoglycosides. In : Ristuccia AM, Cunha BA (eds) Antimicrobial Therapy. Raven Press, New York, USA, pp 305–328
36. Rupp ME, Hamer KE (1998). Effect of subinhibitory concentrations of vancomycin, cefazolin, ofloxacin, L-ofloxacin and D-ofloxacin on adherence to intravascular catheters and biofilm formation by Staphylococcus epidermidis. J Antimicrob Chemother 41(2):155–161
37. Salvati EA, Callaghan JJ, Brause BD et al (1986) Reimplantation in infection. Elution of gentamicin from cement and beads. Clin Orthop Relat Res (207):83–93
38. Soto-Hall R, Saenz L, Tavernetti R et al (1983) Tobramycin in bone cement. An in-depth analysis of wound, serum, and urine concentrations in patients undergoing total hip revisions arthroplasty. Clin Orthop Relat Res (175):60–64
39. Swieringa AJ, Tulp NJ (2005) Toxic serum gentamicin levels after use of gentamicin-loaded sponges in infected total hip arthroplasty. Acta Orthop 76(1):75–77
40. Thornes B, Murray P, Bouchier-Hayes D (2002) Developement of resistant strains of Staphylococcus epidermidis on gentamicin-loaded bone cement in vivo. J Bone Joint Surg (Br) 84(5):758–760
41. Tomasc A (2006) Microbiology. Weapons of microbial drug resistance abound in soil flora. Science 311(5759):342–343
42. Tunney MM, Ramage G, Patrick S et al (1998) Antimicrobial susceptibility of bacteria isolated from orthopedic implants following revision hip surgery. Antimicrob Agents Chemother 42(11):3002–3005
43. Tunney MM, Patrick S, Curran MD et al (1999) Detection of prosthetic hip infection at revision arthroplasty by immunofluorescence microscopy and PCR amplification of the bacterial 16 rRNA gene. J Clin Microbiol 37(10):3281–3290
44. Törholm C, Lidgren L, Lindberg L et al (1983) Total hip joint arthroplasty with gentamicin-impregnated cement. Clin Orthop Relat Res (181):99–106
45. van de Belt H, Neut D, Schenk W et al (2000) Gentamicin release from polymethylmethacrylate bone cement and Staphylococcus aureus biofilm formation. Acta Orthop Scand 71(6): 625–629
46. van de Belt H, Neut D, Schenk W et al (2001) Staphylococcus aureus biofilm formation on different gentamicin-loaded polymethylmethacrylate bone cements. Biomaterials 22(12): 1607–1611
47. von Eiff C, Bettin D, Proctor RA et al (1997) Recovery of Small Colony Variants of Staphylococcus aureus following gentamicin bead placement for osteomyelitis (Brief Reports). Clin Infect Dis 25(5):1250–1251
48. van Raaij TM, Visser LE, Vulto AG et al (2002) Acute renal failure after local gentamicin treatment in an infected total knee arthroplasty. J Arthroplasty 17(7):948–950
49. Wahlig H, Dingeldein E (1980) Antibiotics and bone cements. Experimental and clinical long-term observations. Acta Orthop Scand 51(1):49–56
50. Wahlig H, Dingeldein E, Buchholz HW et al (1984) Pharmacokinetic study of gentamicin-loaded cement in total hip replacements. Comparative effects of varying dosage. J Bone Joint Surg (Br) 66(2):175–179
51. Wininger DA, Fass RJ (1996) Minireview. Antibiotic-impregnated cement and beads for orthopaedic infections.. Antimicrob Agents Chemother 40(12):2675–2679
52. Witsø E, Persen L, Benum P et al (2004) High local concentration without systemic adverse effects after impaction of netilmicin-impregnated bone. Acta Orthop Scand 75(3):339–346

The Role of Suppressive Surgery

E. Concia, A. Tedesco

Department of Infective Disease, University of Verona, Italy

Introduction

The main aim of treating joint prosthesis infections is to eradicate the infection in order to obtain a functional and non-painful joint. Generally, infections are eradicated with a combined surgical and pharmacological treatment, removing the foreign body and prescribing an appropriate antibiotic therapy.

In managing post-prosthetic infections the main treatment options include debridement without removal of the prosthesis, one-stage or two-stage replacement of the prosthesis, permanent removal of the implant, arthrodesis and finally a sole long-term antibiotic therapy.

Main

The sole long-term antibiotic therapy (named suppressive therapy), without the combined surgical intervention in the implant site, is able to control the clinical symptoms but it rarely eradicates the infection. Indeed, in most patients clinical symptoms of infection reoccur after the suspension of the antibiotic therapy [12].

Suppressive antibiotic therapy is considered when the surgical treatment is not advised. This occurs for example if the patient has an intolerance to anaesthesia, if the removal of the prosthesis is technically too difficult, if there is a high morbidity or there are unacceptable risks for the patient or surgeon, if there is no need for the prosthesis to be functional (i.e. the patient is confined to bed or is very old), if the patient refuses the operation, if there are difficulties in removing non-mobile and well-placed prostheses and when the infection is not very virulent and is sensitive to the oral antibiotic therapy [10, 12, 15].

In general, the suppressive antibiotic therapy should be ideally conducted with antibiotics that have a bactericidal action, an antimicrobic activity spectrum against microorganisms that adhere to surfaces, a slow growth and produce biofilm. However, for infections associated to joint prostheses, standard antimicrobial sensitivity tests cannot be used to predict the result in a reliable way [16].

From an etiological point of view, post-prosthetic infections are mainly caused by staphylococci (45–55 %), particularly *S. aureus* (33–43 %) and coagulase-negative staphylococci (17–21 %). However, other microorganisms can be involved such as streptococci (11–12 %) and more rarely Gram-negative bacteria (5–14 %), enterococci and anaerobes. In 5 – 13 % of cases mixed flora is found, while in 5 % of infections no microorganism is isolated [6, 7].

From a pathogenic point of view, the bacterial situation (due to their chronic characteristics and the difficulty of eradication with antibiotic therapies) are similar to typical diseases caused by the local biofilm production. In the biofilm, germs become capable of producing great quantities of polysaccharide polymers (glicocalyx). They reproduce into microcolonies at a very low speed and are aware of their density, triggering off (at very high concentration levels) a synthesis of various virulent factors. For this reason, biofilm is a survival mechanism with which microbes are able to resist the host's internal and external environmental factors, such as antibiotic agents and the immunity system. Due to these physiological situations, which are very different from those that dominate bacterial multiplication in biological liquids and in culture media, sensitivity to antibiotics is very limited thus creating some inconsistencies between the antibiogram data and the real *in vivo* situation [3].

In studies performed on animal infection models in which prosthetic infection was caused by *S. epidermidis* it was analysed the efficacy of different antibiotics. It was noted that fluoroquinolones monotherapy (like Ciprofloxacin) has a low efficacy, but this rises to 90% if combined with rifampicin. It was also noted that during high-dose monotherapy, rifampicin has a high efficacy. Good results were also obtained by the combination of daptomycin and netilmicin, as opposed to daptomycin monotherapy. Poor results were, instead, achieved using glycopeptide monotherapy: however, if vancomycin is combined with netilmicin it becomes more effective [13].

Therefore, among the antibiotics indicated for implant-related staphylococcal infections, rifampicin not only has a good bioavailability and an excellent anti-staphylococcal activity but it also has an excellent penetration of soft tissues, bone, abscesses and polymorphonucleates. It also succeeds in eradicating organisms that adhere to prosthetic surfaces during a steady growth stage. However, the use of rifampicin is limited both by the rapid development of resistance (therefore it must always be combined with another antibiotic) and by patients' poor tolerability to the antibiotic's toxic effects (such as nausea, hepatic disorder) and to the various other pharmaceutical interactions [4].

Last generation fluoroquinolones (such as moxifloxacin and levofloxacin) that have recently been introduced in clinical practice present lower MICs *in vitro* than ciprofloxacin in the presence of Gram-positive microorganisms. However, data regarding their penetration and efficacy in bone infections are still not available. Furthermore, the resistance of nosocomial staphylococci to quinolones has dramatically increased. At the moment, 90% of nosocomial methicillin-resistant *S. aureus* (MRSA) are also resistant to quinolones [4, 12].

Clinical studies show that the use of rifampicin and fluoroquinolones as a monotherapy cure orthopaedic implant infections associated to staphylococci, but most of the treatments fail due to the emergence of antibiotic-resistant isolates. The association of fluoroquinolones and rifampicin is a highly effective in eradicating implant-associated staphylococci and in preventing the emergence of ciprofloxacin-resistant starins. This association has also the advantage of an excellent oral bioavailability of both active principles, which reach serum concentrations comparable to those obtained during intravenous therapy. High levels of intracellular penetration and activity against intracellular staphylococci are also obtained [2, 17].

Fusidic acid is another oral antibiotic used in association with rifampicin, even though It is less effective against oxacillin-resistant and quinolones-resistant staphylococci, but reaches high intracellular concentrations. Bactericidal concentrations have also been obtained in bone infections. However, if used as a monotherapy it rapidly selects resistant bacteria. On the other hand, as shown by *in vitro* studies, the association of fusidic acid and rifampicin seems to prevent the selection of staphylococci resistant to other antibiotics [5].

In case of outpatient treatment of prosthetic infections caused by multi-resistant staphylococci and susceptible only to cotrimoxazole and glycopeptides, high doses of cotrimoxazole were used (trimethoprim 20 mg/Kg/day, sulphamethoxazole 100 mg/Kg/day), obtaining an overall success rate of 66.7% (26 patients out of 39): in knee prosthesis infections the percentage was 62.5 %; in hip prosthesis infections 50 %; 60.7% of patients were treated only with suppressive antibiotic therapy without implant removal. However, home oral treatment with cotrimoxazole is limited to the occurrence of side effects, such as rashes, vomit, diarrhoea, anaemia, thrombocytopenia and neutropenia [11].

Minocycline is another antimicrobial agent that can be used for the treatment of post-prosthetic infections. However, at the moment data regarding the use of this drug in implant-related infections are not available in literature.

Glycopeptides (vancomycin and teicoplanin) are the first choice antibiotics against MRSA. Vancomycin has an antibacterial activity against Gram-positive microorganisms lower than beta-lactam drugs. Furthermore, studies suggest that the administration of vancomycin by continuous i.v. infusion may be more efficient than by intermittent mode. Finally, its use is limited due higher association with nephrotoxicity, lack of oral formulas and cannot be given by bolus injection: all this discourages its use in suppressive therapy. Teicoplanin, instead, has a long half-life that enables its once-a-day administration, with the possibility of discharging the patient from hospital while continuing the parenteral antibiotic therapy at home, with high doses (12 mg/Kg/day). However, its use is limited by the occurrence of toxic effects such as thrombocytopenia, neutropenia, rash and fever [4, 12].

As a consequence of the above considerations, in empirical suppressive therapies of post-prosthetic infections, the association of rifampicin with a fluoroquinolone, or with fusidic acid, or with cotrimoxazole, or a monotherapy with fluoroquinolone could be an optimal solution. The possibility of a monotherapy with cotrimoxazole or minocycline has also been suggested [12].

Conclusion

In conclusion, new antibiotics that could reveal to be effective in the suppressive therapy of these infections are currently being studied. These are quinupristin-dalfopristin, linezolid, daptomycin, tigecycline, dalbavancin, RWJ-416457 (a new oxazolidinone), BP-102 (a new carbapenemic) and new by-products of rifampicin (ABI-0043, ABI-0363, ABI-0699) [1, 12].

Instead, as far as regards infections caused by Gram-negative microorganisms, very few studies are available in literature. Some trials conducted on animal models and *in vitro* have shown that ciprofloxacin is more effective against Gram-negative bacilli with respect to other antibiotics [14].

Finally, the optimal duration of suppressive antibiotic therapies in joint prosthesis infections is still not known [8]. Long-term oral therapy can cause benefits to old-aged patients, where a surgical therapy is not recommended [9, 10]. Important criteria to decide the suppressive therapy must be entrusted to clinical judgement, taking into consideration risk factors, microbiological isolations, drug tolerability, clinical conditions and preferences.

References

1. Bassetti M, Vitale F, Melica G et al (2005) Linezolid in the treatment of Gram-positive prosthetic joint infections. J Antimicrob Chemother 55(3):387–390
2. Bernard L, Hoffmeyer P, Assal M et al (2004) Trends in the treatment of orthopaedic prosthetic infections.J Antimicrob Chemother 53(2):127–129. Review
3. Costerton JW, Stewart PS, Greenberg EP (1999) Bacterial biofilms: a common cause of persistent infections. Science 284(5418):1318–1322. Review
4. Darley ES, MacGowan AP (2004) Antibiotic treatment of gram-positive bone and joint infections. J Antimicrob Chemother 53(6):928–935. Review
5. Drancourt M, Stein A, Argenson JN et al (1997) Oral treatment of Staphylococcus spp. infected orthopaedic implants with fusidic acid or ofloxacin in combination with rifampicin. J Antimicrob Chemother 39(2):235–240
6. Giulieri SG, Graber P, Ochsner PE et al (2004) Management of infection associated with total hip arthroplasty according to a treatment algorithm. Infection 32(4):222–228
7. Laffer RR, Graber P, Ochsner PE et al (2006) Outcome of prosthetic knee-associated infection: evaluation of 40 consecutive episodes at a single centre. Clin Microbiol Infect 12(5): 433–439
8. Marculescu CE, Berbari EF, Hanssen AD et al (2006) Outcome of prosthetic joint infections treated with debridement and retention of components. Clin Infect Dis 42(4):471–478
9. Pavoni GL, Giannella M, Falcone M et al (2004) Conservative medical therapy of prosthetic joint infections: retrospective analysis of an 8-year experience.Clin Microbiol Infect. 2004 Sep;10(9):831–837
10. Segreti J, Nelson JA, Trenholme GM (1998) Prolonged suppressive antibiotic therapy for infected orthopedic prostheses. Clin Infect Dis 27(4):711–713
11. Stein A, Bataille JF, Drancourt M et al (1998) Ambulatory treatment of multidrug-resistant Staphylococcus-infected orthopedic implants with high-dose oral co-trimoxazole (trimethoprim-sulfamethoxazole). Antimicrob Agents Chemother 42(12):3086–3091
12. Trampuz A, Zimmerli W (2006) Antimicrobial agents in orthopaedic surgery: Prophylaxis and treatment. Drugs 66(8):1089–1105
13. Widmer AF, Frei R, Rajacic Z et al (1990) Correlation between in vivo and in vitro efficacy of antimicrobial agents against foreign body infections. J Infect Dis 162(1):96–102
14. Widmer AF, Wiestner A, Frei R et al (1991) Killing of nongrowing and adherent Escherichia coli determines drug efficacy in device-related infections. Antimicrob Agents Chemother 35(4):741–746
15. Zimmerli W, Ochsner PE (2003) Management of infection associated with prosthetic joints. Infection 31(2):99–108. Review
16. Zimmerli W, Trampuz A, Ochsner PE (2004) Prosthetic-joint infections. N Engl J Med 351(16):1645–1654
17. Zimmerli W, Widmer AF, Blatter M et al (1998) Role of rifampin for treatment of orthopedic implant-related staphylococcal infections: a randomized controlled trial. Foreign-Body Infection (FBI) Study Group JAMA 279(19):1537–1541

Basic Research and Local Antibiotic Therapy

PMMA as Drug Delivery System and *in vivo* Release from Spacers

E. Bertazzoni Minelli, A. Benini

Department of Medicine and Public Health, Pharmacology Section, University of Verona

Introduction

Infection is the most serious complication following orthopaedic surgery. The frequency is low, but when present is difficult to treat. Systemic drug administration may not provide inhibitory concentration for a prolonged period, and this is further worsened by the decreased blood supply. The local delivery of antibiotics to the surgical area may may contribute to reduce the infection frequency and the risk of recolonization [16].

In primary prosthetic implants the adequate perioperative antibiotic prophylaxis along with adoption of proper measures of antisepsis seems to be sufficient to contain the risk of infections [10, 19]. 10 % of surgeons utilise antibiotic loaded PMMA in primary hip- or knee- prostheses, increasing to 70 % in the revision surgery in which the risk of septic complications is noticeably increased [10].

The most frequent isolates in orthopaedic surgical infections are Gram-positive cocci. However methicillin-resistant (MRS) and coagulase-negative (CNS) staphylococci are becoming more frequent [35]. In delayed infections (onset 2 to 12 months after prosthesis replacement, according to Cohen classification [10]) CNS and other skin commensals are present and in late infections (onset 12 months after prosthesis replacement) gram-negative and anaerobic bacteria are also isolated [10]. The failure risks are much higher with some "difficult" type of bacteria such as *P. aeruginosa, S. aureus* (methicillin-resistant), *S. epidermidis and* enterococci. Infection commences with adhesion of bacteria to host tissues or prostheses. Biofilm formation, morphological and metabolic modifications (micrococci colonies), combined with reduced host responses in the vicinity of biomaterials, resulting in an active infection around an implant. Organisms within biofilm are difficult to eradicate and will not respond to host defences and antibiotic treatment alone. Removal of the implant, aggressive debridement, local and systemic administration of antibiotics are required [2, 36].

The rationale choice of antimicrobial drugs for local delivery system must take into account the following points: i- microbiological data (micro-organism and its antibiotic susceptibility); ii- bactericidal, wide-spectrum activity of drug; iii- compatibility with cement and other carriers and heat-stability; iv- effects on carrier mechanical resistance, and v- the capacity of elution of the drug from the carrier; vi- drug half-life; vii- capacity of inducing hypersensitivity and adverse drug reactions; and finally, viii- antimicrobial activity at the site of infection.

Drug Delivery Systems

The use of bone antibiotic-containing cements (non-degradable polymethylmethacrylate – PMMA –, beads, spacers) and biodegradable systems is increasing and is an adjunct to current therapy (i.e. surgical debridement and systemic antimicrobial therapy) [19].

Biodegradable carriers loaded with different antibiotics are under investigation and are currently being used in some countries, i.e. collagen-gelatin sponge, hydroxyapatite, polymers-polylactide/polyglycolide and polylactate implants- and bioceramics, cancellous bone, calcium phosphate bone substitutes, etc [20].

All the above systems may release antibiotics at concentrations exceeding the MIC for the most common pathogens of prosthetic infections with limited release in systemic circulation and without adverse effects.

The biodegradable or reabsorbable systems can release high local drug concentrations, do not require surgical removal, but may interfere with biological systems and show different interactions with bacteria. The duration of release of antibiotic is dependent on the characteristics of drug carrier.

Two points are essential for the clinical application and satisfactory outcome:

a) Antimicrobial drug pharmacodynamics (on site drug concentration, wide spectrum of activity microorganism susceptibility – or resistance –, tolerability, stability to heat, pH, organic fluids, and presence of necrosis, foreign bodies, etc.).
b) Cement intrinsic characteristics and capacity to release drug (porosity, surface extension, initial drug concentration, thermostability, good capacity to mix with powder);

Moreover, the drug delivery system should not interfere negatively with bone and tissues.

Bone cement mainly consists of PMMA, because of its excellent biocompatibility and ease of manipulation.

Antimicrobial Drugs

Aminoglycosides (gentamicin, tobramycin, arbekacin) are considered to be the antibiotics of choice, because of their wide-spectrum antimicrobial activity, excellent water solubility, chemical and thermal stability, biocompatibility, low allergenicity and low development of resistance during therapy.

However, due to emerging antibiotic resistance there is now a renewed interest for the addition of other antibiotics (vancomycin, clindamycin, fusidic acid, daptomycin, oxazolidinones, fluoroquinolones, peptides, etc.) to drug delivery systems [15, 28]. Vancomycin exhibits positive physico-chemical characteristics similar to those of aminoglycosides, with some limitation regarding the difficulty of polymerization of cement when used in high doses and shorter period of release [9]. Other antibiotics have also been used as additive to PMMA without satisfactory characteristics *in vivo*. Combinations of antibiotics are also added to bone cements.

The mixing of antibiotics with cement should consider the compatibility of drugs. In Table 1 are summarised the properties of different antibiotics in PMMA. Amino-

Table 1. Comparative properties of antibiotics in PMMA cement utilised in prosthetic surgery

Properties	Amino-glycosides	Vanco-mycin	Betalac-tams	Fluoro-quinolones	Rifam-picin	Clinda-mycin
Delivery	+ + +	+ / + +	+	+ + ?	0	+
Half-life	+ +	+ +	±	+	n.d.	+
Antimicrobial activity	+ +	+ +	+ +	+	0*	+
	-cidal	-cidal	-cidal	-cidal	-cidal	-static
Spectrum of activity	wide	narrow	wide	wide	narrow	narrow
Hypersensitivity	–	–	+ +	+ +	?	?
ADR	–	–	+ +	+ +	?	?
Cement Compatibility	+ + +	+	+	?	– – –	+
Mechanical resistance	+ +	+ ?	+	?	– – –	+ ?

+ + + = very good properties; + + = good properties; + = sufficient properties; ± = insufficient properties; – negative; ? = Controversial or insufficient data; * = Because of no release
ADR = Adverse Drug Reactions

glycosides and vancomycin show good positive characteristics: antimicrobial activity, adequate release, compatibility and mechanical resistance, excellent tolerability. The release of other antibiotics such as betalactams (penicillins, cephalosporins, imipenem) is rapid, elevated but limited overtime (48 hours), while rifampicin shows incompatibility with acrylic cement (PMMA) and loss of antimicrobial effect (our personal data [19]). For this purpose, some negative features should be considered, i.e. short half-life, allergenic capacity, and reduced mechanical resistance of cement (beta-lactam agents) or problems with cement incorporation (liquid preparations of gentamicin and clindamycin) or potential negative effects on muscle-skeletal system (fluoroquinolones) [18].

Modifications in antibiotic release should be considered according to bone cement utilised or the combination of two antibiotics, i.e. gentamicin and clindamycin or fusidic acid [28].

Antibiotics utilized for systemic administration are not all useful for drug delivery systems.

PMMA cements impregnated with aminoglycosides and/or vancomycin are currently utilised as local antibiotic carrier in orthopaedic surgical-site infection to treat prosthetic infections (hip, knee, shoulder, etc) [19].

Several experimental models *in vitro* and *in vivo* (animal) models have been developed to better understand the release kinetics of different antibiotics from cement and to optimise their use in clinical practice.

Release Kinetics of Drugs from PMMA

The release kinetics from PMMA is similar for different antimicrobial drugs tested. Aminoglycosides and vancomycin elution shows a biphasic (bimodal) profile, consisting of an initial high rapid release of drug followed by a much slower but sustained release. The release of gentamicin and vancomycin is prompt (the maximal drug release from beads occurs within few days) and at inhibitory concentrations which are maintained for 4–6 weeks [23, 27]. The bone cement PMMA seems a good carrier material for the protracted release of antibiotic drug by diffusion at the site of infection. Gentamicin and vancomycin are still released from explanted spacers after 3–6 months of implantation; the duration of release is variable [1, 3]. A good inhibitory activity of removed spacers was recorded *in vitro* for two weeks [21]. The release may be maintained for prolonged periods at inhibitory levels in different preparations. The PMMA cement seems maintain release and kinetics properties similar before and after removal. There is little information on long-term release of antibiotics from impregnated bone cement. Furthermore, gentamicin could still be found in tissue surroundings the implant for over five-ten years. This was though to confer long-term protection against haematogenous infections [39]. Gentamicin was detected in joint fluids of patients up to 10–20 years following primary hip or knee arthroplasty, using gentamicin-impregnated cement. Concentrations ranged from 0.06 mg/l to 0.85 mg/l (13/25 patients), while only 1 patient showed infection. Data show that gentamicin is present at significant concentrations and in active form inside the cement for a number of years [13, 31].

Variability of Antibiotic Release

This well-known profile of drugs release kinetics from PMMA may present great variability in terms of drug amounts eluted and modality of elution. There is a great variability in bone cement composition (different components), preparations modalities –i.e. under vacuum or not, hand-made or industrial products-, viscosity and technical characteristics among different brands, different concentrations of antibiotic. Industrial preparations (bone cement, beads and spacers) are considered superior to hand-made preparations because of uniform mixing and standardized procedures [19, 24, 28, 34]. All these factors contribute to variability in drug release and the comparison of data and interpretation of data is very difficult.

Initial drug concentration, cement surface area and porosity are important factors in determining the amount of drug released from beads and spacers [37]. Different mechanisms such as diffusion from cement, surface area and/or cracks and voids in the polymer matrix and bulk porosity are involved in antibiotic release from cement [32]. The release mechanisms are poorly defined and difficult to control. The topic is still debated. The amount of released antibiotic is directly related to cement porosity [37]; the antibiotic release rate of an antibiotic-loaded calcium phosphate bone cement almost tripled on increasing the porosity from 38 % to 69 % [6].

The amount of antibiotic released from cement is different among similar bone cements (gentamicin diffuses from Palacos in larger amounts and for longer period than from Simplex and CMV) [19, 27, 28, 30]. The size is other factor of variability. Beads and mini-beads can release high initial concentrations of gentamicin, but larger beads can maintain a sustained release for more prolonged period in comparison to mini-beads [23, 29].

In our experience, we observed a large variation in gentamicin release from different spacers *in vitro* (Fig. 1). The amounts of gentamicin released from spacers pro-

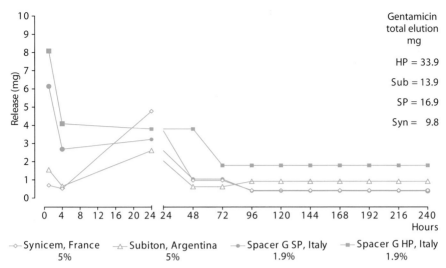

Fig. 1. Release (mg) of gentamicin from different hip spacers produced with PMMA cements utilised in different countries. Values of gentamicin release from 24 to 240 hours are extrapolated as mg/day of elution. (Microbiological method).

duced in France and in Argentina are lower than those released from spacers produced in Italy (Spacer-G & Spacer-K – Tecres Spa, Italy) in spite of higher content of drug. Spacers may present different release according to porosity: spacer HP can release levels of gentamicin (mg 33.9) higher than those of previous models (SP, mg16.9). Moreover, the kinetics of gentamicin release is very different in the first 24 hours of elution: two spacers release *in vitro* very low amounts of drug (1.0 mg and 1.8 mg from Argentina and France products, respectively) after 1 and 4 hours of elution, increasing adequately after 24 hours of elution. This kinetics profile is quite different from that described for aminoglycosides from PMMA cement characterised by a peak release in the first 4 hours of elution. The low initial release of antibiotic can contribute to unsatisfactory antimicrobial effect and risk of selection of resistant bacteria. A high release of antibiotic in the first hours of implant should be considered an important factor in order to reduce the risk of selection of resistant bacteria and biofilm production.

Gentamicin-loaded PMMA constitutes an effective drug delivery system for local antibiotic therapy in bone and soft-tissue infections, and gentamicin concentrations at the site of infection can exceed the MIC for the infecting organisms.

Clinical results report similar rate of eradication of infection for beads and spacers. The comparison of beads (70 patients) versus spacers (58 patients) showed that, the rate of eradication of infection was similar between the groups, with an overall rate of 95.3 % [17]. However, the spacer provided higher hip scores, a reduced hospital stay and enhanced functions between stages. The clinical use of spacers in the hip and knee to help eradicate deep infections is increasing [33, 34].

Concentrations and Antimicrobial Activity of Gentamicin and Vancomycin *in vivo* at the Site of Infection

The release of aminoglycosides and vancomycin from PMMA cement at site of infection seems prompt and effective, presenting high local concentrations above the susceptibility of bacteria and low systemic levels. High intersubject variability was observed, depending on other additional factors such as fluid presence and output, drainage, vascularization, inflammation, repair tissue, and limb mobilisation [7, 8]. Vancomycin release seems more difficult and shorter than that of gentamicin requiring higher drug concentration in cement [7, 9].

Results exhibit high variability among different preparations and assays rendering it difficult to compare data [4, 10].

Combining two antibiotics in bone cement is a common clinical practice, because of increase in gentamicin resistance among bacterial strains responsible for orthopaedic infection. Vancomycin concentrations in drainage fluid following local administration are higher than those obtained with systemic administration and are superimposable to gentamicin release kinetics. The aminoglycosides and vancomycin in combination show synergistic antimicrobial activity [14, 22].

The use of antibiotic in combination requires additional studies. *In vitro* studies showed a reduced release of vancomycin when mixed with gentamicin [5], therefore vancomycin was utilized on the surface of spacer with gentamicin allowing adequate inhibitory concentrations of antibiotics. This activity was maintained also after removal in the majority of spacers [21]. The superficial application of vancomycin seems to favour high concentrations of antibiotic at the site of infection and allows to optimise the antimicrobial drugs selection according to micro-organisms susceptibility and clinical requirements, and "last minute" application maintaining an adequate capacity of antibiotic release from cement. Nonetheless, the preparation of cement in operating room presents the described limitations, i.e unknown mechanical performances and unpredictable antibiotic release.

Antimicrobial Activity at the Site of Infection

In addition to the amount of drug released, another point to be considered in the final drug profile evaluation for an adequate orthopaedic infection treatment is the antimicrobial activity of antibiotics at the site of implant, i.e. in the presence of foreign bodies, fibrin, necrosis, fluids secretion, cellular component (PMNs – granulocytes), different pH, blood perfusion, tissues conditions, and oxygen concentration. pH may modify the antimicrobial activity of some antibiotics.

The gentamicin and vancomycin concentrations achieved at the site of infections are far above the MICs for most common pathogens in orthopaedic infections, in spite of the low percentage of release; systemic levels (serum, urine) are low. The risk of adverse reactions, both local at infection site (hypersensitivity or tissue reactions) and systemic, is very low.

However, biomaterials associated infections are an increasing problem. Major concern is about the bone cement utilised for prostheses fixation in primary implants for infection prophylaxis. The long-term exposure to sub-inhibitory concentrations of antibiotics from cements can increase the risk of resistance [13, 29].

Biofilm and micrococci are present in removed beads after 14 days, beside of high gentamicin release [29] 18/21 patients showed gentamicin-resistant cocci, but 12/18 were free from infection (tissue samples negative). *S. aureus* shows different capacity in biofilm formation and for different PMMA cements [28, 29, 38]. In two-stage revision, the implant of temporary spacers and beads with antibiotic loaded cements has proved effective and the problem of resistance is minimal because of the implant removal after a certain time; in addition, spacers perform both mechanical and biological (antimicrobial) objectives.

The problem of resistant bacteria, in presence of local delivery of antibiotics at sub-inhibitory concentration or in presence of biofilm and inflammation products, remains actually unresolved. However, initial high local concentrations of antibiotics are bactericidal and should reduce the risk of selection of resistant bacteria.

Routine prophylactic use of antibiotic loaded cement remains a subject of controversy and should be restricted to at risk patients. However, the efficiency of gentamicin-loaded cement in THA along with systemic antimicrobial therapy is confirmed, but the risk of selecting bacteria needs to be considered [11, 12].

In vivo Release from Spacers

There is little data available in the literature on antibiotic release *in vivo* [4, 7, 14, 21] at the time of prosthesis implantation as well as after removal. Moreover the high variability in results make the comparison of studies difficult. Another question is related to the evaluation of the effective concentrations and antimicrobial inhibitory activity of antibiotics in the infection site and the duration of the effect.

We determined the concentrations of antibiotics at the prosthetic site after temporary spacer implantation in two-stage revision for infected arthroplasty (hip and knee) and evaluated the inhibitory activity of drainage fluids against clinical isolates [4]. The investigation was carried out in collaboration with the Orthopaedic Clinic of our University Hospital.

Samples from serum and fluids from drainage were collected 1, 4 and 24 hours after implantation from ten patients undergoing two-stage revision surgery with a temporary antibiotic loaded spacers (hip or knee, Spacer-G and Spacer-K, respectively) and treated according to microbiological data.

Currently, the use of spacers is combined with systemic therapy for prosthetic infections treatment. Vancomycin was given intravenously (1 g, bid) or locally in PMMA cement (2.5–5 %).

Antibiotic concentrations were determined by fluorescence polarisation immunoassay. The antimicrobial activity of gentamicin and vancomycin in drainage fluids activity was determined as bactericidal titer [25], against multi-resistant Gram-positive cocci, *P. aeruginosa* and *E. coli*.

The results obtained in 3 representative patients are reported in Fig. 2.

The release of gentamicin from PMMA cement at site of infection seems prompt and effective, presenting high local concentrations (range 40–100 mg/L) in the first

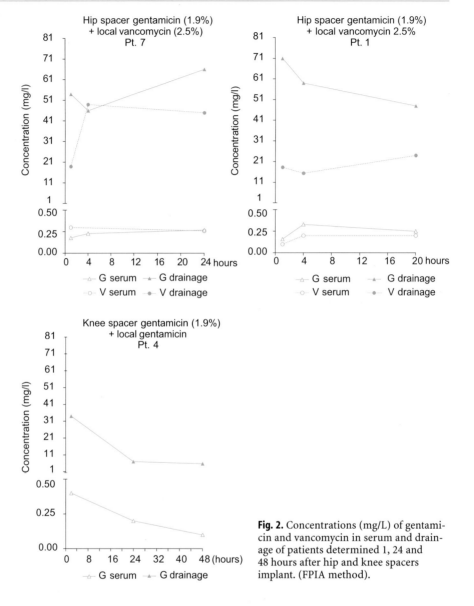

Fig. 2. Concentrations (mg/L) of gentamicin and vancomycin in serum and drainage of patients determined 1, 24 and 48 hours after hip and knee spacers implant. (FPIA method).

24–48 hours after spacer implant. The concentrations are largely above the susceptibility of bacteria. Serum levels are low (<0.2–0.8 mg/L).

Parenteral administration of vancomycin (1 g × 2) allows good local penetration, showing similar range of concentrations (range 15–40 mg/L) in serum and in drainage fluids at different sampling time (1–24 hours).

The local administration of vancomycin (2.5%) produces high concentrations in surgical site (18.3–45.0 mg/L) and low serum levels (<1 mg/L). Higher vancomycin

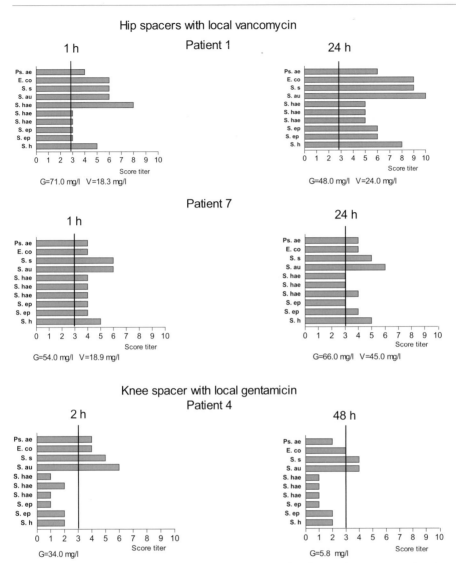

Fig. 3. Bactericidal titer of drainage fluids collected 1, 24 and 48 hours after spacer implant in patients against multi-resistant clinical isolates. Hip spacer (Spacer-G) and local vancomycin are prepared as described in (3) and knee spacer (Spacer-K) is fixed with gentamicin-loaded PMMA cement (2.5 %). The concentrations of gentamicin (G) and vancomycin (V) in drainage fluids are reported for each patient at time of samples collection. The bactericidal titer is defined as the highest dilution achieving 99.9 % bacterial killing (serial two-fold dilutions) and is reported according to following score:

Score = dilution; 1 = 1/2; 2 = 1/4; 3 = 1/8*; 4 = 1/16; 5 = 1/32; 6 = 1/64; 7 = 1/128; 8 = 1/256; 9 = 1/512; 10 = 1/1024

* Lowest bactericidal titer for orthopaedic infections according to (25).

Abbreviations: Ps. ae = *Pseudomonas aeruginosa*; E. co = *Escherichia coli*; S. s = *Staphylococcus* Met- S; S. au = *S. aureus*; S. hae = *S. haemolyticus* (3 different strains); S. ep = *S. epidermidis* (2 different strains); S. h = *S. hominis* concentration (5 %) in cement increased local levels of antibiotic (90 – 150 mg/L) in drains. Vancomycin concentrations in drainage fluid following local administration are higher than those obtained with systemic administration. The release kinetics of gentamicin and vancomycin in the site of implant is superimposable (Fig. 2), allowing to exert an inhibitory combined effect.

The ratio of gentamicin to vancomycin concentrations in drainage fluids was 3:1 and 2:1, but high intersubject variability was observed, depending on other additional factors of the patient.

Drainage fluids showed good inhibitory activity against multi-resistant clinical isolates (*S. aureus, S. epidermidis, S. haemolyticus, E. coli, P. aeruginosa*) (Fig. 2). Drain Bactericidal Titer ranged from 1/8 to 1/64 for bacteria difficult to treat, and from 1/128 to 1/1024 for intermediate and susceptible bacteria in samples collected 1 and 24 hours after implant.

Drugs achieved good bactericidal titer for Gram-positive and Gram-negative pathogens with concentrations in drainage fluids above 2 mg/l and 8 mg/l for vancomycin and gentamicin, respectively. Local gentamicin alone shows inhibitory activity against susceptible microorganisms (knee spacer, patient 4). This is an obvious confirmatory result.

However, the inhibitory effect of the drainage fluids shows large intersubject variability depending on microorganism susceptibility and different concentrations of both antibiotics. We need to define if an optimal concentration ratio of gentamicin to vancomycin is necessary.

The gentamicin and vancomycin in combination show synergistic or summatory antimicrobial activity as defined by FIC determination *in vitro* (Table 2).

Treatments were well tolerated. Gentamicin-containing spacers showed satisfactory clinical results at a follow-up of 5 – 7 years [26].

These results confirm the release characteristics of gentamicin and vancomycin from PMMA *in vivo*. The spacers allow to obtain and maintain inhibitory activity for an adequate local treatment of infection. Spacers seem an adequate system for antibiotic delivery in prosthetic infections in two-stage revision for infected Total Hip and Knee Replacements (THR/TKRs). Our results are in accord with recent data [21, 33].

Vancomycin + Gentamicin			
Strain	FIC Index	MIC (mg/L)	
		Vanco-mycin	Genta-micin
S. epidermidis (8/28)	1.00 A	2.5	R
S. haemolyticus (8/28)	1.00 A	1.25	R
* S. haemolyticus (82/26)	1.00 A	1.25	R
S. haemolyticus (70/26)	1.00 A	1.25	R
* S. epidermidis (137/25)	0.50 A	2.5	R
° S. hominis (126/26)	1.02 A	1.25	I
S. aureus (3A10)	0.15 S	2.5	I
S. aureus (9A28)	0.48 S	1.25	1.25
E. coli (7A27)	0.25 S	156.25	5
P. aeruginosa (4/28)	0.12 S	1250	5

Table 2. *In vitro* activity of gentamicin and vancomycin in combination against multi-resistant clinical isolates. Checker-board method [13].

* Oxacillin Resistant
° Methicillin Resistant
R   = Resistant
I   = Intermediate
FIC ≤ 0.5 Synergism S
FIC = 1 Additivity   A
FIC ≥ 2 Antagonism Ant

Table 3. Release of gentamicin and vancomycin from removed (after 3–6 months of implantation) spacers after ten days of spacers elution. Amounts were determined using FPIA method. Modified from [3].

§ Spacer's surface area 180 cm²

Spacers		Gentamicin		
		Total µg	%	µg/cm²§
Control		15,550	0.82	82.4
Removed mean ± SD (n = 6)		1682.0 ± 530.2	0.07 ± 0.02	9.3 ± 2.9
		Gentamicin + Vancomycin		
		Total µg	%	µg/cm²§
Control	G	14,220	0.75	86.2
	V	24,114	16.1	146.1
Removed mean ± SD (n = 14)	G	3889.6 ± 1806.5	0.2 ± 0.1	23.0 ± 11.1
	V	3484.8 ± 1092.9	2.3 ± 0.8	20.9 ± 6.4

Conclusions

In conclusion the ideal drug delivery system with controlled release of antibiotic is lacking as well as the ideal antibiotic. Different problems must be solved, such as subinhibitory concentrations of antibiotic released from carriers, false negative cultures, ineffective concentrations or activity at site of infection, reduced biocompatibility and mechanical properties and drug utilisation.

Actually the PMMA cement represents the most useful, suitable and studied local antibiotic delivery system in prosthetic infections. The use of antibiotic-containing PMMA cement in the surgery of revision of total hip and knee arthroplasty represents a local antibiotic therapy supplementary to radical debridement and complementary to systemic therapy.

The choice of the appropriate system (cement, beads, spacers, fleeces, or biodegradable carrier) should based on a careful evaluation of risk/benefit and cost/benefit according to different surgical conditions and requests of patient.

Acknowledgements

We thank Chiara Caveiari for her excellent technical assistance.

References

1. Anagnostakos K, Kelm J, Regitz T et al (2005) In vitro evaluation of antibiotic release from and bacteria growth inhibition by antibiotic-loaded acrylic bone cement spacers. J Biomed Mater Res B Appl Biomater 72(2):373–378
2. Berendt RA. (1999) Infections of prosthetic joints and related problems. In "Infectious Disease" (Armstrong D and Cohen J Eds). Mosby, London. Vol. I, Section 2 – p 44.1–44.6
3. Bertazzoni Minelli E, Benini A, Magnan B et al (2004) Release of gentamicin and vancomycin from temporary human hip spacers in two-stage revision of infected arthroplasty. J Antimicrob Chemother. 53(2):329–334
4. Bertazzoni Minelli E, Benini A, Magnan B et al (2005) Release of antibiotics and inhibitory activity in drainage fluids following temporary spacer implants in two-stage revision surgery. J Chemother 17 (Suppl 3):9

5. Bertazzoni Minelli E, Caveiari C, Benini A (2002) Release of antibiotics from polymethyl-methacrylate (PMMA) cement. J Chemother 14(5):64–72

6. Bohner M, Lemaitre J, Van Landuyt P et al (1997) Gentamicin-loaded hydraulic calcium phosphate bone cement as antibiotic delivery system. J Pharm Sci 86(5):565–572

7. Brien WW, Salvati EA, Klein R et al (1993). Antibiotic impregnated bone cement in total hip arthroplasty. An in vivo comparison of the elution properties of tobramycin and vancomy-cin. Clin Orthop Relat Res (296):242–248

8. Bunetel L, Segui A, Cormier M et al. (1989). Release of gentamicin from acrylic bone cement. Clin Pharmacokinet 17(4):291–297

9. Chohfi M, Langlais F, Fourastier J et al. (1998). Pharmacokinetics, uses, and limitations of vancomycin-loaded bone cement. Int Orthop 22(3):171–177

10. Cohen J (1999) Management of chronic infection in prosthetic joints. In "Infectious Disease" (Armstrong D. and Cohen J. Eds). Mosby, London. Vol. I, Section 2 – p 46.1–46.6

11. Diefenbeck M, Mückley T, Hofmann GO (2006) Prophylaxis and treatment of implant-related infections by local application of antibiotics. Injury 37(Suppl 2):S95–104

12. Engesæter LB, Lie SA, Espehaug B et al (2003) Antibiotic prophylaxis in total hip arthro-plasty. Effects of antibiotic prophylaxis systemically and in bone cement on the revision rate of 22,170 primary hip replacement followed 0–14 years in the Norwegian Arthroplasty Reg-ister. Acta Orthop Scand 74(6):644–651

13. Fletcher MAD, Spencer RF, Langkamer VG et al (2004) Gentamicin concentrations in diag-nostic aspirates from 25 patients with hip an knee arthroplasties. Acta Orthop Scand 75(2): 173–176

14. Gonzales Della Valle A, Bostrom M, Brause B et al (2002) Effective bactericidal activity of tobramycin and vancomycin eluted from acrylic bone cement. Acta Orthop Scand 72(3): 237–240

15. Hall EW, Rouse MS, Jacofsky DJ et al (2004) Release of daptomycin from polymethylmetacry-late beads in a continuous flow chamber. Diagn Microbiol Infect Dis 50(4):261–265

16. Henry SL, Hood GA, Seligson D (1993). Long-term implantation of gentamycin-polymethyl-metacrylate antibiotic beads. Clin Orthop Relat Res (295):47–53

17. Hsieh PH, Shih CH, Chang AD (2004) Two-stage revision hip arthroplasty for infection: com-parison between the interim use of antibiotic-loaded cement beads and a spacer prosthesis. J Bone Joint Surg (Am) 86(9):1989–1997

18. Huddleston PM, Steckelberg JM, Hanssen AS et al (2000). Ciprofloxacin inhibition of experi-mental fracture healing. J Bone Joint Surg (Am) 82(2):161–173

19. Joseph TN, Chen AL, Di Cesare PE (2003) Use of antibiotic-impregnated cement in total joint arthroplasty. J Am Acad Orthop Surg 11(1):38–47.

20. Kanellakopoulou K, Giamarellos-Bourboulis E (2000) Carrier system for the local delivery of antibiotics in bone infections. Drugs 59(6):1223–1232

21. Kelm J, Regitz T, Schmitt E et al (2006) In vivo and in vitro studies of antibiotic release from and bacterial growth inhibition by antibiotic-impregnated polymethylmethacrylate hip spacers. Antimicrob Agents Chemother 50(1):332–335

22. Klekamp J, Dawson JM., Haas DW et al (1999) The use of vancomycin and tobramycin in acrylic bone cement: biochemical effects and elution kinetics for use in joint arthroplasty. J Arthroplasty 14(3):339–346

23. Klemm K (2001) The use of antibiotic-containing bead chains in the treatment of chronic bone infections. Clin Microbiol Infect 7(1):28–31

24. Lewis G. and Bhattaram A. (2006) Influence of a pre-blended antibiotic (gentamicin sulfate powder) on various mechanical, thermal, and physical properties of three acrylic bone cements. J Biomater Appl 20(4):377–408

25. Lorian V (1996) Antibiotic in laboratory medicine. Fourth edition. Williams & Wilkins Ed., Baltimore

26. Magnan B, Regis D, Biscaglia R, Bartolozzi P (2001) Preformed acrylic bone cement spacer loaded with antibiotics: use of two-stage procedure in 10 patients because of infected hips after total replacement. Acta Orthop Scand 72(6):591–594

27. Masri BA, Duncan CP, Beauchamp CP (1998) Long-term elution of antibiotics from bone-cement: an in vivo study using the prosthesis of antibiotic-loaded acrylic cement (PROSTA-LAC) system. J Arthroplasty. 13(3):331–338

28. Neut D, de Groot EP, Kowalski RS et al (2005) Gentamicin-loaded bone cement with clinda-mycin or fusidic acid added: biofilm formation and antibiotic release. J Biomed Mater Res A 73(2):165–170
29. Neut D, van de Belt H, Stokroos I, et al. (2001) Biomaterial-associated infection of gentami-cin-loaded PMMA beads in orthopaedic revision surgery. J Antimicrob Chemother. 47(6): 885–891
30. Penner MJ, Duncan CP, Masri BA (1999) The in vitro elution characteristics of antibiotic-loaded CMW and Palacos-R bone cements. J Arthroplasty 14(2):209–214
31. Powles JW, Spencer RF, Lovering AM (1998) Gentamicin release from old cement during revision hip arthroplasty. J Bone Joint Surg (Br) 80(4):607–610
32. Seeley SK, Seeley JV, Telehowski P et al (2004) Volume and surface area study of tobramycin-polymethylmetacrylate beads. Clin Orthop Relat Res 420:298–303
33. Takahira N, Itoman M, Higashi K et al (2003) Treatment outcome of two-stage revision total hip arthroplasty for infected arthroplasty using antibiotic-impregnated cement spacer. J Orthop Sci 8(1):26–31
34. Toms AD, Davidson D, Masri BA et al (2006) The management of peri-prosthetic infection in total joint arthroplasty. J Bone Joint Surg (Br) 88(2):149–155
35. Tunney MM, Ramage G, Patrick S et al (1998) Antimicrobial susceptibility of bacteria iso-lated from orthopaedic implants following revision hip surgery. Antimicrob Agents Chemo-ther 42(11):3002–3005
36. van de Belt H, Neut D, Schenk W et al (2001) Infection of orthopedic implants and the use of antibiotic-loaded bone cements. A review. Acta Orthop Scand 72(6):557–571
37. Van de Belt H, Neut D, Uges DRA et al (2000) Surface roughness, porosity and wettability of gentamicin-loaded bone cements and their antibiotic release. Biomaterials 21(19):1981–1987
38. Van de Belt H, Neut D, Uges DRA, et al (2001). Staphylococcus aureus biofilm formation on different gentamicin-loaded polymethylmethacrylate bone cements. Biomaterials 22(12): 1607–1611
39. Wahlig H, Dingeldein E (1980). Antibiotic and bone cements. Experimental and clinical long-term observations. Acta Orthop Scand 51(1):49–56

11 Antibiotic Cement Spacers in Total Hip and Total Knee Arthroplasty: Problems, Pitfalls, and Avoiding Complications

R.S.J. BURNETT, J.C. CLOHISY, R.L. BARRACK

Department of Orthopaedic Surgery, Washington University School of Medicine
Barnes-Jewish Hospital, Saint Louis, Missouri, USA

Introduction

With the increasing number of total hip (THA) and knee arthroplasties (TKA) performed with expanding indications and at a younger age, there continues to be a low risk of periprosthetic sepsis in association with these surgeries. The incidence of infection in THA/TKA ranges for 0.3 % to 3 %. While sepsis is a rare complication, the management from both patient and surgeon perspective are challenging, often require a prolonged course of treatment, and may lead to complications. The diagnosis and management of periprosthetic sepsis has evolved with the current standard of care and management based upon the useful classification of Gustilo et al [21, 25]. The use of antibiotic impregnated cement beads [19] and spacers as local delivery devices to treat periprosthetic infections in either a single stage [3] or two-stage surgery [12, 17, 18] has evolved and become popular over recent years. Frequently, reports of periprosthetic sepsis do not address antibiotic spacer complications. How-

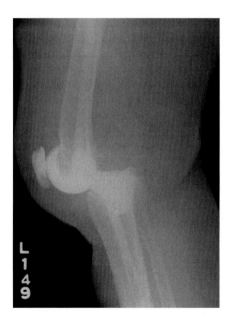

Fig. 1. Dislocation of a mobile AICS of the knee. This patient had poor ligamentous support for an articulating cement spacer.

ever, with increasing number of these surgeries being performed, surgeons have reported new problems and complications [6, 8, 20, 26] (Fig. 1) associated with these cement spacers. Determining who is at risk for complications and what factors are controlled by the surgeon is the purpose of this chapter. In addition to technical aspects of cement spacer surgery, there are multiple risk factors for complications associated with antibiotic impregnated cement spacers (AICS) in infection surgery. This includes patient risk factors, surgical risk factors, organism specific diagnosis and treatment. In addition there are significant treatment costs in association with cement spacer implants, patient morbidity, surgeon frustration, and further outcomes data is necessary in order to establish the success or failure of these devices.

Classification of Periprosthetic Infection

The classification of periprosthetic infection has been defined based on the timing of surgery and the source of infection. Infections may be classified as occurring with a positive intraoperative culture, acute or early postoperative infection (2 – 4 weeks), late chronic infections, and acute hematogenous infections. The focus of this outline is to discuss the use of AICS for late chronic and acute hematogenous infections requiring explantation/removal of a THA / TKA followed by insertion of an AICS.

The treatment options for acute hematogenous or late chronic infections include irrigation and debridement with modular liner exchange if diagnosed at an early stage (less than 2 to 4 weeks); alternatively the option of a single stage versus two-stage reimplantation may be performed. At our institution the two-stage reimplantation procedure is favored for all non-acute infections. This involves implant removal with a thorough irrigation and debridement of bone and soft tissues, placement of an antibiotic impregnated cement spacer for local delivery and elution of antibiotics, and a delayed second stage reconstruction/reimplantation. The results of two-stage reimplantation surgery are favorable, with a 91 to 94 percent eradication rate for infection [14, 15, 27]. At our institution these formal 'two-stages' are frequently insufficient. One initial irrigation debridement is often insufficient to eradicate a purulent infection. In addition, resistant organisms often necessitate a second or third debridement and the soft tissues may often be compromised. A repeat irrigation and debridement, with exchange of the antibiotic spacer is often required, and is frequently a planned procedure at our institution. At the final irrigation and debridement procedure (typically performed over the 7 to 10 day period following the initial explantation), a final definitive antibiotic loaded spacer is placed. In addition we frequently use intramedullary (IM) cement dowels for IM canal local delivery of antibiotics. We have redefined the formal two-stage procedure into a six stage process as follows:

First Stage: diagnosis of infection and removal of infected implant, I&D, and temporary placement of a static non-mobile spacer with or without IM antibiotic impregnated cement dowels. At this stage, if the infection is purulent and the patient is unwell, we will perform a resection ; a planned return to the O.R. for a second I&D is established.

Second Stage: initial postoperative infectious disease consultation with antibiotic directed therapy is started. The patient then typically returns to the OR at 48 to 72 hours for repeat irrigation debridement, exchange of cement spacer, possible exchange of cement dowels. We typically consider a repeat I&D if the infection has significant purulence, unhealthy appearing soft tissues, or a resistant bacterial or fungal organism. At this stage, once the tissues appear healthy, the final definitive AICS (static or mobile) is typically placed. It is at this stage that consideration for a mobile cement spacer is decided, and that the risk factors for complications and avoiding problems with AICS needs to be considered by the surgeon.

Third stage: Antibiotic directed intravenous therapy for a total of six weeks begins following the last I&D. Wound management initially involves immobilization in a cast or brace in order to allow soft tissue healing. Considerations for oral synergistic antibiotics such as rifampin or trimethoprim-sulfamethoxazole (Septra, Bactrim) are considered by the infectious disease specialist in consultation. The nutritional status and parameters of the patient are evaluated and treated.

Fourth Stage: Once the patient has completed a 6 weeks course of IV antibiotics (outpatient), the discontinuation of antibiotics is followed by a 2 to 4 week antibiotic-free interval. The ESR and CRP are followed and wound healing is reevaluated. The patient is medically optimized and undergoes a joint aspiration for cell count and culture specimens in the outpatient clinic.

Fifth Stage: This is the reimplantation/revision THA/TKA procedure. Preoperative planning including the necessity for extensile exposures, intraoperative cultures and cell counts, and intraoperative frozen sections [7] are planned. The reconstruction is planned preoperatively based on underlying bone and soft tissue defects.

Sixth Stage: Following the reimplantation/revision procedure, routine clinical follow-up occurs with monitoring of the ESR, CRP, and clinical observation for any signs of recurring sepsis. We do not typically continue prolonged antibiotics following the second stage, unless there is a concern about chronic infection that requires chronic antibiotic suppression. This occurs in a minority of patients only (less than 10 %).

Antibiotic Cement Spacers: Treatment Goals

The treatment goals with the use of AICS, whether static or mobile, remain the same in all cases of periprosthetic infection. The primary goal of a treatment is to eliminate infection with the adjunctive addition of local antibiotic therapy combined with systemic antibiotic treatment and surgery. The AICS are useful to stabilize or tension the soft tissues, potentially facilitate or make the reimplantation second stage procedure easier [1, 4, 8], and reduce bone loss [11] between stages. The maintenance of appropriate soft tissue tension and joint range of motion may reduce the need for more extensile exposures at the second stage reimplantation surgery, especially during TKA surgery [5]. Despite possible range of motion and second stage advantages, the most important aspect of any AICS treatment therapy remains unchanged: elimination of infection and the local delivery of antibiotic therapy to supplement systemic IV antibiotics, and a thorough surgical irrigation and debridement. With these principles in mind, selection of an AICS plays one part in the role of eradication of periprosthetic sepsis.

Classification of Antibiotic Cement Spacers

New technologies have provided the orthopedic surgeon with several options available for surgery with the use of AICS. A classification of AICS is outlined in Table 1. The advantages of static or simple spacers formed in the operating room include: a simple construct which is easy for the surgeon to make, the surgeon is able to select the antibiotic of choice directed with organism specific therapy. This simple / static spacer may be useful for multiple I&D procedures and to allow delivery of multiple antibiotics from one spacer. The disadvantage of a static / non-mobile spacer is that it does not allow physiologic motion of the joint, which is of secondary importance during infection treatment. In addition, the issue of cement generated exothermic heat, cement shrinkage, and exposure to monomer may be of concern. Similarly, there are complications that may occur with static antibiotic spacers.

The advantages of mobile cement spacers which are preformed include the option of allowing an element of physiologic joint motion [9]. These spacers tend to be simple, 'off the shelf' devices with a fixed antibiotic (and currently single antibiotic) dose. There is evidence that mobile articulating spacers may reduce bone loss in association with a second stage reimplantation surgery [4, 11]. There is no heat or shrinkage that can occur with these preformed implants. The reinforced central core of this type of implant may provide significant biomechanical advantages against catastrophic failure or fracture of the implant. The disadvantages of mobile spacers which are preformed included a limitation in implant sizes and antibiotic dose, often allowing only a single agent delivery of antibiotic. The spacers have little to no inherit constraint and there is a limited number of options for offset restoration with the hip implants. The mobile spacer which is preformed also may be subject to complications with its use.

Mobile spacers which are formed in the O.R. have their own unique advantages and disadvantages. Advantages similar to a preformed spacer include allowing an element of physiologic motion. The option for adjustable antibiotic dosing, a combination of antibiotics [13], and the addition of an antifungal option (amphotericin [22]) may be useful. These implants are available with or without a central reinforced core, may allow for adjustable leg length (PROSTALAC, Depuy, Warsaw, IN, USA), and the option for a semiconstrained articulation. Disadvantages of mobile spacers formed in the O.R. include additional time to construct the implant in the operating room, a limited number of sizes, and complications may similarly occur.

With the option of static preformed cement spacers, mobile preformed spacers, and mobile spacers formed in the operating room, the surgeon and patient have a

Table 1. Classification of Antibiotic Cement Spacers

• Static versus mobile/articulating
• Preformed versus cement spacer formed in the operating room by the surgeon
• Fixed versus variable dose antibiotic in the cement
• Multi agent antibiotic versus single agent delivery
• Reinforced central metallic implant core or all cement implant
• Constrained, conforming, or unconstrained articulating implants
• Exposed metal or polyethylene within the spacer versus non-exposed/entire cement coated

variety of options to treat THA / TKA infections and allow the surgeon to address both bone and soft tissue deficiencies. However, common controversies continue to exist among surgeons with the use of such spacers. The following questions or controversies remain to be answered. Is a mobile spacer better than a static spacer? Does the mobile spacer provide for an easier second stage revision? Can the antibiotic impregnated spacer act as a permanent implant? Do AICS not get re-infected? Is there toxicity to antibiotics/cement in the cement spacer? Is it safe to bear full weight on an AICS? Often the answers to these questions pose challenging decision making options for the surgeon and have allowed us to determine a simple classification of AICS related complications.

Classification of Antibiotic Impregnated Hip Spacer Complications

We have developed a simple classification system to describe the complications that occur in association with an AICS hip implant (Table 2). This simple classification divides the complications into soft tissue or instability related complications, implant related factors, fixation of the antibiotic cement spacer, host bone complications, and pharmacologic toxicity.

1. Dislocation/Instability of Hip Spacers

This is the most common complication in association with a hip periprosthetic infection and antibiotic hip spacers [2, 6, 8, 10, 16]. We have identified several risk factors that occur and may be predictive of instability/dislocation of an antibiotic cement spacer (Table 3). Patients with a prior dislocation (Fig. 2) of a THA may be at higher risk due to underlying soft-tissue tissue deficiencies (muscular and scar tissues). A deficiency of the greater trochanter or abductors should caution the surgeon against using a mobile spacer, which may increase the risk of dislocation. Patients that have undergone multiple prior hip surgeries are specifically at risk for abductor deficiency. It is in these elderly patients that a mobile spacer, while attractive for the surgeon, may result in silent dislocation, with the patient on occasion, unaware that the spacer has dislocated. Similarly, proximal femoral bone deficiency or a prior hip fracture open reduction internal fixation may be associated with increase risk of spacer instability. Acetabular deficiency – specifically in the superior-lateral and posterior-superior region warrant caution with the use of an antibiotic spacer and are high risk for dislocation (Fig. 3). Subsidence of a femoral spacer below the original insertion depth decreases the leg length and offset and increases the risk of dislocation. Unrestored

Table 2. Classification of Antibiotic Impregnated Hip Spacer Complications

- Dislocation/instability
- Fracture of implant
- Subsidence/distal migration
- Periprosthethic femur fracture
- Proximal femoral bone loss/erosion
- Systemic Antibiotic toxicity

Table 3. Risk factors for instability/dislocation of antibiotic hip spacers

- Prior dislocation of THA
- Trochanteric/abductor deficiency
- Multiply operated hip
- Proximal femoral deficiency
- Prior hip fracture open reduction internal fixation
- Acetabular deficiency: superior, lateral, posterior
- Subsidence of femoral spacer
- Unrestored femoral offset
- Preformed spacer head diameter smaller than acetabular diameter (mismatch/undersized head)
- Anteversion of femoral spacer inadequate

native femoral hip offset and a mismatch of the diameter of the spacer with the patient's acetabular diameter increase the risk of dislocation. The anteversion of the femoral cement spacer should attempt to incorporate native host anteversion and a lack of this may increase the risk of instability.

Solutions for avoiding instability and dislocation of hip spacers include identification of preoperative risk factors. Intraoperative accurate match of the acetabular diameter and spacer head diameter are crucial. Restoration of leg length may be achieved by cementing in the cement spacer at the proximal aspect of the implant, and, with the use of a modular head (PROSTALAC) option. Offset restoration will help tension the compromised soft tissues. In patients with extensive proximal femoral deficiency, the use of a proximal femoral cement build-up/proximal femoral replacement type implant will avoid subsidence (Fig. 4). Finally, the use of a Girdlestone procedure or resection arthroplasty should be considered if the intraoperative cement spacer is unstable. Treatment of instability is dependent on the underlying diagnosis and reason for instability, and may include closed reduction, observation, or revision surgery, depending on the patient factors and surgical factors leading to instability of the spacer.

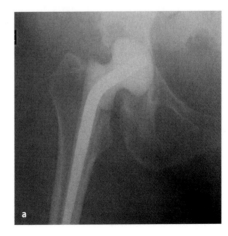

Fig. 2a. This patient underwent placement of a mobile right hip AICS for right THA sepsis (Spacer-G/InterSpace Hip – Exactech, Gainesville, FL, USA). She has a history of recurrent dislocation of her left THA. There is a small superolateral acetabular defect on right hip, which may be a risk factor for AICS dislocation

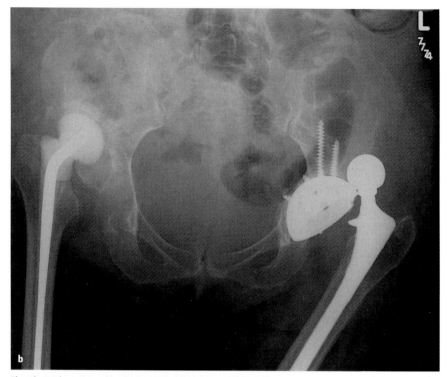

Fig. 2b. Dislocation of both the right hip AICS and the left THA

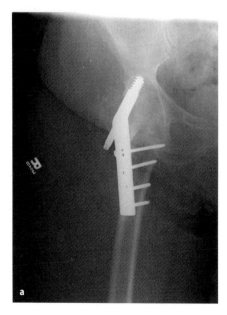

Fig. 3a. Right hip fracture with failure of internal fixation. There is a superolateral acetabular deficiency. The greater trochanter is nonunited. This patient has right hip sepsis

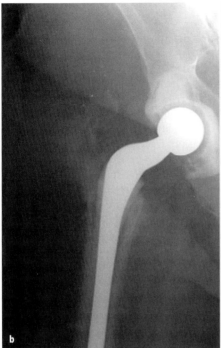

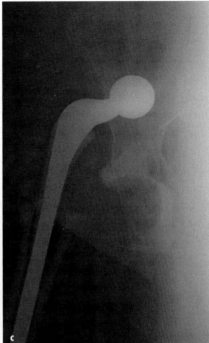

Fig. 3b. The patient underwent I&D, with placement of a semiconstrained AICS of the hip (PROSTALAC, Depuy Orthopedics, Warsaw IN, USA). Note the fragmentation of the greater trochanter and the superolateral acetabular defect

Fig. 3c. At 8 weeks postoperatively, the hip spacer was dislocated, requiring revision surgery to remove the spacer

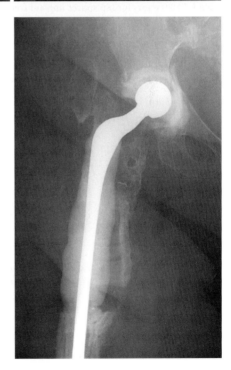

Fig. 4. An AICS (PROSTALAC) with proximal femoral cement buildup was constructed. The implant was cemented into the host femoral canal to provide for stability against subsidence and rotation

2. Implant Fracture of Hip Spacers

The occurrence of an antibiotic impregnated hip spacer implant fracture may be related to several risk factors (Table 4). The loss of proximal femoral bone support may lead to a cantilever on the AICS and result in fracture of the hip spacer. This may occur in conjunction with a loss of proximal femoral bone support or a prior extended trochanteric femoral osteotomy. The risks increase with an implant that lacks a central reinforced metallic core (Fig. 5). Any implant which is loose is at risk for fracture. Preformed spacers (off the shelf) should have more homogeneous cement characteristics and be subject to less risk of fracture than a surgeon-formed implant in the operating room, which may have cement inconsistencies due to mixing. Solutions for avoiding implant fracture include recognizing and treating for risk factors. Cementing the spacer proximally into the femur to avoid instability and subsidence is a useful technique. A long stemmed spacer is indicated to bypass defects such as an extended trochanteric osteotomy site (Fig. 6). Similarly, use of an implant with a central reinforced metallic core such as the Interspace / Spacer-G (Exactech, Gainesville, FL, USA) or PROSTALAC implant provides additional implant strength. Preformed spacers may have improved fatigue cement strength and reduce the risk of cement heterogeneity. The treatment of hip spacer implant fractures may include observation or revision surgery depending on both the patient and implant related factors.

Table 4. Risk factors for hip spacer implant fracture

• Loss of proximal femoral bone support
• Extended Trochanteric femoral Osteotomy
• Absent central reinforce core
• Loose implant
• Cement fatigue with surgeon constructed cement spacers

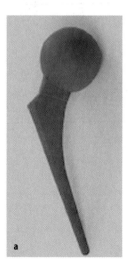

◁
Fig. 5a. A mobile AICS made in the operating room from a mold of antibiotic impregnated cement. This design (Stage One Hip Cement Spacer Mold, Biomet Orthopedics, Warsaw, IN, USA), does not contain a central metallic reinforced core

▷
Fig. 5b. Left hip AICS for periprosthetic sepsis. The surgery required and extended trochanteric femoral osteotomy for removal of the septic femoral component

▷
Fig. 5c. Subsidence and fracture of the AICS implant with a loss of reduction of the extended trochanteric osteotomy. This patient required revision surgery of the AICS

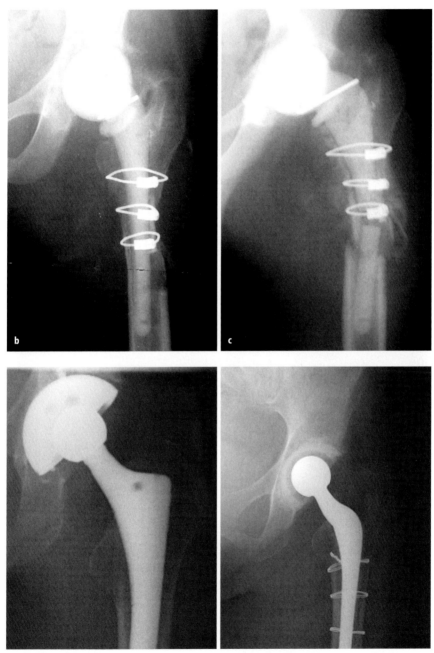

Fig. 6a. Left hip sepsis with Candida albicans – preoperative radiograph prior to implant removal and I&D

Fig. 6b. Left hip insertion of a PROSTALAC spacer. An extended trochanteric osteotomy was required to remove the femoral component. Amphotericin B antifungal powder was added to the cement in the operating room

3. Femoral Subsidence/Periprosthetic Femur Fracture

Risk factors for this complication include a loss of proximal femoral bone support. Similarly, and extended trochanteric femoral osteotomy is a stress-riser and, in addition to an implant fracture risk, is also a risk for proximal femoral fracture. The use of AICS implant which is not cemented proximally is at increased risk for femur fracture. Non compliant patients that are unable to observe protected weight bearing and that attempt bear full weight on an antibiotic spacer are at an increased risk of periprosthetic femur fracture (Fig. 7). Solutions for avoiding femoral subsidence and periprosthetic femur fracture include cementing the spacer proximally in the region of the metaphysis and bypassing an extended trochanteric osteotomy with a long stem spacer. Protected weight bearing is essential and both the patient and surgeon must to have similar goals with a protected weight bearing postoperative course. The treatment of femoral subsidence and periprosthetic femur fracture may include revision surgery, open reduction internal fixation of the fracture, and an implant to bypass the fracture with provisional stabilization during treatment of the infection (Fig. 8).

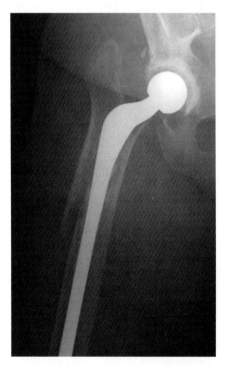

Fig. 7. Right hip AICS subsidence and fracture. This spacer was not cemented in proximally. The patient was medically unhealthy for further surgery, and began to walk with full weight on her hip, resulting in spacer subsidence and fracture of the femur

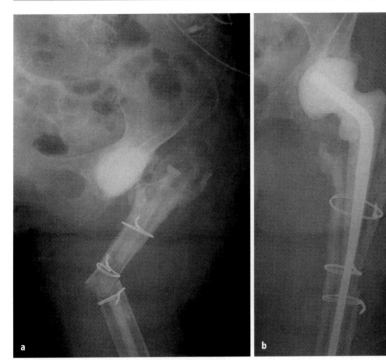

Fig. 8a. Left femur fracture in association with a static antibiotic cement spacer placed for prior periprosthetic chronic left THA sepsis

Fig. 8b. Left hip following removal of the static spacer, open reduction and internal fixation of the fracture, and placement of a long-stemmed articulating cement spacer (Spacer-G/InterSpace Hip)

4. Antibiotic Toxicity

Systemic antibiotic toxicity in association with a local antibiotic spacer delivery implant is a rare complication [13, 17, 23]. This may occur more frequently with surgeon constructed spacer implants and with the addition of high doses of antibiotics to the cement. Other risk factors for toxicity include patients with chronic renal failure. Caution with the use of antibiotic dosing with vancomycin, aminoglycosides, and antifungal agents with surgeon constructed spacers will help avoid this complication. In addition, different brands of cement may have variable antibiotic elution characteristics [24] and the surgeon should be familiar with the elution properties of the cement used in an AICS. The treatment for suspected antibiotic toxicity involves supportive care and following closely the renal function of the patient. Serum levels of antibiotics may be measured to follow antibiotic toxicity. Rarely, more invasive methods such as a renal biopsy (to diagnose acute interstitial nephritis) may be required in order to confirm the diagnosis of this rare complication [26]. If in doubt, and in consultation with the infectious disease and nephrology consultant, consideration for explantation/removal of the cement spacer must be considered by the surgeon (Fig. 9). A high level of suspicion must be considered in patients who present with deteriorating renal function in the postoperative period following insertion of a high dose AICS.

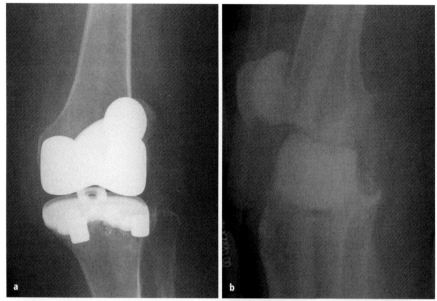

Fig. 9a. Left TKA sepsis (multi-organism) following a minimally invasive TKA surgery. There is loosening of the tibial component

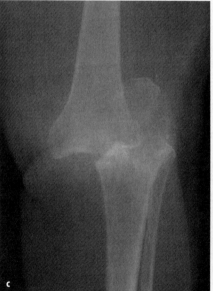

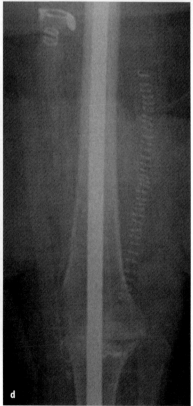

Fig. 9c. Following AICS removal, renal function improved. The patient was not a candidate for a second stage reimplantation and a resection arthroplasty was performed

In summary, there are several patient, surgeon, and implant factors that may help reduce the risk of complications with AICS. The routine interval use of radiographs to follow the patient and AICS implant may be helpful. Restoration of leg length, offset, and anteversion, while not the goal of spacer treatment, will help reduce the risk of hip spacer instability. Minimizing the femoral head spacer-acetabular mismatch reduces the risk of instability. The technique of proximally cementing in the spacer and using longer stems to bypass defects may help reduce the risk of fracture and subsidence. Proximal cement buildup on an antibiotic spacer to substitute for bone loss will additionally prevent subsidence. Careful evaluation of acetabular bone defects and abductor muscle quality will help the surgeon select the appropriate antibiotic delivery device. The option of having a semi-constrained acetabular implant available (PROSTALAC) may provide some increase in stability if bone and soft tissue deficiencies occur. The use of a central reinforced metallic core in the AICS hip spacer may help reduce fatigue fracture of the implant.

Antibiotic Impregnated Knee Cement Spacers: Complications

Complications that occur in association with AICS of the knee may be classified using a similar classification system to that of the hip (Table 5). This section will identify the risk factors, solutions for avoiding knee cement spacers complications, and treatment options for each complication.

1. Dislocation/Instability

The risk factors for dislocation and instability [20] of knee cement spacers relate to both bone and soft tissue defects encountered at the time of removal of the infected TKA. These complications include knee instability, spacer extrusion, and anterior soft tissue impingement of the AICS. Complications may occur with extensive tibial and femoral bone loss, which results in large flexion and or extension gaps of the joint space. The patient with a multiply operated knee and / or multiple incisions may be at increase risk for cement spacer complications (Fig. 10). Similarly, ligamentous insufficiency involving the PCL, LCL or MCL places the patient at increase risk for spacer complications. A disruption of the extensor mechanism may lead to anterior

◁
Fig. 9b. Left knee removal of TKA and insertion of AICS plus intramedullary dowels. The patient developed acute renal failure (acute interstitial nephritis) postoperatively, requiring discontinuation of IV Vancomycin, and removal of the AICS

◁
Fig. 9d. Left knee arthrodesis following a resection arthroplasty

Table 5. Classification of Knee Cement Spacer Complications

- Dislocation/instability
- Implant extrusion:
  - Extensor Mechanism erosion
  - Neurovascular compression
  - Anterior soft tissue compromise
- Overstuffing of patellar femoral or tibial femoral joint
- Fracture of the implant
- Periprosthethic tibial or femur fracture
- Antibiotic Toxicity

extrusion of an AICS. Unsupported cement spacers that have no intramedullary extension and / or that are not cemented in place are at risk for dislocation. The non-compliant patient that is unable to follow a structured restricted postoperative therapy program is at risk for dislocation. Static cement spacers that are placed into the knee with the leg held in full extension with axial distraction are at risk for extruding anteriorly once the patient awakens from anesthesia and in the postoperative course, due to gradual flexion of the knee and anterior extrusion of the spacer. Solutions for avoiding knee instability and spacer extrusion include avoiding overstuffing the extension gap which minimizes the chance of extrusion with postoperative knee flexion. Patients with ligamentous instability should not be considered for mobile / articulating spacers and a static spacer should be implanted. The use of tibial metaphyseal intramedullary cement support when considering a static spacer may help reduce the risk of anterior static spacer extrusion into the soft tissues of the knee (Fig. 11). Treatment of knee antibiotic cement spacer instability complications is directed by the underlying complication and the identified risk factor(s) for this occurrence. At our institution, we delay the range of motion in patients with knee AICS in order to allow soft tissue healing. Prompt decompression of an extruded anterior cement spacer with removal of the spacer should be considered due to impending erosion of the extensor mechanism. Closed reduction and splinting may provide useful treatment for a subluxed spacer, but is usually unsuccessful, with a high recurrence rate of instability. Revision of the cement spacer may be required if the soft tissue impingement is significant. Careful external rotation of mobile articulating cement spacer components will help reduce the risk of component maltracking and extensor mechanism problems. Resection or removal of knee spacers in patients with complications is a useful alternative that may need to be considered in a limited number of patients.

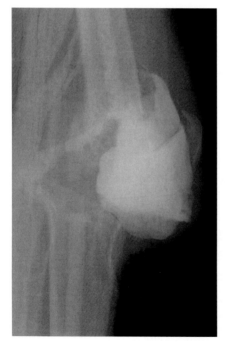

Fig. 10. At four weeks following AICS placement, the spacer has extruded anteriorly, with impingement and anterior soft-tissue compromise. This complication required return to the operating room for removal of the AICS

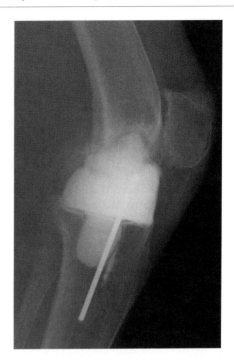

Fig. 11. The use of an adjunctive tibial metaphyseal cement spacer extension with a centrally reinforced core provides for excellent stability with the use of a static knee cement spacer, avoiding anterior spacer extrusion and dislocation

2. Implant and Periprosthetic Fracture

AICS implant and periprosthetic fractures may occur either intraoperatively or postoperatively [20]. Risk factors for implant fracture include several controllable aspects of treatment that require careful intraoperative planning. Surgeon constructed (self made) spacers that are hand mixed in the O.R. may be at higher risk for a fracture – especially with a mobile spacer, due to cement heterogeneity and inconsistencies in mixing. The use of higher antibiotic doses will lead to decreased spacer fracture toughness and increased risk of fracture. A non congruent femoral component fit on host femoral bone may lead to subsidence and fracture of the implant (Fig. 12). The surgeon should avoid impacting the mobile cement spacer during cementing due to the brittle consistency of these implants. In the patient that has a flexion contracture following insertion of the mobile cement spacer, forced extension of the knee and cement spacer may lead to femoral implant fracture. Non compliant patients similarly are at risk of implant fracture with a knee cement spacer. Periprosthetic fractures of the distal femur and proximal tibia may occur in association with loose spacer implants, malalignment of the knee (varus or valgus deformity), notching of the anterior femur, and extensive bone loss or poor bone quality in the region of the spacer. Solutions for avoiding implant fracture at the knee include the use of a preformed implant with more homogeneous cement consistency. Antibiotic dosing and the effect on cement strength and fatigue is a consideration. The surgeon should aim for a congruent femoral fit and size of the AICS on the distal femur. Avoiding impaction of the implant during cementing and not attempting forced extension of a cement spacer will help reduce implant and periprosthetic bone fracture risk. In the

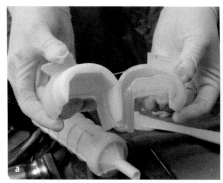

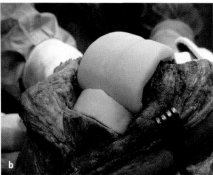

Fig. 12a. A mobile articulating articulating spacer (Stage One Knee Cement Spacer Mold, Biomet Orthopedics, Warsaw, IN, USA) was constructed in the O.R. using a mold and surgeon mixed cement

Fig. 12b. The AICS femoral implant was over-sized and had a non-congruent fit on the distal femur. The knee was unable to be fully extend-ed due to over-stuffing of the extension gap

Fig. 12c. During an attempt at improving the flexion contracture, femoral AICS fractured

Fig. 12d. A smaller size femoral AICS was constructed, and the articulating implants were then cemented onto the host bone

Fig. 12e. The articulating femoral implant loos-ened at 8 weeks postoperatively, rupturing the extensor mechanism (quadriceps) as it dislo-cated anteriorly. The patient required removal of the AICS and is awaiting a knee arthrodesis

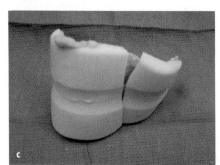

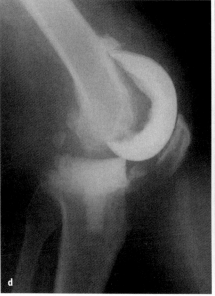

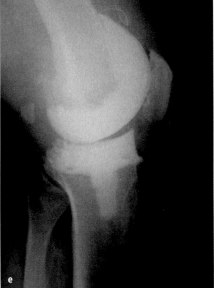

event that there is a flexion contracture and the anterior soft tissue retinaculum is unable to be closed, removal of the femoral mobile spacer while maintaining the tibial spacer has been a successful option performed at our institution.

3. Overstuffing of the Tibio-femorall and Patello-femoral Joints

Overstuffing the tibio-femoral or patello-femoral joint occurs not uncommonly with the use of antibiotic knee spacers. In patients with history of prolonged immobility and extensive scar tissue, the AICS implant often 'overstuffs' one or both of these joints. Risk factors include patients with prolonged immobilization with the knee in extension, and the multiply operated knee with extensive scar tissue. A prior anterior rough cut with inadequate thickness may overstuff the patello-femoral joint once the spacer is inserted. If the patellar composite (remaining host patella) is too thick, this will overstuff the patello-femoral joint. Similarly, if the femoral component is extended or not seated on the distal femur, the patello-femoral joint may be compromised with difficulty closing the anterior soft tissues over the cement spacer. A tibial spacer that is too thick or over-fills the flexion and extension gap will lead to a flexion contracture and difficulty closing the anterior soft tissues. Solutions for overstuffing the patello-femoral and tibio-femoral joints include identifying the above risk factors and appropriately avoiding them. Mobile spacers should be avoided if the patient has had a prolonged history of immobilization in extension or in the multiply operated knee. The prior anterior rough cut should be assessed intraoperatively and, if necessary, lowered down to the flush anterior level of the femur by the surgeon. The patellar composite thickness or remaining patella must be assessed and, if necessary, the patella may be required to be recut to help reduce the patello-femoral gap. Ensuring that the femoral component is well seated and that the tibial spacer is not of excessive thickness will help reduce a knee flexion contracture and facilitate closure of the soft tissues. Cementing the knee AICS in place with generous cement that enters the metaphyseal region will help reduce AICS instability.

In summary, complications with knee AICS are predictable. With the identification of risk factors and surgical technique modifications by the surgeon, most complications are avoidable. With the advent of new mobile articulating knee AICS that allow antibiotic delivery, this option has become a new alternative for maintenance of range of motion while providing local antibiotic delivery in TKA sepsis. In order to avoid complications with the use of these mobile cement knee spacers, certain technique highlights should be adhered to. Cementing the mobile cement spacer at the implant-host bone interface will provide stability during range of motion and reduce the risk of implant loosening and dislocation. Avoiding overstuffing the patello-femoral and tibio-femoral joints will facilitate soft tissue closure over the spacer. Careful attention to external rotation of the femoral and tibial components of the spacer will facilitate extensor mechanism tracking. Observing a graduated conservative physical therapy protocol which allows early soft tissue healing and at a later date active range of motion will avoid soft tissue complications. Contraindications for mobile AICS of the knee include patients that have extensive bone loss at the knee, ligamentous instability, extensor mechanism deficiency, or prior prolonged immobilization with extensive scarring of the anterior soft tissues and extensor mechanism.

Conclusions: Knee and Hip Antibiotic Impregnated Cement Spacer Complications

In summary, the options for delivery of local antibiotics to the surgical site of periprosthetic THA/TKA infections have provided useful adjuncts to the treatment of periprosthetic sepsis. The gain in both high-dose local antibiotic delivery and functional improvements may be of benefit to these patients. The gain in function with mobile spacers is associated with newer patient functional achievement and higher patient demands. Articulating spacers may provide improved range of motion and prevent bone loss in association with a second-stage reimplantation procedure. Component removal with surgical irrigation and debridement is still the primary treatment for periprosthetic THA/TKA sepsis. In order to avoid complications with antibiotic cement spacers, the surgeon must carefully assess for and identify patient factors that may be associated with cement spacer problems. This includes identifying intraoperative risk factors to reduce complications, and following conservative postoperative therapy and weight bearing protocols in this group of patients. Preoperatively, predicting which patients are at risk for complications, and the early recognition and treatment of antibiotic cement spacer complications in the hip and knee will help reduce bone and soft tissue complications which may occur with the use of these devices.

References

1. Barrack RL, Engh G, Rorabeck C et al (2000) Patient satisfaction and outcome after septic versus aseptic revision total knee arthroplasty. J Arthroplasty 15(8):990–993
2. Bertazzoni Minelli E, Benini A, Magnan B et al (2004) Release of gentamicin and vancomycin from temporary human hip spacers in two-stage revision of infected arthroplasty. J Antimicrob Chemother, 53(2):329–334
3. Callaghan JJ, Katz RP, Johnston RC (1999) One-stage revision surgery of the infected hip. A minimum 10-year followup study. Clin Orthop Relat Res (369):139–143
4. Calton TF, Fehring TK, Griffin WL (1997) Bone loss associated with the use of spacer blocks in infected total knee arthroplasty. Clin Orthop Relat Res (345):148–154
5. Comley A, MacDonald S, McCalden R et al (2004) Articulating Spacers versus Static Spacers in Infected Total Knee Arthroplasty: A Retrospective Matched Series. Presented at the Combined Meeting of Orthopedic Surgery, Sydney, Australia, September 2004
6. D'Angelo F, Negri L, Zatti G et al (2005) Two-stage revision surgery to treat an infected hip implant. A comparison between a custom-made spacer and a pre-formed one. Chir Organi Mov 90(3):271–279
7. Della Valle CJ, Bogner E, Desai P et al (1999) Analysis of frozen sections of intraoperative specimens obtained at the time of reoperation after hip or knee resection arthroplasty for the treatment of infection. J Bone Joint Surg (Am) 81(5):684–689
8. Durbhakula SM, Czajka J, Fuchs MD et al (2004) Antibiotic-loaded articulating cement spacer in the 2-stage exchange of infected total knee arthroplasty. J Arthroplasty 19(6): 768–774
9. Emerson RH, Jr, Muncie M, Tarbox TR et al (2002) Comparison of a static with a mobile spacer in total knee infection. Clin Orthop Relat Res (404):132–138
10. Evans RP (2004) Successful treatment of total hip and knee infection with articulating antibiotic components: a modified treatment method. Clin Orthop Relat Res, (427):37–46
11. Fehring TK, Odum S, Calton TF et al (2000) Articulating versus static spacers in revision total knee arthroplasty for sepsis. The Ranawat Award. Clin Orthop Relat Res (380):9–16
12. Haleem AA, Berry DJ, Hanssen AD (2004) Mid-term to long-term followup of two-stage

reimplantation for infected total knee arthroplasty. Clin Orthop Relat Res (428):35–39

13. Hsieh PH, Chang YH, Chen SH et al (2006) High concentration and bioactivity of vancomycin and aztreonam eluted from Simplex cement spacers in two-stage revision of infected hip implants: a study of 46 patients at an average follow-up of 107 days. J Orthop Res 24(8): 1615–1621

14. Kendall RW, Masri BA, Duncan CP, Beauchamp CP et al (1994) Temporary antibiotic loaded acrylic hip replacement: a novel method for management of the infected THA. Semin Arthroplasty 5(4):171–177

15. Leone JM, Hanssen AD (2005) Management of infection at the site of a total knee arthroplasty. J Bone Joint Surg (Am) 87(10):2335–2348

16. Magnan B, Regis D, Biscaglia R et al (2001) Preformed acrylic bone cement spacer loaded with antibiotics: use of two-stage procedure in 10 patients because of infected hips after total replacement. Acta Orthop Scand 72(6):591–594

17. Masri BA, Duncan CP, Beauchamp CP (1998) Long-term elution of antibiotics from bone-cement: an in vivo study using the prosthesis of antibiotic-loaded acrylic cement (PROSTALAC) system. J Arthroplasty 13(3):331–338

18. Meek RM, Masri BA, Dunlop D et al (2003) Patient satisfaction and functional status after treatment of infection at the site of a total knee arthroplasty with use of the PROSTALAC articulating spacer. J Bone Joint Surg (Am) 85(10):1888–1892

19. Nelson CL, Evans RP, Blaha JD et al (1993) A comparison of gentamicin-impregnated polymethylmethacrylate bead implantation to conventional parenteral antibiotic therapy in infected total hip and knee arthroplasty. Clin Orthop Relat Res (295):96–101

20. Pietsch M, Hofmann S, Wenisch C (2006) Treatment of deep infection of total knee arthroplasty using a two-stage procedure. Oper Orthop Traumatol 18(1):66–87

21. Segawa H, Tsukayama DT, Kyle RF et al (1999) Infection after total knee arthroplasty. A retrospective study of the treatment of eighty-one infections. J Bone Joint Surg (Am) 81(10): 1434–1445

22. Silverberg D, Kodali P, Dipersio J et al (2002) In vitro analysis of antifungal impregnated polymethylmethacrylate bone cement. Clin Orthop Relat Res (403):228–231

23. Springer BD, Lee GC, Osmon D et al (2004) Systemic safety of high-dose antibiotic-loaded cement spacers after resection of an infected total knee arthroplasty. Clin Orthop Relat Res (427):47–51

24. Stevens CM, Tetsworth KD, Calhoun JH et al (2005) An articulated antibiotic spacer used for infected total knee arthroplasty: a comparative in vitro elution study of Simplex and Palacos bone cements. J Orthop Res 23(1):27–33

25. Tsukayama DT, Estrada R, Gustilo RB (1996) Infection after total hip arthroplasty. A study of the treatment of one hundred and six infections. J Bone Joint Surg (Am) 78(4):512–523

26. van Raaij TM, Visser LE, Vulto AG et al (2002) Acute renal failure after local gentamicin treatment in an infected total knee arthroplasty. J Arthroplasty 17(7):948–950

27. Younger AS, Duncan CP, Masri BA et al (1997) The outcome of two-stage arthroplasty using a custom-made interval spacer to treat the infected hip. J Arthroplasty 12(6):615–623.

12 The Preformed Spacers: From the Idea to the Realization of an Industrial Device

R. Soffiatti

Research & Development, Tecres Spa, Sommacampagna (VR), Italy

Medical Work of Art

At the beginning of the nineties visiting the operation theatres, it was possible to see the surgeons modelling with their hands bone cement in order to obtain handmade devices with a prosthesis-like geometry. The device was created to replace temporarily the removed septic prosthesis. The positioning in the septic site of an antibiotic-loaded bone cement device aimed at strengthening the systemic antibiotic therapy. As a matter of fact systemic antibiotic therapy is not always able to guarantee optimal antibiotic concentration in the infected site. After some months from implantation, the device was removed replacing it with a new prosthesis, giving back to the patient an healed joint and a certain functional recovery. This devices were called "spacers" [1, 7, 13, 14].

Mechanical Failure

Unfortunately in many cases it was possible to see also bad situations, determined by the mechanical failure of the hand-made devices. If on one side breakage was a fearsome and undesired complication, on the other side surgeons were very satisfied with the anti-septic effectiveness of the device. In other words the "spacer " and the systemic treatment increased the probability of infection healing compared to systemic antibiotic therapy alone.

Spacer-G

The positive results described led Tecres to start the research and study systematically the spacers made by the surgeon in order to design a device which could be at a time mechanically safe and pharmacologically effective: in other words a "reproducible effective device". A device which could also give the patient a better quality of life.

With these key features the Spacer-G was designed (Fig. 1). Its geometry was studied to permit an optimal interaction between the acetabulum and the femur: anatomical stem-neck angle chosen to limit as much as possible dislocation; saddle shape neck to limit the possible acetabular protrusion; extreme smoothness of the head to reduce the possible generation of debris. An inner stainless steel bar (Fig. 2) was

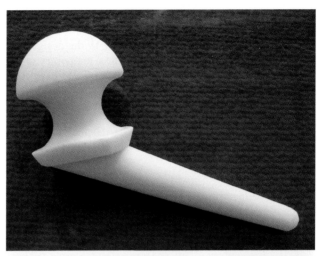

Fig. 1. Spacer-G, hip spacer

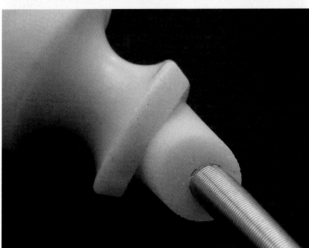

Fig. 2. Inner core present in Spacer-G

inserted to provide high mechanical strength and gentamicin was chosen as antibiotic due to the wide spectrum of activity and the good properties of release from PMMA.

Mechanical and pharmacological testing confirmed the good performances of the device which is solid and allows partial weight-bearing and releases effective amount of antibiotic in the infected site [2, 3, 4, 5, 9]. Soon after the first positive cases, the one-size spacer was joined by a smaller and a bigger head size, which permitted to improve the head-acetabulum coupling and reducing dislocation. Then the long-stem version was introduced which allowed to use the device also in the absence of a proximal support, in the presence of large metaphyseal defects and after a trans-femoral approach [12].

Knee, Shoulder and Elbow Spacers

The clinical success of the Spacer-G lead to the design of a knee spacer, Spacer-K (Fig. 3), with the same performances. These temporary spacer are CE marked as class III devices and are the first device of this type to have obtained the FDA clearance (InterSpace™ for Hip; InterSpace™ for Knee; InterSpace™ for Shoulder). On the basis of these experiences and taking advantage of the same principles the shoulder (Spacer-S) and the elbow spacer were designed (Figs 4–5).

Nail Clothing

The current management of infected nails has two main objectives: infection control, which is generally achieved by hardware removal with debridement and local deliv-

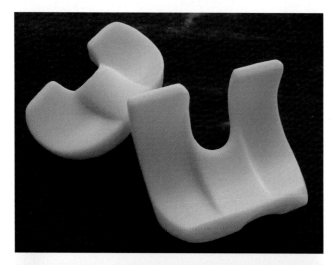

Fig. 3. Spacer-K, knee spacer

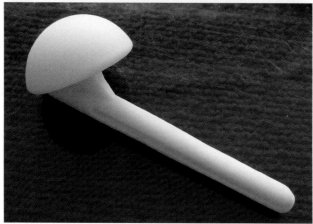

Fig. 4. Spacer-S, shoulder spacer

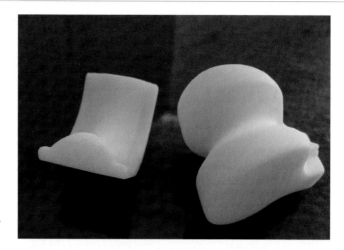

Fig. 5. Spacer-E, elbow spacer

ery of antibiotics by antibiotic beads [8], an irrigation-perfusion technique [6], or an antibiotic cement nail beads [11], and fracture union, which is usually accomplished by providing alternative fixation, mostly external fixation.

The infective problems induced by endomedullar nails have also been faced with the same principle of the local release of antibiotic bone cement-mediated. In this case the system has been designed with a different approach: for mechanical and dimensional reasons, the supporting internal structure is the nail itself onto which a cement clothing is placed. Everything is assembled in the operating theatre in a few minutes. The device (Nail Clothing) is made of industrially preformed tubular antibiotic-loaded bone cement segments (Fig. 6a): the surgeon inserts the segments onto the nail till to cover it all and with a special glue, fix them on the nail itself (Fig. 6b).

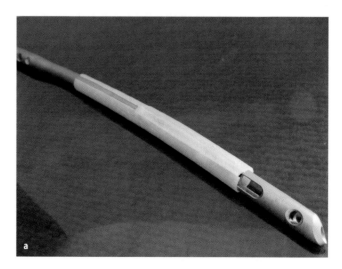

Fig. 6a. Nail clothing

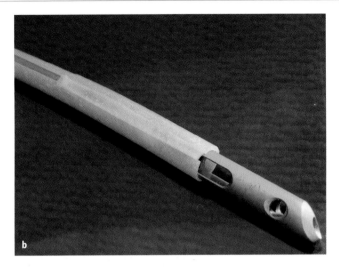

Fig. 6b. Nail clothing glued to nail

Bone Cement Elution from PMMA

The mechanism or the mechanisms of elution of antibiotic from PMMA are not so clear yet. Therefore it is more correct to speak of experimental observations which show the conditions which lead to an increase or the decrease in the release of antibiotic. Synthetically, keeping fixed solvent and temperature, the increase of the release occurs when:

- increases the concentration of the antibiotic in PMMA;
- increases the surface at the interface cement-solvent;
- increases the permeability of the cement matrix.

Permeability = porosity + chemical/physical properties (of matrix)

A reduction in the release will occur when in the opposite situation (Fig. 7).

Fig. 7. Factors influencing the release of antibiotic from a PMMA matrix

As an example, the preparation of bone cement under vacuum determines a reduction in the cement porosity and therefore a reduction in the antibiotic release [10].

In addition to the above mentioned parameters, other experimental observations show that the antibiotic (drug) molecule is able to migrate in the cement matrix even in the absence of a solvent following a diffusion behaviour (Fig. 8). The relation which better satisfies such experimental observations is the Fick's equation:

$$J = D \frac{(C1 - C2)}{X}$$

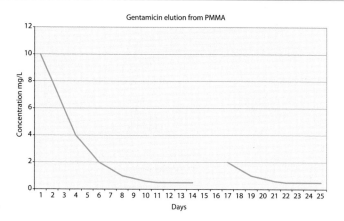

Fig. 8. Elution kinetics of an antibiotic loaded cement: after an elution period in saline, the specimen is dried and left in the open air. A second elution period is then started showing an initial release higher than expected: the migration of the antibiotic in the PMMA matrix occurs also in absence of a liquid solvent.

J is the molecular flux which is directly proportional to the diffusion coefficient (**D**), which depends from antibiotic, matrix and temperature; interface area (**A**); concentration difference (**C1 – C2**) where **C1> C2**, and inversely proportional to the distance between C1 and C2 (**X**).

If we consider to keep C and X constant, the formula becomes:

$$J = D \, A \, K$$

Therefore if we want to increase the antibiotic release it is sufficient to increase the diffusion coefficient **D** and the interface area **A**. This has been the route followed to design the new spacers.

High-release Matrix for the Spacers

In 2006 the distribution of the spacers with increased antibiotic release started. The absolute amount of antibiotic in the devices is identical, but the new spacers have an increased release capacity. The release can be as high as 4 – 5 times the release of the previous spacers. This result has been achieved in two ways: 1) the external surface, e.g. the interface area with the biological liquids, has been increased thanks to a special finishing which increases the interface area. Figure 9 shows the surfaces of Spacer-G stem before and now; 2) the bone cement matrix which includes the antibiotic is made with a new generation of polymers which are structured in a way to increase permeability.

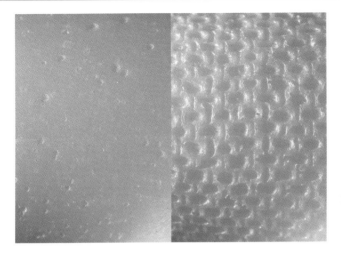

Fig. 9. Spacer-G stem: left, old version with smooth surface; right, new version with textured surface

Microscopy of the High-porosity Spacers

Before turnig into a compact and solid structure, the spacer is a powder of spheroidal particles made of a mixture of PMMA, barium sulphate and gentamicin sulphate. Only with a colorimetric method it is possible to discriminate the components. Figure 10 shows a group of spheroidal particles which constitutes the powder used to manufacture the spacers. The colourless particles are PMMA, the blue ones are gentamicin. When the liquid monomer, MMA, is added to the powder a mouldable dough is obtained which in a few minutes gets hard and solid. In the hardened mass the spheroidal particles of PMMA cannot be distinguished any more, but the gentamicin ones can. Figure 11a shows the particles of gentamicin coloured in red. Actually these spheroidal particles act as micro-reservoirs from which gentamicin flows outside the

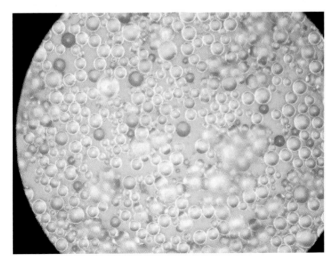

Fig. 10. Bone cement powder: PMMA pearls are colourless, gentamicin sulphate pearls are blue

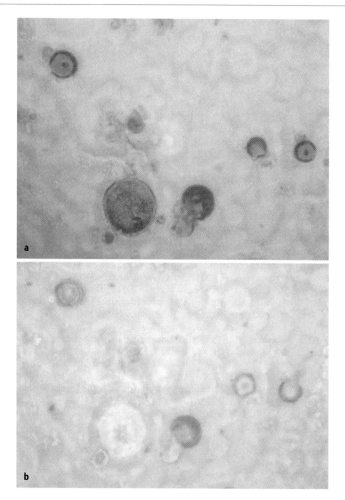

Fig. 11. Cured genta-
micin bone cement:
a reservoir with gentamicin in red; **b** empty
reservoir (after con-
tact with solvent)

cement mass. Figure 11b shows the empty micro-reservoir of gentamicin after the
contact with the solvent.

Conclusions

The constant work carried out over the years has led towards an extension of the use
of bone cement in fields hardly immaginable a few years ago. Today it is possible to
manufacture with this material medical devices with different properties which can
be modulated at pleasure. Bone cement as a drug delivery system can be designed and
specific elution kinetics can be achieved.

This aspect expands the concept of cementation and if the right synergy among
specialists of different disciplines it will be possible to strengten the surgical and therapeutical tools and increase the healing expectances of the patient.

References

1. Abendschein W (1992) Salvage of infected total hip replacement: use of antibiotic/PMMA spacer. Orthopedics 15(2):228–229
2. Affatato S, Mattarozzi A, Taddei P et al (2003) Investigations on the wear behaviour of the temporary PMMA-based hip Spacer-G. Proc Inst Mech Eng [H] 217(1):1–8
3. Baleani M, Traina F, Toni A (2003) The mechanical behaviour of a preformed hip spacer Hip International (13):159–162
4. Bertazzoni Minelli E, Benini A, Magnan B et al (2003) Release of gentamicin and vancomycin from temporary human hip spacers in two-stage revision of infected arthroplasty J Antimicrob Chemother 53(2):329–334
5. Bertazzoni Minelli E, Benini A, Magnan B et al (2005) Release of antibiotics and inhibitory activity in drainage fluids following temporary spacer implants in two-stage revision surgery Proceeedings of ECCI 2005 Florence, Italy 19–22 October 2005
6. Boda A (1979) Antibiotic irrigation-perfusion treatment for chronic osteomyelitis. Arch Orthop Trauma Surg 95(1–2):31–35
7. Cohen JC, Hozack W, Cuckler JM et al (1988) Two-stage reimplantation of septic total knee arthroplasty. Report of three cases using an antibiotic-PMMA spacer block. J Arthroplasty 3(4):369–377
8. Henry SL, Ostermann PA, Seligson D (1990) The prophylactic use of antibiotic impregnated beads in open fractures. J Trauma 30(10):1231–1238
9. Magnan B, Regis D, Biscaglia R et al (2001) Preformed acrylic bone cement spacer loaded with antibiotics: use of two-stage procedure in 10 patients because of infected hips after total replacement. Acta Orthop Scand 72(6):591–594
10. Neut D, van de Belt H, van Horn JR et al (2003) The effect of mixing on gentamicin release from polymethylmethacrylate bone cements. Acta Orthop Scand 74(6):670–676
11. Ohtsuka H, Yokoyama K, Higashi K et al (2002) Use of antibiotic-impregnated bone cement nail to treat septic nonunion after open tibial fracture. J Trauma 52(2):364–366
12. Romanò C, Meani E (2004) The use of preformed long stem antibiotic loaded cement spacers and modular non-cemented prosthesis for two-stage revisions of infected hip prosthesis Proceedings of the AAOS 2004 San Francisco (USA)
13. Wilde AH, Ruth JT (1988) Two-stage reimplantation in infected total knee arthroplasty. Clin Orthop Relat Res (236):23–35
14. Zilkens KW, Casser HR, Ohnsorge J (1990) Treatment of an old infection in a total hip replacement with an interim spacer prosthesis. Arch Orthop Trauma Surg 109(2):94–96.

Fatigue and Wear Characterization of the Preformed Hip Spacer

M. Baleani[1], S. Affatato [1], F. Traina[1,2], A. Toni[1,2]

[1] Medical Technology Laboratory, Rizzoli Orthopaedic Institutes, Bologna, Italy
[2] 1st Division of Orthopaedic-Traumatologic Surgery, Rizzoli Orthopaedic Institutes, Bologna, Italy

Introduction

The management of infected total hip arthroplasties is a complex issue. Depending on patient characteristics, infecting organisms and personal opinion of the surgeon, treatment options include antibiotic therapy, debridement of surrounding tissues, complete removal of the implant, irrigation and re-implantation of a new prosthesis [4, 5, 8 – 10, 16, 18].

The re-implantation of the prosthesis may be performed during a second surgical session – a procedure called two-stage revision. The two-stage revision involves the removal of the infected prosthesis and usually the implantation of a temporary hip spacer made of antibiotic loaded polymethylmethacrylate (PMMA) [11, 12]. Once the antibiotic therapy is completed and diagnostic analyses indicate the eradication of the infection, the spacer is removed and a new prosthesis is implanted.

The temporary hip spacer should assure local delivery of antibiotics as well as the preservation of the anatomical configuration of the hip joint [6, 21]. If the hip spacer can also act as a temporary implant, prolonged immobilisation of the patient can be avoided, reducing morbidity especially in elderly. However, in these cases the hip spacer must withstand wear and resist loads generated during the daily activities of the patient.

This study investigated the wear and the mechanical behaviour of a preformed hip spacer made of antibiotic loaded polymethylmethacrylate (PMMA).

Materials and Methods

A commercially available preformed hip spacer (Spacer-G – Tecres S.p.A., Verona, Italy) was studied in the present work. Currently, no standardised procedures are available to investigate the wear or the mechanical behaviour of preformed hip spacers. Therefore, two different test protocols were designed to investigate the fatigue strength of the entire device and the wear of the head of the device.

Fatigue Testing

Fatigue testing aims to assess the behaviour of a device under cyclic loads. Generally, severe loading conditions are selected for these tests to evaluate the safety of the device. For this reason in this study the device was considered a provisional hemiarthroplasty for the draft of a fatigue testing protocol for hip spacers. This assumption implies that the patient has no limitation in daily activities in the period between the two surgical sessions. It has been demonstrated that about one million load cycles is the load history that a hip prosthetic stem undergoes yearly *in vivo* [15]. Assuming the duration of an in-vivo service of six months [14] the loading history of the hip spacer could be roughly estimated as 0.5 million cycles.

On the basis of this rationale, the fatigue testing was performed following the recommendations of the international standard for assessment of fatigue strength of hip stem (ISO 7206/4). The hip spacer was fixed distally at 80 mm from the head centre at 9° in flexion and 10° in adduction (Fig. 1). A compressive sinusoidal load (300 – 2300 N) was applied at a frequency of 4Hz to the head of the spacer until failure of the stem or up to 0.5 million cycles. The test was performed in saline solution at 37 °C. Three test repetitions were performed on spacers with the largest head size (60 mm).

Wear Testing

Wear testing investigates the wear process of a joint in simulated working conditions. Since the hip spacer was assumed to be a temporary hemi-arthroplasty, the wear tests were carried out in a hip joint simulator (Shore Western manufacturing, Monrovia, CA, U.S.A.). In this simulator the joints were assembled in a non-anatomical position (upside-down) with the cup mounted with an inclination of 23° from the horizontal plane (Fig. 2). A vertical sinusoidal load was applied at a frequency of 1 Hz to the joint while a relative angular motion occured simulating patient walking. The load value was adjusted to simulate partial or full bearing conditions. To compensate the unfavourable effects of the third-body wear due to the non-anatomical position, the lubricant was changed washing and cleaning also the specimen at regular intervals.

To investigate the wear behaviour of the spacer, the head was coupled to the acetabulum of human cadaver pelvis. The hemi-pelves was cut to allow the fixation into

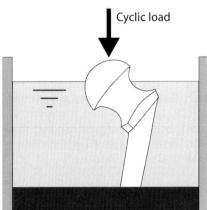

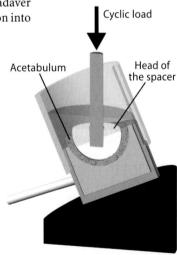

Fig. 1. Fatigue testing set-up according to the recommendations of the ISO 7206/4 standard.

Fig. 2. Wear testing set-up showing the non-anatomical position (upside-down) of the articular joint.

the test chambers, obtained using acrylic resin. Before testing the acetabula were immersed in a 4 % formalin solution for two weeks and then reamed hemispherically, leaving the subchondral bone. The size of the spacer head was selected to fit correctly the articular surface of the pelvis. The wear tests continued for 0.2 million cycles. A maximum load of about 1.0 kN, simulating partial weight bearing, was applied during the first 0.1 million cycles. Then the peak load was raised to 2.0 kN simulating unconstrained walking condition [2, 3]. This load history was selected to simulate the rehabilitative phase in which the surgeon allow partial wear bearing during the first half of the period between the two surgical sessions. The joint surfaces were lubricated during the test with a lubricant similar to the synovial fluid (30 % sterile bovine calf serum, 70 % deionised water plus sodium azide). The articular surfaces were removed from the simulator at 0.1 million cycles, cleaned and controlled for fracture before restarting the test with fresh lubricant solution. The lubricant was collected for debris analysis. Five test repetitions were performed on spacers with a head size ranging from 46 mm to 54 mm.

Wear debris found in the lubricant was isolated from the fluid. A previously validated procedure [1] allowed the separation of the bone debris from the PMMA debris. The collected material was analysed microscopically. Finally, the head of the spacer underwent microscopical analysis (Scanning Electron Microscope, Cambridge Stereoscan 200, UK) to investigate the morphology of the worn surface.

Results

Fatigue testing

Two spacers failed during the fatigue test at 0.40 and 0.45 million cycles, respectively. The third spacer completed the test. In the failed spacers, the fracture propagated from the anterior-lateral side to the internal metallic rod (Fig. 3).

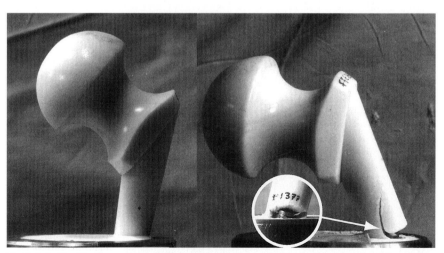

Fig. 3. *Left:* The hip spacer that completed the fatigue test. *Right:* A hip spacer that failed during the fatigue test. The enlargement shows the lateral side of the fractured stem.

Wear testing

Two out of five wear tests were stopped at 0.1 million cycles due to acetabulum fracture (Fig. 4). The remaining three joints completed the test. Unfortunately, in one of these three joints the head of the spacer was fractured by the loading device due to fixation failure. Since the coupling surface was partially damaged as well, this specimen was also discarded from the analyses.

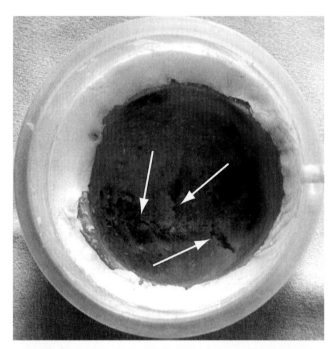

Fig. 4. An acetabulum fractured during the wear test. The white arrows indicate the fracture on the articular surface.

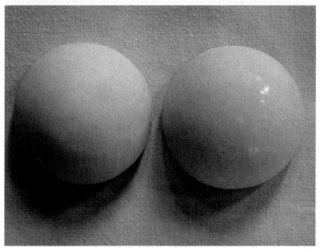

Fig. 5. *Left:* The head of the untested spacer. *Right:* The head of the spacer which completed the wear test. This head appeared smoother than the untested one due to polishing of the matching surface caused by abrasive wear.

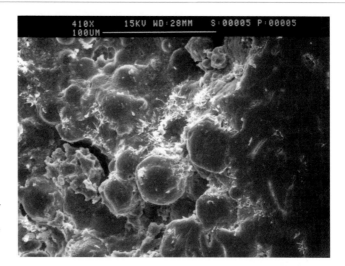

Fig. 6. On the left a surface cavity containing wear debris. On the right the morphology of the worn surface is visible.

The two remaining spacer heads, which completed the test, showed polished zones that could not be found on the untested surfaces (Fig. 5). At high magnification these zones appeared smooth while wear debris was found in the surrounding pores (Fig. 6). This debris, consisting of both PMMA and bone tissue, was also found in the lubricant.

Discussion

In this study the hip spacer was considered a temporary hip hemi-prosthesis which may undergo full physiological loads – the worst working condition which can be supposed for this device – therefore neglecting problems such as spacer stability, risk of dislocation or bone fracture [7, 14]. The experimental procedures developed to investigate the fatigue and wear behaviour of the spacer were designed based on this rationale.

The loading history, applied in the fatigue testing, implies that: 1) the period between the two surgical sessions is six months; 2) the patient is active during the entire period; 3) the patient is allowed to place load upon the operated hip without restrictions. The hip spacer showed finite fatigue strength under the above described conditions. However, this loading history is hardly experienced by the hip spacer *in vivo*. Additionally, in clinical practise only partial load bearing is allowed to the patient between the two surgical sessions if the spacer is stable [7, 14]. Since decreasing the load level increases the fatigue life of a device, the mechanical failure of the spacer stem seems unlikely, taking into account the above mentioned recommendation.

The wear test was designed in an attempt to replicate a probable loading history. The following assumptions distinguished this loading history form the previous one: 2') the patient is partially active between the two surgical sessions; 3') the patient is allowed to load partially the operated hip. Only during the last phase of in vivo service the spacer undergoes full load. Abrasive wear of the spacer head occurred under this condition. It was roughly estimated that the coupling releases about half a gram of PMMA debris in one million cycles. Although this phenomenon did not affect the functionality of the articular surface, the estimated wear rate was at least one order of magnitude greater than that measured for hip prosthesis with the acetabular cup made of polyethylene (UHMWPE) [13, 17].

PMMA debris has been recognized to promote tissue reactions and finally osteolysis, in a similar way that UHMWPE debris do [19, 20]. However, the short duration of the *in vivo* service of the spacer and the lavage of the periprosthetic tissue – or even better the reaming of the bone cavities – should reduce the biological effect of the PMMA debris. Conversely, damage of the acetabulum by the spacer head is a reason for concern. Although this phenomenon may be affected by the mechanical behaviour of the chemically fixed bone tissue, the risk of progressive damage of the acetabulum and, in the worst scenario, the protusion of the spacer head through the acetabulum can not be ignored when full weight bearing is allowed. Therefore the recommendation of partial weight bearing between the two surgical sessions is a precaution to avoid the risk of wear of the acetabulum and/or bone fracture more than the risk for damage of the hip spacer.

Conclusions

The spacer showed finite fatigue strength under the above-described loading conditions but failure was achieved only at the end of a severe loading history, hardly experienced by the spacer in vivo. Additionally, at the end of the wear test the head of the spacer appeared slightly polished on the matching areas due to abrasive wear but fracture of the acetabulum occurred in two out five couplings. Although these outcomes may be affected by the mechanical behaviour of the chemically fixed bone tissue, damage on the acetabulum caused by the spacer head is a reason for concern. However, since decreasing the load level leads to an increase in the fatigue life and a decrease in the wear rate – and the risks of acetabulum fracture are also reduced – the surgeons can safely implant the spacer if the patient is constrained to a reduced activity and partial weight bearing, as in existing standard clinical practice.

Acknowledgements

This study was funded by Tecres S.p.A. The authors thank Luigi Lena for the illustrations, Cecilia Persson and Paolo Erani for their help in drafting the manuscript.

References

1. Affatato S, Fernandes B, Tucci A et al (2001) Isolation and morphological characterisation of UHMWPE wear debris generated in vitro. Biomaterials 22(17):2325–2331
2. Bergmann G, Graichen F, Rohlmann A (1993) Hip joint loading during walking and running, measured in two patients. J Biomech 26(8):969–990
3. Bergmann G, Deuretzbacher G, Heller M et al (2001) Hip contact forces and gait patterns from routine activities. J Biomech 34(7):859–871

4. Bittar ES, Petty W (1982) Girdlestone arthroplasty for infected total hip arthroplasty. Clin Orthop Relat Res (170):83–87

5. Buchholz HW, Elson RA, Engelbrecht E et al (1981) Management of deep infection of total hip replacement. J Bone Joint Surg (Br) 63(3):342–353

6. Duncan CP, Beauchamp C (1993) A temporary antibiotic-loaded joint replacement system for management of complex infections involving the hip. Orthop Clin North Am 24(4): 751–759

7. Durbhakula SM, Czajka J, Fuchs MD et al (2004) Spacer endoprosthesis for the treatment of infected total hip arthroplasty. J Arthroplasty 19(6):760–767

8. Fehring TK, Calton TF, Griffin WL (1999) Cementless fixation in 2-stage reimplantation for periprosthetic sepsis. J Arthroplasty 14(2):175–181

9. Hanssen AD, Spangehl MJ (2004) Treatment of the infected hip replacement. Clin Orthop Relat Res (420):63–71

10. Hofmann AA, Goldberg TD, Tanner AM et al (2005) Ten-year experience using an articulating antibiotic cement hip spacer for the treatment of chronically infected total hip. J Arthroplasty 20(7):874–879

11. Hsieh PH, Shih CH, Chang YH et al (2004) Two-stage revision hip arthroplasty for infection: comparison between the interim use of antibiotic-loaded cement beads and a spacer prosthesis. J Bone Joint Surg (Am) 86(9):1989–1997

12. Ivarsson I, Wahlstrom O, Djerf K et al (1994) Revision of infected hip replacement. Two-stage procedure with a temporary gentamicin spacer. Acta Orthop Scand 65(1):7–8

13. Liao YS, McKellop H, Lu Z et al (2003) The effect of frictional heating and forced cooling on the serum lubricant and wear of UHMW polyethylene cups against cobalt-chromium and zirconia balls. Biomaterials 24(18):3047–3059

14. Magnan B, Regis D, Biscaglia R et al (2001) Preformed acrylic bone cement spacer loaded with antibiotics: use of two-stage procedure in 10 patients because of infected hips after total replacement. Acta Orthop Scand 72(6):591–594

15. Morlock M, Schneider E, Bluhm A et al (2001) Duration and frequency of every day activities in total hip patients. J Biomech 34(7):873–881

16. Nestor BJ, Hanssen AD, Ferrer_Gonzalez R et al (1994) The use of porous prostheses in delayed reconstruction of total hip replacements that have failed because of infection. J Bone Joint Surg (Am) 76(3):349–359

17. Saikko V, Ahlroos T, Calonius O et al (2001) Wear simulation of total hip prostheses with polyethylene against CoCr, alumina and diamond-like carbon. Biomaterials 22(12):1507–1514

18. Salvati EA, Gonzalez Della Valle A, Masri BA et al (2003) The infected total hip arthroplasty. Instr Course Lect (52):223–245. Review

19. Schmalzried TP, Jasty M, Harris WH (1992) Periprosthetic bone loss in total hip arthroplasty. Polyethylene wear debris and the concept of the effective joint space. J Bone Joint Surg (Am) 74(6):849–863

20. Shardlow DL, Stone MH, Ingham E et al (2003) Cement particles containing radio-opacifiers stimulate pro-osteolytic cytokine production from a human monocytic cell line. J Bone Joint Surg (Br) 85(6):900–905

21. Yamamoto K, Miyagawa N, Masaoka T et al (2003) Clinical effectiveness of antibiotic-impregnated cement spacers for the treatment of infected implants of the hip joint. J Orthop Sci 8(6):823–828

14 Fatigue Characterisation of the Preformed Knee Spacer

T. Villa, D. Carnelli, R. Pietrabissa

Laboratory of Biological Structure Mechanics, Department of Structural Engineering, Politecnico of Milan, Italy

Introduction

Infection is one of the most severe complications that can arise after the implant of a knee prosthesis [2, 7]. Late infections are usually treated by removing the infected prosthesis and reimplanting a new one, following either the one or two stages technique: in order to avoid persistent and recurrent infections that have been reported when using the one-stage technique [8, 10] the two-stage technique has been introduced, consisting in the removal of the infected prosthesis in a first operation stage and in the reimplantation of a new one after adequate treatment of the infection in a second stage, usually performed six to twelve weeks after the first procedure [7, 10, 12, 14].

In the interim period the usage of a knee spacer is suggested in order to avoid patient immobilization and soft tissues contracture with consequent shortening of the operated leg and difficulty of reimplantation [11, 12]. In cases of knee spacers made of antibiotic addicted bone cement, a locally focused therapy to prevent colonization [9] is achieved.

The knee spacer can be static or mobile, the difference laying in the possibility of knee flexion during the interim period: static spacers have shown difficulties in the exposure at the time of reimplantation due to quadriceps shortening and soft tissues adherences, a poor range of motion postoperatively, instability and bone erosion [4]: these drawbacks moved the surgeons to the usage of mobile articulating spacers that have improved reimplantation and a better range of mobility of the knee after the second operation stage [5, 10, 13].

Considering that six to twelve weeks must pass between the two operating stages and that the patient is often allowed to bear weight in order to prevent soft tissue contracture, the assessment of the mechanical performances of mobile knee spacers made of polymethyl methacrylate (PMMA) bone cement is a key issue to evaluate their reliability before the clinical use.

In particular the loads that act on the spacer come from the walking activity of the patient that can be defined as a cyclic activity, requiring a repetition of a high number of cycles of load. The fatigue performances of the device must be investigated in order to prevent failures during the clinical usage.

In this work the fatigue performances of Tecres Spacer-K knee spacer were investigated through two types of tests: (i) resistance tests on the whole device (condyles + tibial plate) run on a four degree of freedom knee simulator basically following the prescription of ISO 14243 standard; *(ii)* fatigue tests on the tibial tray run according to ASTM F 1800 – 04 standard.

Materials and Methods

The knee spacer that has been subjected to tests (Fig. 1) is made of a tibial component consisting in a flat base upon which a femoral component articulates, thus permitting the flexion of the knee. Both the components of the device are made of PMMA containing 2.5 % w/w gentamicin and are fixed to the bone using antibiotic addicted bone cement. The spacer is made in three different sizes (small-S, medium-M and large-L) and is manufactured by Tecres S.p.a., Sommacampagna (VR), Italy with the commercial name of Spacer-K.

All the tests have been performed at the Laboratory of Biological Structure Mechanics of the Politecnico di Milano, Milan, Italy.

Cyclic Tests on the Whole Spacer

Cyclic tests consisted in applying to the knee spacer 500,000 loading cycles in order to assess its mechanical resistance during a period of time corresponding to a six month walking activity, which could be the period of implant of the spacer.

The tests were carried out on three spacers of different size (small-S, medium-M and large-L) and were performed on a four degrees of freedom MTS knee simulator (MTS Systems, Minneapolis, MN, USA) (Fig. 2) mounted on a MTS Bionix 25kN-250Nm axial-torsional testing machine. The knee simulator allows to impose simultaneously with the axial force three kinematic conditions, namely the flexion-extension and the internal-external rotation of the femoral condyles and the antero-posterior (A-P) shear of the tibial plate: the axial force simulates the action of the bodyweight during walking on the knee while the three kinematic conditions are the basic components in which the multidirectional movement of the knee during the gait cycle can be divided.

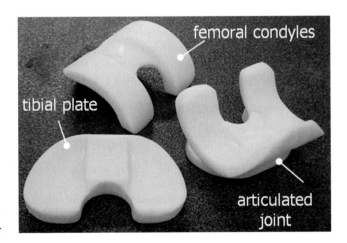

Fig. 1. Components of the Tecres knee spacer

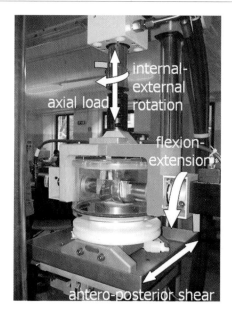

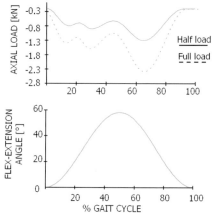

Fig. 3. Load waveform applied to the spacer (*upper*), flexion-extension angle waveform (*lower*)

◁

Fig. 2. The MTS knee simulator

The patterns and ranges of the axial force and of the flexion-extension conditions are reported in Figure 3: the internal-external rotation has been set to a fixed value because the knee spacer does not allow any rotation about the vertical axis while the lower sliding block has been left free to move in order to adapt its movement to the one imposed by the femoral condyles during flexion-extension. The maximum value of the imposed load was set to 1300 N, half of the load that normally acts during walking, considering that the patient, during the rehabilitation period that follows the implant of the spacer, should walk with the aid of crutches, thus reducing the total amount of the load that acts on the knee. In order to asses the mechanical reliability of the device even in case the patient should not follow the prescription of using crutches, three more tests have been performed on the S-size device imposing a vertical load equal to 2600 N corresponding to the full bearing condition. In both the conditions, the test frequency was set to 0.5 Hz.

In order to mimic the in vivo environmental conditions of the tissues that surround the spacer, on the MTS knee simulator the device was located into a sealed chamber and kept constantly lubricated by means of a mixture of water and 25 % bovine serum at the temperature of 37°C. This mixture is recognized as having lubricating properties similar to those of sinovial fluid [3].

Fatigue Tests on the Tibial Tray

The test goal was determining the fatigue behavior of the tibial plate of the spacer, basically following the prescription of ASTM F 1800 – 97 standard: this set-up suggests to place the specimen on the testing machine in the configuration of a cantilever beam by cementing it to the lower grip and fixing to its centerline through a clamp as illustrated in Figure 4.

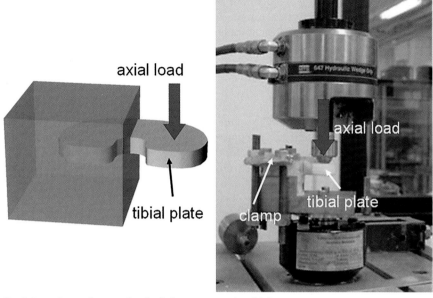

Fig. 4. Experimental set-up for the fatigue tests on the tibial tray

Table 1. Fatigue tests parameters

Minimum load [N]	Maximum load [N]	Frequency [Hz]
60	600	2.5
50	500	3
40	400	4
32.5	325	4.5

In order to determine which of the three sizes of the spacer could be the weakest, previously to the fatigue tests, three static tests were performed on a plate of the S- size, on a plate of the M-size and on a plate of the L-size under displacement control at the speed of 2 mm/min until break was detected.

In the fatigue tests a sinusoidally variable load was applied with maximum and minimum values corresponding to those reported in Table 1; tests were performed until either break was detected or 500,000 cycles were run, accordingly to the expected time of use of the spacer (test frequency is reported in Table 1 as well).

Tests have been repeated on three samples of the tibial tray for each load value.

Results

Cyclic Tests on the Whole Spacer

As concerns the mechanical resistance of the whole spacer, this has been assessed by the fact that no failure was recorded for any spacer at the end of the loading sessions: half of the normal load acting on the knee during walking has been applied on the spacer, due to the fact that the patient is supposed to walk in the interim period with the aid of crutches, and the frequency of testing was half the normal one, too, considering that the same patient should walk slower than a normal person does. Even the eventuality of a patient that does not follow medical prescription of using crutches has been investigated by doubling the applied load with the good result of absence of failure in this case too.

Fatigue Tests on the Tibial Tray

As regards the tests on the reliability of the tibial plate of the spacer, results of the preliminary static tests are reported in Figure 5: the plate of S-size spacer, as expectable, has turned out to be the weakest and, for this reason, the fatigue tests have been performed on plates of that size. Results from fatigue tests (Wöhler curve) are reported in Figure 6: such a curve reports on the x-axis the number of cycles reached for each tested spacer and on the y-axis the maximum load at which the spacer has been tested. The plot reports also the 95 % and 99 % confidence bands, that represent, in case one hundred specimens should be tested, the interval containing 95 and 99 failure points, respectively. The arrow rising from the three coinciding points at 325 N load level means that the tests have been stopped after 500,000 cycles, in accordance to the expected lifetime of the device.

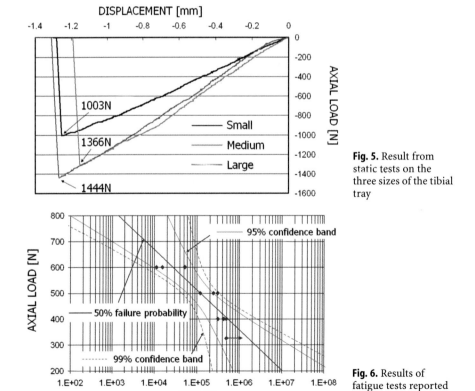

Fig. 5. Result from static tests on the three sizes of the tibial tray

Fig. 6. Results of fatigue tests reported in the Wöhler curve

Discussion

At the time the infection arises, the surgeon must face three main problems, here reported in chronological sequence: *i)* the infection must be defeated as soon as possible and without risk of recurrences together with an immediate relief of pain; *ii)* in the interim period before the new prosthesis is implanted, the patient should live as much as possible a "normal" life, in terms of possibility of movements and deambulation; *iii)* the reimplantation of the new prosthesis must be facilitated, trying to avoid any factor that may cause bone loss or difficulties in exposure at surgical time.

The three above described requirements stimulated the surgeons to move from the use of static spacers to mobile spacers, in particular after assessing the reliability of the latter as regards the efficacy of the infection treatment [5, 6].But the great advantages that may come from the use of a mobile spacer must be searched in the possibility of movement for the patient in the interim period, resulting in an increase of the range of motion (ROM) of the knee after the second implant [5, 10, 13] , in a lower incidence on bone loss due to resorption [6] and in an easier operating act at the time of reimplantation [10].

Different mobile spacers have been proposed with different materials for the articulating components, either antibiotic addicted PMMA on PMMA or metal on Polyethylene (PE): metal on PE implants do not have the ability of antibiotic release and may increase the risk of reinfection due to the presence of additional surface area for bacteria to adhere; on the other hand, the proposed PMMA on PMMA mobile spacers have been manufactured by means of intraoperatively moulds, that means a non-controlled manufacturing procedure with the risk of unknown mechanical resistance properties.

Some authors have implicitly asked the knowledge of these properties. For example, Fehring et al.[6], who found little differences in ROM between static and mobile spacers, lamented that the conservative formal physical therapy in the interim period may have influenced this poor result and suggested that a more aggressive rehabilitation should improve the mobility of the knee. On the other hand, the increase of such rehabilitation facility could be responsible for any mechanical failure of the implanted device and so the *in vitro* evaluation of the mechanical performances of the mobile spacer turns out to be a key issue to assess its suitability in a pre-clinical phase: the six month period of permanence inside the knee of the patient can easily be considered long enough to assign the spacer the name of "prosthesis" with the consequent need of a complete experimental procedure that takes into account the problems that can arise in the long run, particularly related to fatigue.

This study has been made possible thanks to the fact that the spacers were industrially manufactured, with a controlled manufacturing procedure, thus allowing to have specimens whose characteristics do no depend (differently from those proposed in literature) on the particular parameters under which they have been obtained: quantity of antibiotic in the PMMA mass, temperature and humidity of the environment in which they have been moulded (operating theatre), moulding technique. In particular, having a controlled percentage of antibiotics is an advantage both for the infection healing capacity of the spacer and for its mechanical resistance performances, that are strongly influenced by this factor.

In order to assess the mechanical reliablity in time of the device both cyclic tests on the whole spacer and fatigue tests on the tibial tray have been performed and some considerations can be drawn when evaluating the above reported results. In the cyclic tests on the whole spacer, the choice of using over-loading factors (very high load, great number of cycles, wide range of motion) are a commonly used procedure in the designing phase of an experimental set-up used to assess the mechanical reliability of an endoprosthesis. In fact, the biological response of the host tissue to the insertion of the device and the complexity of the anatomy and physiology of the prosthetic joint are two factors that are definitely very difficult to simulate in *in vitro* tests: our experimental set-up, for example, is able to take into account, as a biological factor, only the lubricating mixing composition and its temperature that are similar to those found *in vivo* in the prosthetic knee. As a consequence, in order to give consistence to the results coming from the tests, a sort of "safety factor" is introduced by applying mechanical conditions that are surely much more severe than the one the device will be *in vivo* subjected to (in our case we increased the magnitude of the mechanical input parameters such as load, number of cycles, flexion-extension ROM).

Also in the case of the fatigue tests on the tibial tray, the same consideration above expressed on the testing experimental conditions that are applied to the device can be valid and some factors must be taken into account when examining the results. The loading configuration proposed by ASTM F 1800–04 is defined in literature as an exaggeration of reality as it prescribes to load the tibial tray as if either in the medial or in the lateral side the bone support should completely lacks: this condition is far from reality where a resorption of the tibial bone as well as the formation of fibrous tissue between the bone and cement may cause inadequate support to the tray, but the complete absence of one tibial emi-plate has never been observed. Therefore, the load that is applied to the spacer cannot surely be the physiological one (about 2000 N), that would produce failure of the tibial plate due to the particular prescribed testing configuration: the choice of the right load to apply has been discussed in literature [1] with the final suggestion of a 500 N vertical load repeated for five million cycles (corresponding to five year waking of the patient) as the preferred loading condition to assess the fatigue reliability of the tibial tray of a total knee arthroplasty (TKA): considering that the patient bearing a knee spacer has an activity level well below the one of a patient bearing TKA, the value of the vertical load of 325 N assessed for a life of 500,000 cycles could be high enough to ensure the fatigue reliability of the knee spacer tibial tray.

As a conclusion of this study, even if the tested spacer can be defined as a "temporary" device, the authors' consideration is that, in the pre-clinical phase, the experimental procedure that is run in order to assess its biomechanical reliability must be as much complete as possible and very close to the one that is usually applied to a "permanent" device: in this light, the spacers that have been tested have shown a good behaviour, with a consequent high enough degree of suitability for the clinical use.

References

1. Ahir SP, Blunn GW, Haider H et al. (1999) Evaluation of a testing method for the fatigue performance of total knee tibial trays. J Biomech 32(10):1049–1057
2. Bengston S, Knutson K, Lidgren L (1989) Treatment of infected knee arthroplasty. Clin Orthop Relat Res (245):173–178
3. Bigsby RJ, Hardaker CS, Fisher J (1997) Wear of ultra-high molecular weight polyethylene ace-

tabular cups in a physiological hip joint simulator in the anatomical position using bovine serum as a lubricant. Proc Inst Mech Eng [H] 211(3):265–269

4. Calton TF, Fehring TK, Griffin WL (1997) Bone loss associated with the use of spacer blocks in infected total knee arthroplasty. Clin Orthop Relat Res (345):148–154

5. Emerson RH, Muncie M, Tarbox TR et al (2002) Comparison of a static with a mobile spacer in total knee infection. Clin Orthop Relat Res (404):132–138

6. Fehring TK, Odum S, Calton TF et al (2000) Articulating versus static spacers in revision total knee arthroplasty for sepsis. Clin Orthop Relat Res (380):9–16

7. Goldman RT, Scuderi GR, Insall JN (1996) 2-stage reimplantation for infected total knee replacement. Clin Orthop Relat Res (331):118–124

8. Hanssen AD, Trousdale RT, Osmon DR (1995) Patient outcome with reinfection following reimplantation for the infected total knee arthroplasty. Clin Orthop Relat Res (321):55–67

9. Henry SL, Seligson D, Mangino P et al (1991) Antibiotic-impregnated beads. Part I: Bead implantation versus systemic therapy. Orthop Rev 20(3):242–247

10. Hofmann AA, Kane KR, Tkach TK et al (1995) Treatment of infected total knee arthroplasty using an articulating spacer. Clin Orthop Relat Res (321):45–54

11. Insall JN (1996) Infection of total knee arthroplasty. Instr Course Lect (35):319–324

12. Insall JN, Thompson FM, Brause BD (1983) Two-stage reimplantation for the salvage of infected total knee arthroplasty. J Bone Joint Surg (Am) 65(8):1087–1098

13. Siebel T, Kelm J, Porsch M et al. (2002) Two-stage exchange of infected knee arthroplasty with an prosthesis-like interim cement spacer. Acta Orthop Belg 68(2):150–156

14. Wilde AH, Ruth JT (1988) Two-stage reimplantation in infected total knee arthroplasty. Clin Orthop Relat Res (236):23–35

Surface Analysis of the Spacer Before and After the Clinical Use

A. Cigada, M.F. Brunella

Department of Applied Phisical Chemistry, Politecnico of Milan, Italy

Introduction

Various studies have been conducted on the preparation of hip and knee spacers for the local treatment of infections in terms of choosing the right antibiotic and dose and designing the components. [2, 3, 7]. In fact, in addition to releasing the drug to treat the infection, the spacer's goal is to enable joint movement [8] and to support a partial load without further bone loss. The advantage of the two-stage technique is that the patient is not obliged to stay in bed for the period in which the infection is being treated and the shortening of his extremity is preserved [5]. The efficacy of the two-stage treatment using the spacer has given positive results in more than 90 % of cases [3, 4] with an average follow-up of 36 months. In some cases the stems broke [6], Failure has not been directly related to the use of the spacer except in a small number of fatigue failure of the stem [2]. Even the process of wearing, tested *in vitro* with acetabular corpse cups, seem to indicate the hip spacer's improved performance with a limited release of wear particles [1].

In general, the spacer is a preformed device, covered in bone cement loaded with antibiotic. There are examples, as in the spacer shown in Fig. 1, in which the antibiotic

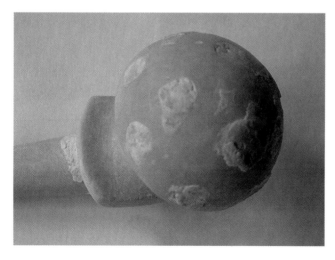

Fig. 1. Hip spacer with antibiotic insertions

was added by the surgeon directly before the implant by inserting it in the preformed spacer. For a better distribution of the drug the loading should take place before the cement's polymerization. For the hip joint, the device is composed of the femoral stem and head which can be obtained from a mould (Spacer-G – Tecres Spa, Italy) and a hollow stainless steel cylindrical rod is inserted in the stem.

The design of the knee spacer is similar to a normal prostheses but the material modified as an antibiotic-loaded acrylic cement. The tibial component is composed of a flat base and the femoral component matching automatically. This enables repeated rotation movements between the distal femur and the proximal tibia during flexion and extension. Both components are secured to the bone with bone cement. Acrylic cement is prone to wearing and degradation and therefore will require a second stage revision when the infection has been controlled [2].

The aim of this paper is to evaluate the wear characteristics of acrylic cement in spacers. They were evaluated at different stages after cycling and the breakdown of areas in contact were recorded.

Experimental

Two hip Spacer-G and two knee Spacer-K (Tecres Spa, Italy) were analysed. The knee spacers were removed after having functioned *in vivo* for 5 and 6 months, while the two hip spacers were removed at 3 – 6 months. They were compared to new implants to evaluate wear characteristics. The composition of the acrylic cement used in Spacer-G and the Spacer-K is indicated in Table 1. The removed implants were cleaned of organic residue prior to evaluation. Initial evaluation was carried out with an optical microscope. A macroscopic survey using a stereomicroscope (WILD M8) was then utilized in areas that wear was identified. A stereoscan microscope (Cambridge Stereoscan 360) and a microanalysis with X-ray spectrometer (Oxford INCA 200) was then carried out. The surfaces' wearing conditions were evaluated through a laser section measurement (UBM microfocus) to further determine the amount of acrylic wear.

The Spacer-K was also submitted to Gel Permeation Chromatography in order to determine the degradation of the acrylic polymer.

Table 1. Chemical composition of the antibiotic cement of Spacer-G and Spacer-K

Liquid component:	
Methylmethacrylate	98.20 % w/w
N-N Dimethyl-p-Toludine	1.80 % w/w
Hydroquinone	75 ppm
Powder component:	
Polymethylmethacrylate	82 % w/w
Barium Sulphate Ph.Eur.	10 % w/w
Gentamicin Sulphate	Max: 5 % w/w*
Benzoyl Peroxide	3 % w/w

* Equivalent always to 2.5 % Gentamicin base.

Results and Discussion

Macroscopical Examination

The macroscopical examination of the new Spacer-K highlighted the fact that the surface of the two parts that compose the spacer is completely opaque. No particular finishing touches were observed. However, a certain porosity distributed over the whole surface, even at the back of the parts, with big pores of different dimensions even one-millimetre wide, were clearly observed. These are typical of acrylic cement (Figs 2a, 2b).

The surfaces of the Spacer-K, after explantation, are characterised by the existence of very shiny areas with respect to the remaining opaque surface. These areas were different both in shape and extension in the two explants. Contact areas between the flat shinbone and the thigh bone component are indicative. Therefore in these areas the wearing conditions of the material was observed. It was noticed that in the smaller spacer (5 months) the shiny part extended to almost the whole area covering the two surfaces that were in contact with the thighbone, including an area on the surface of the central part in relief. In the bigger Spacer-K, it was instead noticed that the shiny areas were located on the component sides and this was more noticeable on one side (Fig. 3).

The hip Spacer-G, used as a reference, is smaller than the two explants. But even in this case, like the previous one, it was used as a reference to compare the surface of the cement after *in vivo* functioning.

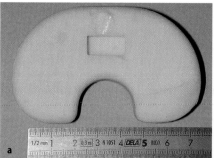 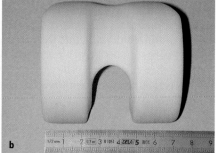

Fig. 2. Blank Spacer-K: **a** tibial component; **b** femoral component

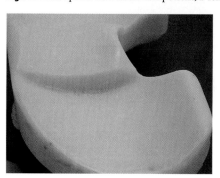

Fig. 3. Explanted Spacer-K: glossy areas on the tibial component

Similarly to the knee spacer, the surface of the new Spacer–G was totally opaque. It had macroscopic imperfections, such as open and closed pores. The latter were barely seen underneath a cement film, identified as whiter spots. The line joining the two parts of the mould could also be seen and, in particular, the head showed signs of mechanical workmanship that increased the surface's roughness. Explanted devices were distinguished for the different dimensions of the head, which was bigger in the spacer explanted after 6 months. In one of the two stems, following the breakage of the cement at the end, the metallic rod could be seen inside. Both stems showed a breakage of the cement coating in the distal area. Observing the heads enabled the identification of contact areas, which were particularly shiny with respect to the rest of the surface which, instead appeared just like the new sample of reference. The shiny areas no longer had the mechanical workmanship that was identified on the new spacer and that was still visible on the rest of the heads' surface. The shinier areas developed along a circular crown towards the side of the head (Fig. 4). These had more or less the same extension. In the bigger head, the smooth surface extended partly even over the side while in the other one it was mainly distributed on the same cap. The location with respect to the stem was also different. It was towards the upper end in the first and sideways in the second. A summary of the observations conducted during this first stage of analysis is contained in Table 2.

Microscopical Examination

The SEM observation of spacers was conducted on the less bulky parts, in order that these would be better moved inside the instrument's chamber. In particular, the heads of the Spacer-G devices were tested, after having been cut from the stem and shinbone plates of the Spacer-K devices.

The common aspect found in all new spacers, which characterises their surface, is the existence of prepolymer beads (generally in relief) and the existence of a powder compound, in the polymerized matrix, based on radiopacifying barium sulphate, as shown in the EDS spectrum obtained from an accurate analysis of the area (Fig. 5). It was not possible to highlight even an eventual presence of the Gentamicin sulphate antibiotic, since there were no discriminating elements to detect this additive with respect to the polymer and the radiopacifying agent. On the Spacer-G heads the prepolymer beads were quite noticeable on the ridges of the holes left by the mechanical workmanship (Fig. 6) and flatter on the plains. This was already highlighted by the macroscopical observation.

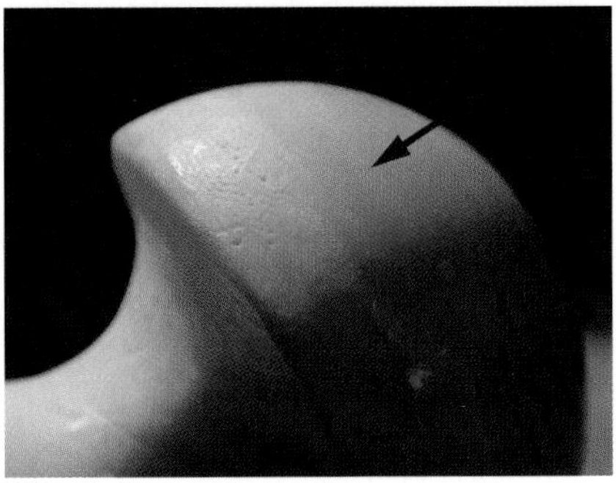

Fig. 4. Explanted Spacer-G: glossy areas on the head

Table 2. Summary of the macroscopical and microscopical examination results

	Surface	Site	Spacer type
Macro-scopical exami-nation	Opaque Presence of open and close pores Signs of mechanical finish-ing	Head Stem	Spacer-G
	Opaque Presence of pores, even in the order of mm	Femoral component Tibial component	Spacer-K
	Very smooth areas on the remaining opaque surface	Femoral component Tibial plate • Extended smooth areas in the planes of coupling with the femoral component • Limited smooth areas and localized at the borders of the components	Spacer-K 5M Spacer-K 6M
	Fracture in the acrylic cement coating	Stem in distal zone	Spacer-G 3M
	Very smooth areas respect the remaining opaque sur-face and absence of mechanical finishing signs	Head The areas develop in a circu-lar crown shifted towards the rim Extension of the smooth area beyond the head border	Spacer-G 6M Spacer-G 6M
Microscop-ical exami-nation by SEM and EDS micro-analysis	Emerging pre-polymer spheres inside a matrix mainly composed of $BaSO_4$ particles	Head Tibial component	Spacer-G Spacer-K
	Flattened pre-polymer spheres	Head, bottom of mechanical finishing grooves	Spacer-G
	As above + cracks	Opaque areas of head and tibial component	Spacer-G 3M Spacer-G 6M Spacer-K 5M Spacer-K 6M
	Polishes pre-polymer spheres. Reduction pow-dery material made of $BaSO_4$	Smooth areas in head and tibial component (more in head)	Spacer-G 3M Spacer-G 6M Spacer-K 5M Spacer-K 6M
	Several cracks	Smooth and opaque (in lesser size) areas Head and tibial plate	

Spacer-G = Spacer-G new; Spacer K = Spacer-K new; Spacer-G 3M = implanted 3 months; Spacer-G 6M = implanted 6 months; Spacer-K 5M = implanted 5 months; Spacer-K 6M = implanted 6 months

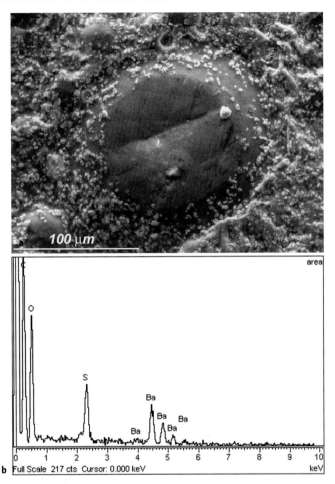

Fig. 5. a BaSO$_4$ powder in the polymerized matrix on the groove throat **b** EDS spectrum of the compound in the matrix among the spheres

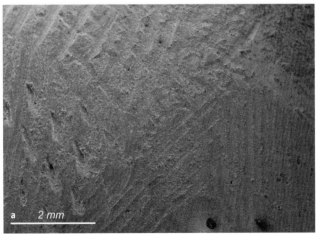

Fig. 6. SEI-BSE mix signal images of the blank Spacer-G: **a** grooves due to mechanical finishing

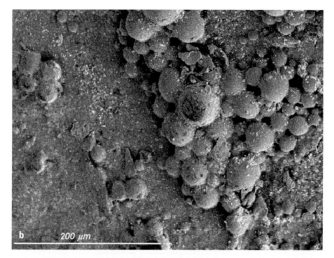

Fig. 6b. Prepolymer spheres on the groove top

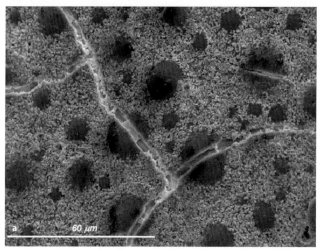

Fig. 7. Explanted Spacer-K, SEM micrographs of: **a** the smooth area

The rough areas observed on the spacers after explantation have a similar shape to the ones of reference on the new spacers, except for the existence of cracks that are particularly numerous and evident in the more worn out areas, that appear shiny under macroscopic observation. The worn out areas are characterised not only by a series of cracks but also by the smoothing out of the prepolymer beads and the absence of the powder compound between the beads which actually tends to transform into islands between the small spheres (Fig. 7). The same figure also shows how the cracks are not only distributed over the polymerized matrix, but they also cross the same prepolymer beads. The worn out surfaces of Spacer-G heads, have another peculiarity. They show a general flattening out of workmanship signs. It was also noticed that some prepolymer beads (especially those in relief on the ridges of the workmanship signs) have been moved to other areas, implanted in the matrix, with

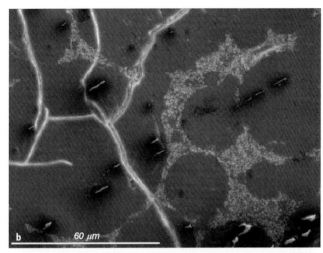

Fig. 7b. The rough area

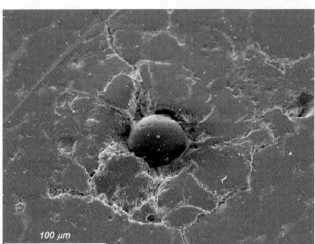

Fig. 8. Explanted
Spacer-G: SEM micro-
graph of the smooth
area with a sphere
implanted in the
matrix

clear formation of little new cracks on the sides (Fig. 8). As in previous observations, the most significant results are indicated in Table 2.

Roughness Measurements

Roughness measurements carried out on spacers have given results expressed in average roughness Ra, assessed according to regulation DIN4768, indicated in Table 3 and in Figures 9 to 11. The average roughness of non implanted spacers has been indicated as a reference. Average roughness values measured in opaque areas are very close to the non implanted spacers, which in any case show a different surface finish between the Spacer-G (R_a = 3.37 µm) and the Spacer-K. The surface roughness of the latter is actually considerably lower, both on the femoral component (R_a = 0.97 µm)

Spacer	Average roughness R_a (μm)	
	Rough areas	Smooth areas
New Spacer-K (Fem Comp)	0.97	–
New Spacer-K (Tib Comp)	1.25	–
Spacer-K 5M (Fem Comp)	1.52	0.35
Spacer-K 5M (Tib Comp)	1.52	0.24
Spacer-K 6M (Fem Comp)	1.31	0.69
Spacer-K 6M (Tib Comp)	1.31	0.66
New Spacer-G	3.37	–
Spacer-G 3M	3.55	0.21
Spacer-G 6M	3.45	0.48

Table 3. Average roughness R_a of the spacer's surface

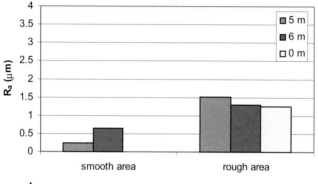

Fig. 9. Average roughness R_a of the smooth and rough areas of the Spacer-K tibial component. For comparison the average roughness of the blank spacer surface is reported

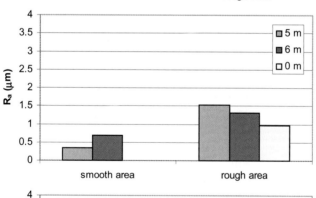

Fig. 10. Average roughness R_a of the smooth and rough areas of the Spacer-K femoral component. For comparison the average roughness of the blank spacer surface is reported

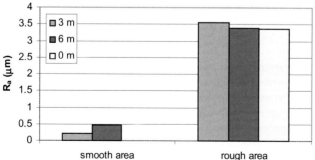

Fig. 11. Average roughness R_a of the smooth and rough areas of the Spacer-G head. For comparison the average roughness of the blank spacer surface is reported

Table 4. Molecular weights of the material of the new Spacer-K and after 6 months of implantation

Spacer-K	Mw	Mn	DPM
New	35,6890	66,318	5.381
Implanted for 6 M	23,5856	41,992	5.616

and on the tibial one (R_a = 1.25 µm). It can be noted that the shiny areas found are actually less rough than the opaque ones. This difference is even more noticeable in the Spacer-G rather than the Spacer-K. The former varies between a maximum roughness of over 3 µm to a minimum of less than 0.5 µm, while the latter has a difference of barely 1 µm. Even if there have been difficulties in evaluating the roughness of the femoral component of Spacer-K devices, there is no substantial difference between the wearing of the shinbone plate and the thighbone component. The differences between roughness values measured on glossy areas and rough ones for the explanted devices are 3.34 µm and 2.97 µm for Spacer-G respectively after 3 and 6 months of *in vivo* functioning. The analogous differences are 1.28 µm and 0.65 µm for Spacer-K tibial component respectively after 5 and 6 months of *in vivo* functioning.

Molecular Weight

In order to obtain an average evaluation of the cement's deterioration conditions, the molecular weights of the new Spacer-K cement was compared to the one of the Spacer-K cement explanted after 6 months.

The values obtained were indicated in Table 4. The $\overline{M_w}$ (weight-average molecular weight) decreased from 356,890 to 235,856 and the $\overline{M_n}$ (number-average molecular weight) from 66,318 g/mol to 41,992. The polydispersity index (DPM) increased from 5.381 to 5.616.

Discussion

Analyzing the observation results summarized in Table 2 some consideration can be drawn.

From the macroscopical point of view the opaque appearance of the new spacers surfaces allowed to identify more easily the worn areas on the spacers *ex vivo*. In fact it was observed that the areas that came in contact during the *in vivo* functioning appear glossy. This aspect can be usefully utilized to evaluate the positioning and the loading conditions of the device. On the spacer-K explanted after 5 months the shiny part extended to almost the whole area covering the two surfaces that were in contact with the thighbone, including an area on the surface of the central part in relief, which indicates an imperfect matching between the two components but, in any case, a good distribution of the load on the surface. In the Spacer-K explanted after 6 months, the different location of the shiny areas at the edges of the components indicates that the surfaces that were in contact were less extensive and therefore the load was concentrated on a limited surface of the spacer.

The smoothing of the contact areas observed on the heads' surfaces of the Spacer-G devices and the consequent disappearing of the mechanical workmanship that was identified on the rough surface suggests that a large amount of cement could be worn out during the *in vivo* functioning. The presence of the glossy areas developed along a circular crown towards the side of the head on both the spacers-G shows that the spacer was partly loaded and surely articulating, even if it was not able to support the natural load of a thighbone. The glossy areas extension and the different location on the head and with respect to the stem observed on the two explanted devices suggests a different matching with the acetabulum.

Microscopical observations, carried out by SEM, have not highlighted any detail that shows different wearing conditions of the surfaces of spacers explanted after different functioning times. A slight difference was found on the Spacer-K, which was explanted after 5 months with respect to the same type of spacer explanted after 6 months. It consists in the existence of fewer microcracks which, however, could also be caused by the material's different load conditions as argued also by macroscopical observations. A greater difference can be seen between knee and hip spacers. The latter actually show a more consistent smoothing out effect of the prepolymer beads and a reduction in the radiopaque areas. This fact suggests that if the powder compound based on radiopacifying agents is associated to the antibiotic, the worn out areas are less efficient in releasing the drug, since it is moved or absorbed more deeply by the cement and therefore less available. This adds to the evident wear, even if it is distributed to limited areas of contact, with extirpation and consequent release of waste that can increase the inflammatory response thus reducing the device's efficacy. The presence of cracks can increase this phenomenon since these can lead to the breakage of small fragments of cement.

Roughness measurements confirmed the microscopical observation results. In fact the extension in time of the device *in vivo* functioning does not seem to be highlighted by roughness measurements. If we consider, for example, the two Spacer-G devices explanted after 3 and 6 months you cannot notice a substantial difference in roughness values of the shiny areas. However, apart from not knowing the exact functioning conditions that the spacers were submitted to during the time they were implanted, it should also be noted that roughness measurements on the spacer head after 6 months were not taken in the area that appeared shinier after a macroscopical observation. This is because the position could not be reached by the analysis system.

The major roughness values difference between implanted and new devices has been revealed for spacer-G. One should keep in mind, though, that even if the spacers were completely loaded, the weight on the knee is not as heavy as that on the hip joint. Moreover the spacer-G head surfaces are rougher than the spacer-K ones and rougher surface wears out more easily.

Another effect of the *in vivo* functioning of the spacer has been highlighted by the polymer molecular weight measurements. Results show that the polymer, which spacer-K is made of, has suffered from deterioration during the 6 months of *in vivo* functioning. In actual fact, apart from the reduction of the $\overline{M_w}$ (weight-average molecular weight), and the $\overline{M_n}$ (number-average molecular weight), there was also an increase in the DPM (polydispersity index). This shows there has been a degradation of part of the molecules with the formation of smaller molecules.

References

1. Affatato S, Mattarozzi A, Taddei P et al (2003) Investigations on the wear behaviour of the temporary PMMA-based hip Spacer-G. Proc. Instn Mech Engrs part H: J Engineering in Medicine 217(1):1–8
2. Durbhakula S M, Czajka J, Fuchs M D et al (2004) Spacer endoprosthesis for the treatment of infected total hip arthroplasty. J Arthroplasty 19(6):760–767
3. Durbhakula S M, Czajka J, Fuchs M D et al (2004) Antibiotic-loaded articulating cement spacer in the 2-stage exchange of infected total knee arthroplasty. J Arthroplasty 19(6): 768–774
4. Evans R P (2004) Successful treatment of total hip and knee infection with articulating antibiotic components: a modified treatment method. Clin Orthop Relat Res (427):37–46
5. Hsieh PH, Shih CH, Chang YH et al (2004) Two-stage revision hip arthroplasty for infection: comparison between the interim use of antibiotic-loaded cement beads and a spacer prosthesis. J Bone Joint Surg (Am) 86(9):1989–1997
6. Hsieh PH, Shih CH, Chang YH et al (2005) Treatment of deep infection of the hip associated with massive bone loss: two stage revision with an antibiotic-loaded interim cement prosthesis followed reconstruction with allograft. J Bone Joint Surg (Am) 87(6):770–775
7. Takahira N, Itoman M, Higashi K et al (2003) Treatment outcome of two-stage revision total hip arthroplasty using antibiotic-impregnated cement spacer. J Orthop Sci 8(1):26–31
8. Yamamoto K, Miyagawa N, Toshinori M et al (2003) Clinical effectiveness of antibiotic-impregnated cement spacers for the treatment of infected implants of the hip joint. J Orthop Sci 8(6):823–828

16 Bone Loss: Does Use of the Spacer Affects it?

H. Ferrer Escobar, R. Torres Romaña, A. Matamala Pérez,
J. Asunción Márquez

Department of orthopaedics, Hospital Mutua de Terrassa, Spain

Introduction

Total hip replacement revision has always been an interesting and difficult challenge for surgeons. This challenge is even bigger in presence of an infected revision, since the control of infection is one of the key element for the implant final result.

Debates are still going on today on the modalities and timing (one- or two-stage) that surgeons should adopt in infected revision surgery, since several factors have to be considered before taking this decision.

In our experience, two-stage surgical treatment is used in 90 % of revisions, when there is a clear pre-clinical diagnosis of infection and when there is a strong clinical suspicion of infection.

The choice of the two-stage revision technique gives the surgeon the possibility to choose (between the first and second operation) if a resection arthroplasty according to Girdlestone [3] or the use of a spacer is required [2, 9].

If resection arthroplasty is chosen, the first operation involves a considerable shortening of the limb and requires long admittance periods due to the application of continuous traction forces. The subsequent formation of muscle/ligament adhesion and retraction makes more complicated the second operation increasing the blood loss and prolonging its duration.

Studies on the use of antibiotic-loaded PMMA-spacers, published by Clive P. Duncan in 1993 [2], marked a turning point in prosthetic revision surgery of the hip and the knee.

Following the experience proposed by Duncan, between 1994 and 1998 our group started to use an intra-operatively prepared spacer made with cement and gentamicin. The results achieved in terms of infection eradication were positive, but mechanical failure of the device was observed in some cases. From 1998 till today, being aware of the advantages of the use of a spacer in revision surgery of infected implants, we started to use a preformed hip spacer, Spacer-G (Tecres Spa, Italy). Initially the device was available only with a short stem (Fig. 1a), and in some cases a varus positiong was noted, moreover in case of absence of proximal support, in the presence of large methaphyseal defects or after a trans-femoral approach for implant removal the device could not be used. This problem was overcome when the long stem version was introduced in the market (Fig. 1b).

One of the problem still debated is the possibility of increasing bone loss with the use of the spacer, and this was the aim of this retrospective study.

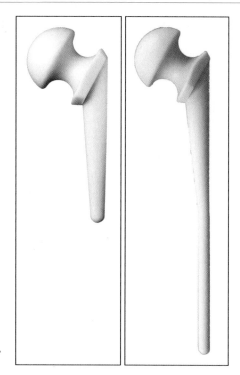

Fig. 1. a Spacer-G (short stem); **b** Spacer-G XL (long stem)

Materials and Methods

Between 1998 and 2005 forty-six patients (22 M, 24 F) underwent a two-stage revision procedure for the treatment of infected THA. In all patients Spacer-G was implanted for a mean period ranging from 2 to 20 weeks.

The diagnosis of infection was based on clinical history, bio-humoral parameters (ESR, CRP), imaging studies (X-rays, scintigraphy), microbiological and histological assay [6].

The mean age of the patients at the time of surgery was 62 years (range 42–83).

The infecting pathogen was *Staphylococcus epidermidis* (19), *Staphylococcus aureus* (16), methicillin-resistant *Staphylococcus aureus, MRSA* (2), *Streptococcus* (2), *Peptostreptococcus* (1) and *Mycoplasma hominis* (1). Polymicrobial infection was diagnosed in 4 cases. In one patient the pathogen was not detected.

In 24 patients Spacer-G was implanted after having carried out an extended trochanteric osteotomy [5].

There are no defined methods for evaluating the loss of bone mass. Since only radiological data were available for all the patients, we decided to analyze and compare the X-rays taken after the implantation of the spacer and the X-rays taken a few days before its removal.

At acetabular level it was evaluated the possible presence of pelvic perforation or lifting of the spacer head; at femoral level it was evaluated the femoral endomedullar cavity.

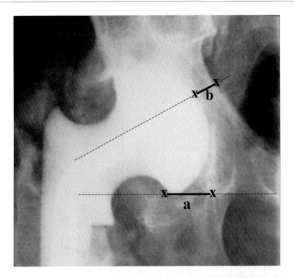

Fig. 2. Measurement of the bone loss at acetabular level **a** lifting, **b** penetration

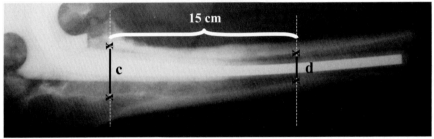

Fig. 3. Measurement of the bone loss at femoral level **c** level of the minor trocanter, **d** at 15 cm from the minor trochanter

As measurable parameters, at acetabular level we established: 1) the distance between the spacer head perimeter and the unnamed line; 2) the distance between the lower edge of the radiological "U" and the lower part of the spacer head. This enabled us to record the bone loss as lifting of the spacer head (a) and/or as intrapelvic perforation (b) (Fig. 2). At femoral level, we measured the distance from the medullary space on two levels: 1) at the minor trochanter level (c); 2) 15 cm below the first measurement (d) (Fig. 3).

Moreover where an extended trochanteric osteotomy had been performed, it was verified that the osteotomy was radiologically visible and consolidated at the time of the second surgical operation.

Results

No bone loss, according to the criteria selected, was found in 44 patients out of 46 (95.6 %). Bone loss was seen only in two patients.

Acetabular level: in the first case the spacer head lifted by 4 mm (a) with a pelvis

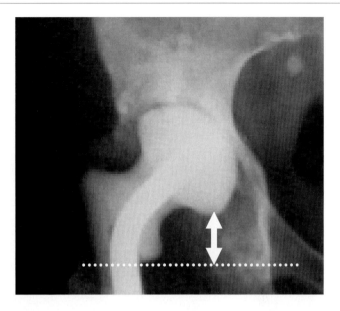

Fig. 4. Lifting of the spacer head at the acetabulum level

perforation of 3 mm (b); in the second case the spacer head lifted by 3 mm (a) without any measured perforation (Fig. 4).

Femoral level: in both cases an increase of the endomedullar cavity diameter was found. In the first case the sinking of the spacer caused a fracture of the trochanter and extended the higher femoral measurement by 5 mm (c). In the second case, instead, even without any sinking, the higher measurement had enlarged by 3 mm (c) and the lower one by 5 mm (d).

As concerns the cases which underwent an extended trochanteric osteotomy, in 21 cases the osteotomy consolidated before the final prosthesis reimplantation (Fig. 5), and 3 developed into pseudo-arthrosis.

We observed 2 spacer dislocations and 1 major trochanter fracture.

Discussion

Revision surgery of total hip prostheses always involves considerable problems for surgeons. Firstly, it is not always easy to determine the cause of the pain [1] and secondly, once a second operation on the patient has been decided, it is important to know if the cause of pain is an aseptic or a septic loosening.

The diagnosis of a septic or aseptic loosening has clear consequences on the type of treatment adopted. Today, the debate on the treatment options of infected hip prostheses continues. There are two traditional approaches: one-stage revision or two-stage revision [4] broken up by a period in between the two operations that is influenced by various factors.

In this period there are two options: the first is the application of the Girdlestone technique, which was designed for the treatment of articulated tuberculosis of the hip [3], which is considered an intermediate solution while waiting for the second opera-

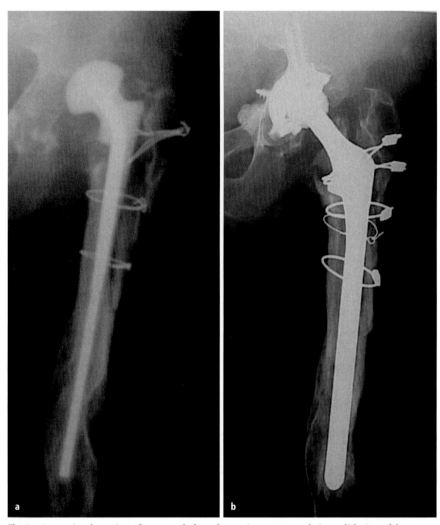

Fig. 5. a Spacer implantation after extended trochanteric osteotomy; **b** Consolidation of the osteotomy

tion (implant of the new prosthesis). Resection arthroplasty implies a treatment of continuous traction that increases the patient's stay in bed, thus lengthening admittance times. However, what is really important is that with this procedure the retraction of soft tissues and formation of muscle adhesions play an unfavourable role in the prosthetic reimplant operations. They make it difficult to approach the hip again, thus hindering the correct identification of the various levels, causing the retraction of important structures such as the abductor system increasing the surgical times and complications.

The second option is the positioning of a spacer, as described by Duncan in 1993 [2]. The spacer has a mechanical function, as it keeps the space between the bone segments, providing a certain degree of joint mobility, and a biological function, as it realeses locally high concentration of antibiotic [8, 9]. The patient quality of life is considerably improved: few days after the removal of the infected prosthesis and the implantation of the hip spacer, the patient can get out of bed and freely deambulate without load but with the use of two crutches. On the other hand, the surgeon highly benefits from the use of the spacer: the surgeon can operate a hip without the retraction of soft tissues, with an excellent identification of the different access levels, without fibrous scars and without any shortening of the limbs nor of the abductor system. This contributes to reduce surgical times and blood loss, and avoid intra-operation complications.

The aim of our work was to study if the use of a preformed hip spacer may increase bone loss both at acetabular and femoral level. Several factors may influence theoretically such a phenomenon: patient bone condition, spacer stability, length of implantation, patient correct behaviour (partial weight-bearing).

Patient bone condition influences the decision of the surgeon of allowing or not partial weight-bearing to the patient; the stability of the spacer depends on the congruency between the spacer head and the acetabulum and can be increased by using the long-stem spacer, which avoids the possible varus positioning of the short-stem spacer, and by performing a proximal cementation of the spacer neck. The average length of spacer implantation is nowadays between 8–12 months, but in some case due to contingent reasons can be much longer. Eventually the behaviour of the patient cannot be controlled: it cannot be excluded that patients will walk with full weight-bearing when at home.

Notwithstanding all these possible negative effects, we found a condition of increased bone loss only in two patients. It can be concluded that, according to the criteria selected, the preformed hip spacer does not affect bone loss.

References

1. Duffy PJ, Masri BA, Garbuz DS et al (2005) Evaluation of patients with pain following total hip replacement. J Bone Joint Surg (Am) 87(11):2566–2575
2. Duncan CP, Beauchamp C (1993) A temporary antibiotic-loaded joint replacement system for management of complex infections involving the hip. Orthop Clin North Am 24(4):751–759
3. Horan FT (2005) Robert Jones, Gathorne Girdlestone and excision arthroplasty of the hip. Historical notes. J Bone Joint Surg (Br) 87(1):104–106
4. McDonald DJ, Fitzgerald RH Jr, Ilstrup DM (1989) Two-stage reconstruction of the total hip arthroplasty because of infection. J Bone Joint Surg (Am) 71(6):828–834
5. Morshed S, Huffman R, Ries MD (2005) Extended trochanteric osteotomy for 2-stage revision of infected total hip artrhroplasty J Arthoplasty 20(3):294–303
6. Spangehl MJ, Masri BA, O'Connell JX et al (1999) Prospective analysis of preoperative and intraoperative investigations for the diagnosis of infection at the sites of two hundred and two revision total hip arthroplasties. J Bone Joint Surg (Am) 81(5):672–683
7. Williams JL, Norman P, Stockley I (2004) The value of hip aspiration versus biopsy in diagnosing infection before exchange hip arthroplasty surgery. J Arthroplasty 19(5):582–586
8. Bertazzoni Minelli E, Benini A, Magnan B et al (2004) Release of gentamicin and vancomycin from temporary human hip spacers in two-stage revision of infected arthroplasty. J Antimicrob Chemother 53(2):329–334
9. Magnan B, Regis D, Biscaglia R et al (2001) Preformed acrylic bone cement spacer loaded with antibiotics. Use of two-stage procedure in 10 patients because of infected hip after total replacement. Acta Orthop Scand 72(6):591–594

17 Antibiotic Impregnated Bone Grafts – What Do We Know?

E. Witsø

Department of Orthopaedic Surgery, St. Olavs University Hospital; Norwegian University of Science and Technology; Trondheim, Norway

Introduction

The Dutch surgeon, Door M. De Grood, who worked at St. Elisabeth-Ziekenhuis in Tilburg, was the first to report on mixing penicillin with cancellous bone when filling bone defects [9]. Two patients were successfully treated for residual cavities due to osteomyelitis. During the 1980's Alex McLaren presented several studies on bone graft as an antibiotic carrier at different scientific meetings [23, 24, 26]. In 26 patients treated with cancellous bone impreganted with tobramycin and vancomycin, sub-toxic serum levels (6 and 9 µg/mL, respectively) were registered at 12 hours postoperatively. Antibiotic concentration in the drain fluid was very high: 185–1690 µg/mL of tobramycin and 230–2345 µg/mL of vancomycin [25].

During the last decade several *in vitro* and *in vivo* studies have been published on cancellous and cortical bone as antibiotic carriers, and also clinical studies [5, 6, 7, 8, 27, 35, 36, 37, 38, 39, 40].

Cancellous Bone

In vitro and in vivo Studies

Different antibiotics can be adsorbed to and subsequently released from a morcellized cancellous bone *in vitro*. The release of antibiotics is characterized by a high early release and exponential decay. The decay of the curve is antibiotic specific (Fig. 1). Studies on aminoglycosides indicate that there is a complete release of antibiotics from impregnated cancellous bone. Different techniques have been used when cancellous bone allograft is impregnated with antibiotics. Antibiotic powder has been mixed with the bone graft, or the bone graft has been impregnated in an antibiotic solution. *In vitro*, antibiotic-impregnated cancellous bone elutes aminoglycoside and vancomycin for five to six weeks. Generally, the amount of vancomycin released from cancellous allograft is not inferior to that of an aminoglycoside. This is contrary to other studies on the release of aminoglycosides and glycopeptides from bone cement and PMMA beads [1, 19, 22]. There is a more rapid release of aminoglycosides compared to vancomycin. The fraction of the total amount eluted during the first 24 hours of an aminoglycoside and vancomycin, are 80 % and 30 %, respectively [38]. The release of antibiotics from cancellous bone is influenced to varying degrees by vari-

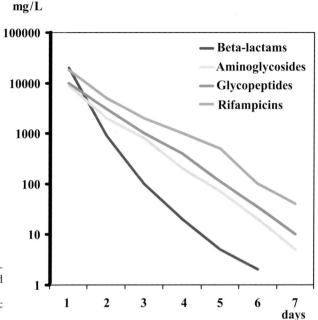

mg/L

Fig. 1. The elution profile of antibiotics from cancellous bone is characterized by an exponential decay, specific for each antibiotic

ables employed when the bone is impregnated with antibiotics, such as a) the concentration of antibiotics in the impregnating fluid, b) the time used to impregnate the bone, c) the pH of the impregnating fluid, d) the degree of bone morcellizing and e) antibiotic combination. Under optimal conditions, more than 70 mg of aminoglycoside and 100 mg of vancomycin are released from one gram of cancellous bone, *in vitro*.

In *vivo*, the release of beta-lactams from cancellous bone is so fast that it is difficult to compare the elution profile from *in vitro* and *in vivo* processed bone. However, the elution profiles of aminoglycosides, vancomycin, clindamycin and rifampicin are similar, *in vitro* and *in vivo* [37].

Clinical Studies

Bone graft impregnated with either aminoglycoside or vancomycin results in extremely high local concentrations when impacted in the femur canal or acetabulum (Fig. 2). The local antibiotic concentration is above MIC of vancomycin against most strains of *S. aureus* and *S. epidermidis* for at least 48 hours [8]. The antibiotic concentration in the wound drainage fluid in patients receiving cancellous bone impregnated with aminoglycoside is considerably higher than that recorded when using gentamicin-containing bone cement [3, 4, 20, 30, 32, 33, 39].

Very few studies on clinical results when using antibiotic-impregnated cancellous bone have been published in peer-reviewed medical journals, or presented at scientific meetings. Buttaro [6] presented a study on two-stage revision of infected total hip arthroplasties. Culture results at first stage revision included Gram- positive and

mg/L

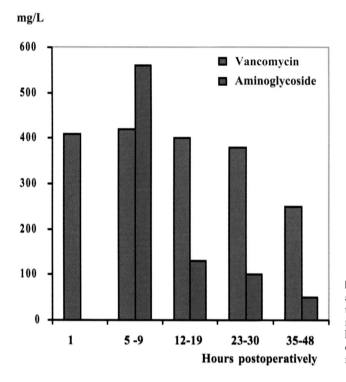

Fig. 2. Very high local antibiotic concentrations have been recorded in revision hip surgery with use of antibiotic-impregnated cancellous bone

Gram-negative bacteria. At second stage procedure vancomycin-loaded allograft (500 gram vancomycin per femoral head) was impacted in the actebulum and femur. All patients received a cemented femoral stem (without added antibiotics). At latest follow up (mean 32 months) there was no sign of reinfection or prosthetic loosening in 29 out of 30 hips.

Cortical Bone

With cortical allografts, graft-host non-union, graft fracture and graft infection occurs [2]. Infection rates of 4–12 percent have been reported [2, 13, 14, 21, 31]. Webb et al. [34] studied antibiotic resistance in *S. aureus* adherent to polyethylene, polymethylmetacrylate and cortical bone allografts *in vitro*. Compared to bacteria growing on the surface of polyethylene and polymethylmetacrylate, bacteria from the surface of cortical allograft were associated with the highest degree of antibiotic resistance. A cortical allograft may serve as a dead, foreign body that is not protected by the local cellular defense mechanisms. Hence, a prolonged period with prophylactic antibiotics has been recommended after implantation of large allografts [2, 21]. There are many reports on contamination of bone allografts during the process of procurement [10, 16, 18]. Rinsing a large bone allograft with an antibiotic solution after removal from the donor does not effectively eradicate microorganisms [10, 16]. The exposure time may bee too short for the antibiotics to be effective [10]. However, due to long and extensive surgery, multiple operations, problems with wound healing and haematogenous spread of bacteria, large bone allografts are probably more often contaminated during and after the operation [21, 31]. Moreover, many of these patients have malignant tumors and are concomitantly treated with adjuvant radiation or immunosuppressive chemotherapy.

In vitro studies have documented that cortical bone can act as an antibiotic carrier [35, 40]. When a cortical allograft is impregnated with aminoglycoside, vancomycin, ciprofloxacin or rifampicin the amount of antibiotics subsequently released from the bone is highly influenced by the time used for impregnation of the bone. Cortical allografts impregnated with netilmicin, vancomycin or rifampicin eradicate peroperative contamination with *S. aureus* in an experimental osteomyelitis model [40].

Local Antibiotics and Incorporation of Bone Allograft

Antibiotic impregnation of bone graft could have a detrimental effect on osteogenesis [15]. Ciprofloxacin reduces fracture healing when injected subcutaneously in rats, and topically applied chloramphenicol and methicillin powder diminishes the osteogenesis in corticocancellous graft [12, 17]. Miclau [28] showed that tobramycin concentration < 200 mg/L had no effect on osteoblast replication, while concentrations > 400 mg/L impaired osteoblast replication, *in vitro*. Vancomycin and cefazolin concentrations less than 1000 and 100 mg/L, respectively, have little or no effect on osteoblast replication, *in vitro* [11]. *In vivo*, the effect of vancomycin on osteogenesis has been studied thoroughly. Vancomycin-supplemented bone allograft in pigs has the same osteogenic activity as non-supplemented bone [29]. Vancomycin-supplemented bone allograft used for the treatment of tibia defects in pigs did not radiographically, histologically or immunohistochemically differ from the healing process occurring with non-supplemented allograft [5]. In a case report, the histology of vancomycin-supplemented impacted allograft has been studied in two patients. Due to periprosthetic fracture the patients were operated 14 and 20 months after a septic revision with the use of vancomycin-supplemented allograft. Histological examination of biopsies showed viable new bone formation, similar to what has been reported in allografts without antibiotics [7].

Conclusion

The release of antibiotics from antibiotic-impregnated bone allograft is characterized by a high early release and an exponential decay. The decay of the curve is antibiotic specific. When antibiotic-impregnated cancellous bone has been employed in revision hip surgery, extremely high local antibiotic concentrations have been recorded. Cancellous bone is an effective vehicle for local antibiotic delivery. However, the long time effects of antibiotic impregnation on bone regeneration have not been studied.

References

1. Adams K, Couch L, Cierny G et al (1992) In vitro and in vivo evaluation of antibiotic diffusion from antibiotic-impregnated polymethylmethacrylate beads. Clin Orthop Relat Res (278): 244–252
2. Aro HT, Aho AJ (1993) Clinical use of bone allografts. Ann Med 25(4):403–412. Review
3. Bunetel L, Segui A, Cormier M et al (1989) Release of gentamicin from acrylic bone cement. Clin Pharmacokinet 17(4):291–297
4. Bunetel L, Segui A, Cormier M, Langlais F (1990) Comparative study of gentamicin release from normal and low viscosity acrylic bone cement. Clin Pharamcokinet 19 (4):333–340
5. Buttaro M, Della Valle AMG, Piñeiro L et al (2003) Incorporation of vancomycin-supplemented bone allografts. Radiographical, histopathological and immunohistochemical study in pigs. Acta Orthop Scand 74(5):505–513
6. Buttaro M, Pusso R, Piccaluga F (2005). Vancomycin-supplemented impacted bone allografts in infected hip arthroplasty. Two-stage revision results. J Bone Joint Surg (Br) 87(3): 314–319
7. Buttaro M, Morandi A, Garcia Rivello H et al (2005) Histology of vancomycin-supplemented impacted bone allografts in revision total hip arthroplasty. J Bone Joint Surg (Br) 87(12): 1684–1687
8. Buttaro M, Gimenez MI, Greco G et al (2005). High local levels of vancomycin without nephrotoxicity released from impacted bone allograft in 20 revision hip arthroplasties. Acta Orthopaedica 76(3):336–340
9. De Grood DM (1947) Het plomeren van restholten na osteomyelitis met "bone-chips". Ned Tijdschr V Gen 91.III.32: 2192–2196. (In Dutch)
10. Deijkers RLM, Bloem RM, Petit PLC et al (1997) Contamination of bone allograft. Analysis of incidence and predisposing factors. J Bone Joint Surg (Br) 79(1):161–166
11. Edin ML, Miclau T, Lester GE et al (1996). Effect of cefazolin and vancomycin on osteoblasts in vitro. Clin Orthop Relat Res (333):245–251
12. Gray JC, Elves MW (1981) Osteogenesis in bone grafts after short-term storage and topical antibiotic treatment. An experimental study in rats. J Bone Joint Surg (Br) 63(3):441–445
13. Gross AE, Hutchison CR, Alexeeff M et al (1995) Proximal femoral allografts for reconstruction of bone stock in revision arthroplasty of the hip. Clin Orthop Relat Res (319):151–158
14. Haddad FS, Spangehl MJ, Masri BA et al (2000) Circumferential allograft replacement of the proximal femur. Clin Orthop Relat Res (371):98–107
15. Hanssen AD (2005) Local antibiotic delivery vehicles in the treatment of musculoskeletal infection. Clin Orthop Relat Res (437):91–96
16. Hirn MYJ, Salmela M, Vuento RE (2001) High-pressure saline washing of allografts reduces bacterial contamination. Acta Orthop Scand 72(1):83–85
17. Huddleston PM, Steckelberg JM, Hanssen AD et al (2000) Ciprofloxacin inhibition of experimental fracture-healing. J Bone Joint Surg (Am) 82(2):161–173
18. Journeaux SF, Johnson N, Bryce SL et al (1999) Bacterial contamination rates during bone allograft retrieval. J Arthroplasty 14(6):677–681
19. Klekamp J, Dawson JM, Haas DW et al (1999) The use of vancomycin and tobramycin in acrylic bone cement. Biomechanical effects and elution kinetics for use in joint arthroplasty. J Arthroplasty 14(3):339–346
20. Lindberg L, Önnerfält R, Dingeldein E et al (1991) The release of gentamicin after total hip replacement using low or high viscosity bone cement. Int Orthop 15(4):305–309
21. Lord CF, Gebhardt MC, Tomford WW et al (1988) Infection in bone allografts. J Bone Joint Surg (Am) 70(3):369–376
22. Mader JT, Calhoun J, Cobos J (1997) In vitro evaluation of antibiotic diffusion from antibiotic-impregnated biodegradable beads and polymethylmethacrylate beads. Antimicrob Agents Chemother 41(2):415–418
23. McLaren A (1988) Antibiotic impregnated bone graft: Post-op levels of vancomycin and tobramycin. Orthopaedic Trauma Assoc Annual Meeting. Pp: 758–759. (Abstract)
24. McLaren A (1989) Antibiotic impregnated bone graft. J Orthop Trauma 3(2):171 (Abstract)
25. McLaren AC (2004) Alternative materials to acrylic bone cement for delivery of depot antibiotics in orthopaedic infections. Clin Orthop Relat Res (427):101–106

26. McLaren AC, Miniaci A (1986) In vivo study to determine the efficacy of cancellous bone graft as a delivery vehicle for antibiotics. Proceedings of 12th Annual Meeting Society for Biomaterials. Minneapolis-St.Paul, Minnesota, USA. p:102
27. Miclau T, Dahners LE, Lindsey RW (1993) In vitro pharmacokinetics of antibiotic release from locally implantable materials. J Orthop Res 11(5):627–632
28. Miclau T, Edin ML, Lester GE et al (1995) Bone toxicity of local applied aminoglycosides. J Orthop Trauma 9(5):401–406
29. Petri WH (1984) Osteogenic activity of antibiotic-supplemented bone allografts in the Guinea pig. J Oral Maxillofac Surg 42(10):631–636
30. Salvati EA, Callaghan JJ, Brause BD et al (1986) Reimplantation in infection. Elution of gentamicin from cement and beads. Clin Orthop Relat Res (207):83–93
31. Tomford WW, Thongphasuk J, Mankin HJ et al (1990) Frozen musculoskeletal allografts. A study of the clinical incidence and causes of infection associated with their use. J Bone Joint Surg (Am) 72(8):1137–1143
32. Wahlig H, Dingeldein E (1980) Antibiotics and bone cements. Acta Orthop Scand 51(1):49–56
33. Wahlig H, Dingeldein E, Buchholz HW et al (1984) Pharmacokinetic study of gentamicin-loaded cement in total hip replacements. Comparative effects of varying dosage. J Bone Joint Surg (Br) 66(2):175–179
34. Webb LX, Holman J, Araujo B de et al (1994) Antibiotic resistance in staphylococci adherent to cortical bone. J Orthop Trauma 8(1):28–33
35. Winkler H, Janata O, Berger C et al (2000) In vitro release of vancomycin and tobramycin from impregnated human and bovine bone grafts. J Antimicrob Chemot 46(3):423–428
36. Witsø E, Persen L, Løseth K et al (1999) Adsorption and release of antibiotics from morselized cancellous bone. Acta Orthop Scand 70(3):298–304
37. Witsø E, Persen L, Løseth K et al (2000) Cancellous bone as an antibiotic carrier. Acta Orthop Scand 71(1):80–84
38. Witsø E, Persen L, Benum P et al (2002) Release of netilmicin and vancomycin from cancellous bone. Acta Orthop Scand 73(2):199–205
39. Witsø E, Persen L, Benum P et al (2004) High local concentration without systemic adverse effects after impaction of netilmicin-impregnated bone. Acta Orthop Scand 75(3):339–346
40. Witsø E, Persen L, Benum P et al (2005) Cortical allograft as a vehicle for antibiotic delivery. Acta Orthopaedica 76(4):481–486

18 Antibiotic-loaded Bone Allograft: Personal Experience

G. Gualdrini, L. Amendola, R. Ben Ayad, A. Giunti

7th Division of Orthopaedic and Traumatology, Rizzoli Orthopedic Institutes, Bologna, Italy

Introduction

In 1996 a new method for the production of morcellized bone allograft (MB) was described by Ullmark and Hovelius [3]. According to the clinical research of Ullmark [4] new bone formation surrounding the bone allograft was histologically demonstrated after 4 weeks. After 6 months allograft chips were still evident and surrounded by large quantity of growing bone tissue and vessels; after 4 years, the histological sections of stemmed proximal femur in revision hip prosthesis showed a normal bone tissue in the site of the bone loss stock: allograft chips were not evident anymore, and only new bone tissue growth with plenty of regenerated blood vessels were present. It was also demonstrated that defatted graft reduces bone-integration time and homologous tissue bio-compatibility [2].

Following these experiences, since 1998 the Musculoskeletal Tissue Bank of the Rizzoli Institute [1] produces morcellized defatted bone allograft in conformity with Ullmark and Hovelius experience. The bone allograft is utilized for different pathological lesions to replace bone loss stock. Witso [7, 8] and Winkler [6] experience showed that morcellized bone allograft is a good antibiotic carrier *in vitro*. We used antibiotic-loaded morcellized bone graft (AMB) to refill debrided septic bone loss stock. In such cases, a surgical debridement was always performed in the first stage to eradicate infection, whereas in the second stage the restoration of bone loss was performed with ABM (Figures 1a, b, c). Recurrence of a deep local infection with chronic fistula, without a septic involvement of the bone graft, was observed in some cases (Figures 1d, e). In some cases it has been possible to see significant roentgengraphic growth into a solid bone mass and satisfactory remodelling of bone allograft into new bony tissue (Figures 1f).

ABM has shown to be a promising composite for the treatment of septic bone loss stock even in presence of chronic infection. Nonetheless, the poor mechanical strength of this composite has led us to study *in vitro* and *in vivo* the pharmacological and mechanical behaviour of ABM mixed with PMMA cement (CAMB).

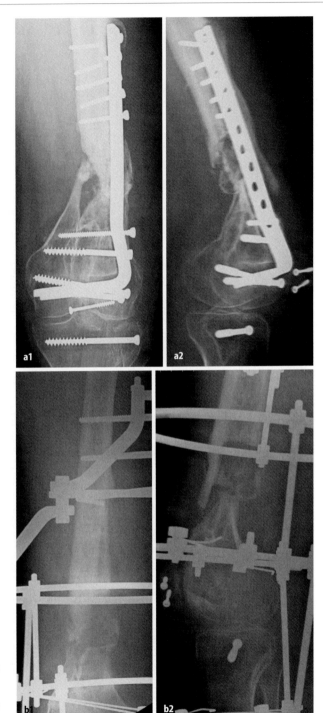

Fig. 1a. Septic non-union of the distal femur. Patient BS IV (UTMB Stage System). Fistula

Fig. 1b. X-ray after surgical debridement of septic tissue and stabilization with an Ilizatov frame. The original length of the femur is restored. Fistula

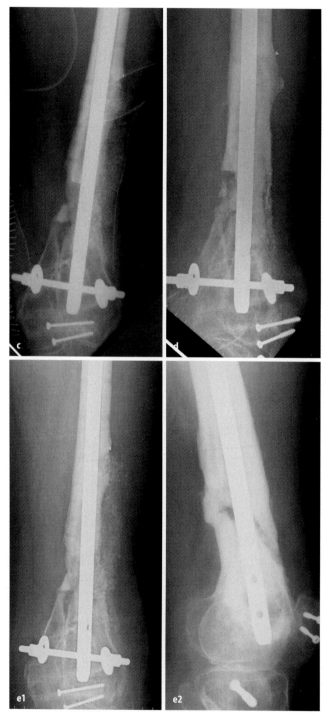

Fig. 1c, d. After two months the external fixator is removed. **c** Stabilization with a locked nail. The bone loss stock is filled with AMB. Fistula. AMB has an important X-ray evidence. **d** Two months later. Fistula. AMB is going into new bone

Fig. 1e. One year later. Fistula

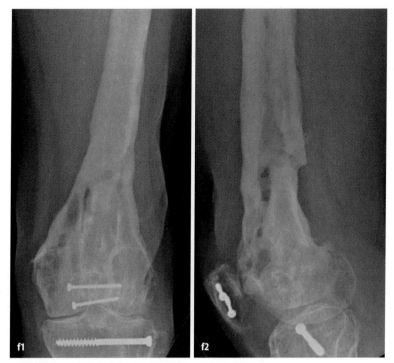

Fig. 1f. Four years later. No signs of deep infection

Clinical Section

From 1998 to 2002 at the Rizzoli Orthopaedic Institutes 249 patients were operated for different local bone pathologies using morcellized defatted bone allograft: 82 hips prosthesis revisions; 6 knee prosthesis revisions; 13 post-traumatic hip prostheses; 51 spinal fusions; 50 curettage and filling of pathological lytic bone lesions (6 aneurysmatic bone cysts and 7 giant cell tumours); 47 fracture non-unions of long bones (morcellized allograft was used to fill debrided gap at the fracture site augmented with cortical allograft and plates).

Morcellized bone graft is prepared mainly of spongy bone by removing fibrous tissue, cartilage and cortical layers. The cancellous bone is then grinded with a bone mill (Hovex Bone Mill, Orthologic Ltd) obtaining 3 mm bone chips. Morcellized allograft is then washed with warm saline solution and defatted. Eventually the material is gamma-sterilized at 25 kGy and then stored at −80 °C.

In 15 patients morcellized bone graft was mixed with antibiotic dry powder (AMB). Six patients had a septic non-union of the forearm, five a septic non-union of the femur and four had septic knee prosthesis (five knees). A two-stage technique was always performed and AMB was essentially used to fill residual empty space after the complete resolution of the infective process.

Forearm: in the 1st stage a bone and soft tissue debridement was performed, followed after 30 – 40 days, by the 2nd stage in which the functional restoration of the

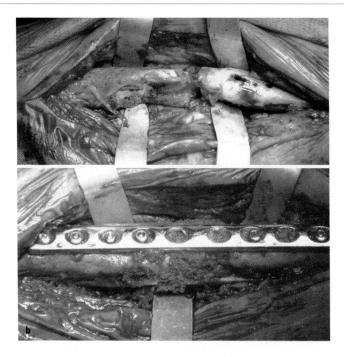

Fig. 2a. Septic non-union of the forearm at the second stage. **b** AMB is surroundig the nonunion site with the cortical and full bone graft

forearm bones was achieved using cortical full bone graft augmented by AMB (Figure 2a, 2b).

Femur: in the 1st stage an extensive bone and soft tissue debridement, and the application of an Ilizarov fixator to restore the original length was performed. This was followed, after 60–90 days, the 2nd stage in which the Ilizarov fixator was replaced by a locked intramedullary nail. The space of lost bone was filled with AMB in one case (Figure 1c, d), and with full cortical bone graft augmented by AMB in the others.

Knee: the patients presented a peri-prosthetic wide bone gap. The defects were all classified as Engh Type 3. In the 1st stage the knee prosthesis was removed and replaced with an antibiotic-loaded spacer. This was followed, after 50–90 days, by the implantation of a revision knee prosthesis and AMB in the lost bone space.

The 15 patients underwent intravenous (1 week) and oral (4 weeks) antibiotics administration, based on micro culture and antibiotic sensitivity assay from the tissue biopsy.

Results

At a mean follow-up of five years, in 14 patients no relapse of the septic process was present with good bone stock restoration. In only one patient with a septic fracture non-union of the femur, the treatment was failed.

Forearm: the resolution of septic nonunion was obtained in the 6 cases. The functional restoration has been related to the local conditions at the beginning of the treatment.

Femur: in 3 patients resolution of the septic process and bone segments union was achieved; in one patient we had a failure: a 58 year-old man treated with a full-bone graft, AMB and a locked nail developed a severe infection 30 days after the second surgical stage and underwent amputation. This was the only failure in our experience.

Knee: the 4 patients regained a satisfactory range of motion (0°- 50°), good joint stability. The long-term postoperative radiographic control revealed a good bone density of grafted bone defect and, in our opinion, is the character of a new bone tissue growth.

Discussion

In our experience the use of morcellized defatted bone graft has become an usual opportunity for the treatment of bone defects. When a septic complication is combined to a bone defect, a two-stage technique is preferred. The use of AMB is still a further care for the treatment of bone defect with a former septic complication.

Some Authors describe positively their experience with antibiotic loaded allograft [9], but other suppose that local antibiotic is not necessary when bone grafts are used [5]. Our opinion is that an accurate selection of the patients and more experience is necessary to understand the effectiveness and indications of AMB for the treatment of septic bone defects.

Experimental section

The more frequent use of AMB and the observation of its poor mechanical strength, stimulated a research of a new composite similar to human bone: morcelized bone allograft with vancomycin and PMMA.

In our Institute Lab, with a specific mould of 1 cm diameter and 1 cm height, cylinders (CAMB) were made with a mixture of morcellized bone graft (0.8 g), vancomycin (0.1 g), PMMA powder (0.5 g) plus PMMA liquid (0.3 ml) and others control cylinders (CA) made of vancomycin (0.1 g), PMMA powder (0.5 g) plus PMMA liquid (0.3ml). Both groups were tested for *in vitro* antibiotic release in two different media: saline solution and human plasma.

5 CAMB cylinders were immersed into 30 ml of human plasma (Group I) and 5 CAMB in 30 ml of physiological saline solution (Group II). 3 CA cylinders were immersed into in 30 ml of human plasma (Group III) and 3 CA in physiological saline solution (Group IV).

All cylinders were incubated at 35–37 °C. Human plasma and saline solution were refreshed at every taking: every day for the first 7 days, and then once a week for the next 3 weeks. Human plasma derived from different donors.

Vancomycin (μg/ml) was measured using a fluorescent immunological method (Tdx, Abbott Lab). Data were analysed with the *Mann-Whitney's test* and non-parametrical data with *Montecarlo.*

Results

The total antibiotic release measured in the four weeks of immersion is shown in Table 1: Group I showed the highest release (1515 $\mu g/ml$), slightly lower values were measured for Group II and Group IV, the minimum release was measured for Group III (719 $\mu g/ml$).

Similar kinetics of antibiotic release was observed in all groups, i.e. peak quantity of release in the first day of immersion followed by gradual decrease of release in the following days. Group II and IV, elueted in saline, showed a burst release in the 1st day followed by a sudden release drop in the next days.

Another observation which related to group II and IV immersed in saline that showed a burst quantity release in 1st day followed by sudden drop of the curve

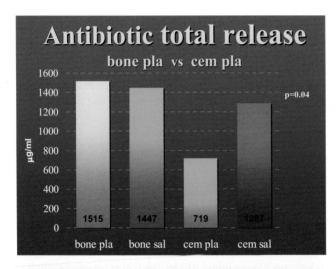

Table 1. Total vancomcyin release in 4 weeks: Group I CAMB in plasma; Group II CAMB in saline; Group III CA in human plasma; Group IV in saline

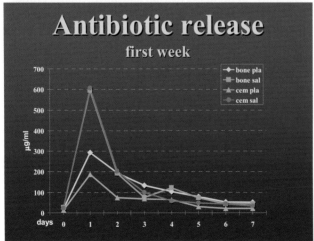

Table 2. Vancomycin release in the first week

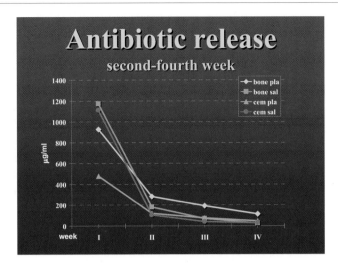

Table 3. Vancomycin release (second-fourth week)

(Table 2). Furthermore in the first week of immersion (Table 2), Group II and IV eluted in saline showed higher release compared to Group I and III, which were eluted in plasma. In the following three weeks of immersion (Table 3), Group I kept a relatively higher and constant antibiotic release (588 μg/ml), whereas Group II and III 50 % less (275 μg/ml and 241 μg/ml respectively), eventually Group IV released the lowest amount (174 μg/ml) 75 % lesser.

Discussion

During the preparation of the samples we tried to preserve the most similar physiological conditions. The amount of PMMA used was the minimal to obtain component stability, whereas the amount of antibiotic was the highest amount which could be mixed.

Human plasma from different donors was used to limit the effect of mono-donor variable. Control samples (CA), which did not contain bone allograft, were treated in the same manner, i.e. same quantity of antibiotic and PMMA cement. The material was incubated in a thermostatic incubator with limited temperature change.

Vancomycin was preferred as it can be easily mixed with the other components and it is an antibiotic effective against aerobic and non-aerobic bacterial pathogens in bone infections. Samples with morcellized bone allograft (CAMB) eluted in human plasma showed a constant antibiotic release, markedly superior to all the other groups.

The lowest standard error was found in Group I which indicated a constant quantity release in relation with the time. The total vancomycin release from CAMB is higher than from CA.

CAMB has the property to maintain a more constant and higher antibiotic release when eluted in human plasma. These combinations have been promise group I (CAMB plasma) as a most favourable group, because it maintains an effective local therapeutic level of antibiotic for sufficient duration.

The CA Groups have a fast release, offering an immediate therapeutic level, but for short duration. The amount released from the samples were superior to the MIC for streptococcal species (MIC $\leq$ 1 μg/ml) and enterococcal species (MIC < 4 μg/ml), but not for bacterial species (MIC $\geq$ 32 μg/ml).

Mechanical testing

Preliminary tests were performed on CAMB and CA cylinders. Tensile strength showed very low values (0,8 $\pm$ 0,6 MPa) compared to pure PMMA (30 MPa), while the compressive strength was about 1/10 (13,6 $\pm$ 3,7 Mpa) compared to pure PMMA (80 MPa). This value is comparable to the compressive strength measured for human cancellous bone.

In vivo biocompatibility

Following the Italian Law on animal experiments, cylindrical specimens of CAMB (8 mm in diameter, 10 mm in length) were implanted in the trabecular iliac crest of 6 sheep.

After 3 months, a histological and morphometric study showed the direct apposition of new bone to the composite material surface and matrix. The fluorescent light test showed bone growth marked with tetracycline all over the section of CAMB.

Conclusion

AMB has high osteoconductive properties and enables to recover of septic lost bone stock with a high resistance to local chronic infections. It has a good antibiotic release rate and a good bone induction. As a carrier, we think that it is necessary to have a longer experience to evaluate its real efficacy. The disadvantage of AMB is the low mechanical strength. For this reason we studied the *in vitro* release of vancomycin from the composite CAMB which showed good release properties. In addition, the mechanical characterization showed that the composite of CAMB has a compressive strength comparable to human cancellous bone. The biocompatibility testing confirmed that CAMB has a good bone induction property demonstrated by growth of new bone after 3 months.

In conclusion, due to these results, CAMB could be considered as a new bio-synthetic opportunity to minimize the morbidity of chronic bone infection.

References

1. Fornasari PM, Bassi A, Poluzzi V (1999) La banca dell'osso degli istituti ortopedici rizzoli: Storia e Attività. XXV Congresso Nazionale SITO, E 12
2. Thoren K (1994) Lipid extracted bone graft. Thesis University of Lund, Sweden
3. Ullmark G, Hovelius L (1996) Impacted morsellized allograft and cement for revision total knee arthroplasty. Acta Orthop Scand 67(1):10–12

4. Ullmark G, Linder L (1998) Histology of the femur after cancellous impaction grafting using a Charnley prosthesis. A case report. Archiv Orthop Trauma Surg 117(3):170–172

5. Vilalta I, Tibau R, Tubau J (2006) Is it necessary local antibiotic when bone allograft is used? Abstract Booklet of the 25° EBJIS Meeting, Budapest 25–27 May

6. Winkler H, Berger C, Kristen KH et al (2000) Vancomycin-Tobramycin composite grafts. A new treatment for chronic osteomyelitis of the neuropatic food. Abstract Booklet of the 19° EBJIS Meeting, Berlin 25–27 May

7. Witsø E, Persen L, Løseth K, Bergh K (1999) Adsorption and release of antibiotics frommorse-lized cancellous bone. Acta Orthop Scand 70(3):298–304

8. Witsø E, Persen L, Løseth K et al (2000) Cancellous bone as an antibiotic carrier. Acta Orthop Scand 71(1):80–84

9. Witsø E, Persen L, Egeberg T (2006) Two-Sstage revision of infected total hip arthroplasties, 6 (2–12) years follow up in 46 patients operated with impaction of allograft impregnated with antibiotics and implantation of a HA coated prosthesis. Abstract Booklet of the 25° EBJIS Meeting, Budapest 25–27 May.

19 Antibiotic Loaded Cement: From Research to Clinical Evidence

GEERT H.I.M. WALENKAMP

Department of Surgery and Orthopaedics, University Hospital Maastricht, the Netherlands

Introduction

The defect created by the osteomyelitic destruction and its debridement has always been seen as an important cause of non-healing. Surgeons therefore have tried to fill these cavities with all kinds of autogenous tissues and allogenic materials: patients own skin or muscle, plaster of Paris or gauzes. Since antiseptics were introduced, they have been mixed with these fillers, e.g. plaster of Paris with carbolic acid or cod liver oil [4, 8]. And the same happened with antibiotics, which were admixed with plaster of Paris, as well as to bone grafts or patient's own blood.

Antibiotics have been increasingly used for prevention of infection, in open fractures but also in joint replacement, in addition to the treatment of established infections. Buchholz used antibiotic-containing solutions for regular lavage during operation, and sutured cloths soaked in antibiotics to the fascia [3]. In his search for more effective reduction of the postoperative deep infections of hip prostheses (as high as 3 %), he was shown by chemists that bone cement was able to release various substances, as the residual monomer and CuS. So in a pilot study he admixed four heat-stable antibiotic powders with bone cement and found that, except for tetracycline, the antibiotics indeed were released by a diffusion process for at least 2 weeks in a bactericidal concentration. In 1969 studies started by Merck GmbH (Darmstadt, Germany) to develop an antibiotic loaded bone cement, resulted in the gentamicin containing bone cement Refobacin-Palacos® [15, 16].

Pharmacokinetic Studies

Bone cement is based on methyl methacrylate and made by mixing the liquid monomer with the polymer powder (PMMA). During the curing process a network of newly formed PMMA chains is formed. Various substances, as for example antibiotics, can be admixed and are incorporated in between these PMMA chains. When PMMA absorbs water, these substances are released by diffusion, a process determined by the hydrophobicity of the cement. The antibiotic release is influenced by the porosity and roughness of the cement [1]. It has been demonstrated that antibiotics incorporated into a bone cement can be released, but this is limited to a depth of 100 µm [10]. The initial high release is a surface phenomenon, which is then followed by a reduced, but sustained release, which depends on bulk porosity, i.e. it depends on the penetration of fluids through connected pores in the cement [1].

Many brands of PMMA have been tested with many kind of antibiotics showing similar kinetics of release. As regards gentamicin, Palacos® bone cement shows the higher release [9, 12, 14, 18].

Release of antibiotics from a carrier is a diffusion process, with exchange of the antibiotics to water. The maximum release is in the very beginning when the gradient between the carrier and the surrounding hematoma and tissues is the highest. The release then deminishes over time, and this is reflected in the local concentration of the antibiotic in the exudate. [15].

The antibiotic concentration in the tissues depends of the concentration reached in the exudate around the bone cement. The tissue concentration decreases with the increase of the distance from the carrier, but also with time. The penetration of the antibiotic is also influenced by the tissue properties itself: cortical bone can accumulate a lower concentration then spongious bone, which can accumulate a lower concentration than the haematoma [15].

Newer carriers have been studied in the last decade, and special interest is given to resorbable carriers, and to the possibility of customized antibiotic choices, eventually in combinations. Resorbable carriers available now are e.g. collagen, $CaSO_4$, hydroxyapatite, tricalciumphosphate, polylactides. The main problem in these newer products is to create a slow release, often a too quick release is caused by insufficient binding of the antibiotic to the carrier [13], or a burst release when the carriers dissolves. A good prolonged release of many antibiotics is also realised by admixing antibiotics to bone grafts *in vitro* as well as *in vivo* [19, 20].

The optimal period to maintain a high local antibiotic concentration would be about 4 weeks, although no hard data are available. This period seems to be necessary for the diffusion process of the antibiotics in the tissues, especially in presence of dense structures, such as in scarred soft tissues and sclerotic bone [15].

The concentration that can be achieved with an optimal use of gentamicin beads is 300 – 400 ug/ml in the exudate, with an accumulation at day 2 or 3 (Fig. 1). For achieving these concentration it is necessary the application of as many beads as possible in

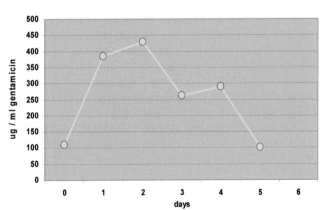

Fig. 1. Gentamicin concentration in the exudate of a patient after extraction of an infected knee prosthesis and implantation of 180 gentamicin PMMA beads. The concentration increases with a maximum level of more then 400 microgram per millilitre, about 400 times higher then the MIC value of the causative *S. aureus*. The maximum is achieved due to accumulation in the first 2 – 3 days

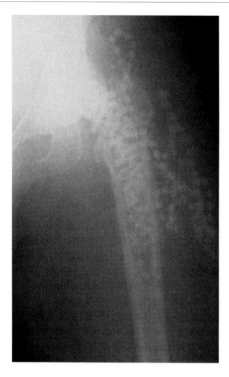

Fig. 2. Gentamicin PMMA beads used in a hip after removal of an infected total hip prosthesis: 360 beads are implanted in the whole area

the cavity, and a haematoma that is as small as possible and with a volume similar to the volume of the implanted beads. For example, after the removal of a non-hinged knee prosthesis about 180 beads can be implanted, after removal of a total hip 360 beads (Fig. 2).

An increase in the surface of the beads is reflected by an increase in the release of antibiotic too [11]. Minibeads can release an amount of gentamicin which is seven times higher than standard Septopal beads [17].

There are some very important differences between the pharmacokinetic properties of beads and spacers. Commercially available gentamicin PMMA beads have a higher porosity, compared with hand made beads or spacers. This decreases the gentamicin release per cement surface. Even more important is the large difference in surface, when beads are compared with spacers. Since the antibiotic release is a surface related diffusion process, the release of spacers largely decreased as compared with beads with the same total volume.

This is the reason why spacers, which have a reduced surface as compared to beads, cannot reach such high local antibiotic concentrations [6]. As a personal experience, after the implantation of a spacer an exudate concentrations not higher than 50 ug/ml and decreasing after the operation was measured (Fig. 3).

So a better release of antibiotic from a carrier at the infected site can be achieved by: 1) a large surface of the carrier; 2) a more porous structure of the carrier; 3) a carrier that dissolves and so releases its content completely; 4) a higher antibiotic concentration in the carrier; 5) the election of a carrier with good release properties

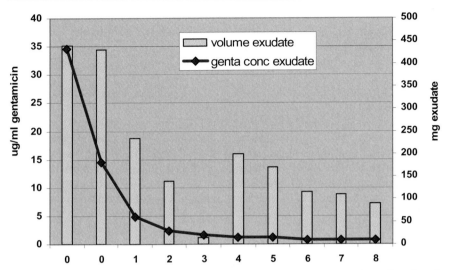

Fig. 3. Gentamicin concentration in the exudate of a patient after extraction of an infected total hip and implantation of a spacer. The concentration decreases after implantation of the spacer in 1 – 2 days to a low level

Conclusion

Nowadays the use of antibiotic-loaded acrylic cement (ALAC) in total joint proce-dures is widespread and a substantial body of evidence demonstrates its efficacy in infection prevention and treatment [5, 7]. In the management of the of infected implant sites the use of ALAC has reduced reinfection rates in one-stage exchange revision. The use of ALAC in the form of beads and spacers in two-stage revision has also demonstrated to reduce the infection rate [7].

Spacers are helpful in revision of infected arthroplasties in technical point of view. They maintain the space for the prosthesis in case of delayed reimplantation, as in two-stage revisions. That is more important in knees then in hips. The release of the scarred tissue of the hip in case of a Girdlestone situation, and restoration of length is not easy after a year, but can be achieved. In knees however, after removal of the prosthesis weight-bearing is not possible without damaging the bone surfaces, and the ligaments are definitely shortened. Reimplantation of total knee prostheses would result generally in a knee with a bad function, so without much advantage over a knee fusion. That is why at our Institute in the past reimplantation was done immediately after infection treatment, so only a short-term two-stage procedure was possible, and not a long-term interval procedure. Therefore mostly we preferred an artrodesis. This has changed since the introduction of the spacers, giving more time to wait and see if the infection has healed.

The above mentioned pharmacokinetic considerations, and the experience with gentamicin beads as a powerful and surgeon-friendly instrument in the treatment of infected prostheses has resulted in the following approach of deep infected arthro-plasties:

1. removal of prostheses and all cement, debridement, implantation of gentamicin beads (as much as possible in the whole infected area), i.v. antibiotics
2. after 2 weeks repeated debridement if necessary, again beads, otherwise step 3
3. if healing seems appropriate: extraction of beads, implantation of a preformed spacer
4. 1 week after the last operation: switch to oral antibiotics until 6–12 weeks post-operative.
5. 6 weeks after stop of antibiotics punction of the joint cavity, culture. Attention in the laboratory to slow growing bacteria, also caused by the local antibiotics
6. If culture is negative: reïmplantation of the prosthesis. If any doubt as a short-term two stage procedure with again a 2 week gentamicin bead treatment. This offers the opportunity to re-debride and to take many deep tissue samples for culture, and to individualize eventually the bone cement to be used in the reïm-plantation.

Although the literature is rather positive about the clinical results in the use of spacers [7] , there is probably a considerable publication bias, non-publication of bad results, as usual in new treatments. Moreover, as in the beginning period of the beads in the seventies, spacers as a new approach are again used as a magic tool in the treatment of infections, used by surgeons without many experience in the treatment of infections, and without realizing the limits of the treatment on the basis of the pharmacokinetic properties.

References

1. Belt van de H, Neut D, Uges DR et al (2000) Surface roughness, porosity and wettability of gentamicin-loaded bone cements and their antibiotic release. Biomaterials 21(19):1981–1987
2. Bengtson S, Knutson K (1991)The infected knee arthroplasty. A 6-year follow-up of 357 cases. Acta Orthop Scand 62(4):301–311
3. Buchholz HW, Gartmann HD (1972) Infektionsprophylaxe und operative Behandlung der schleichende tiefen Infektion bei der Totalen Endoprothese. Chirurg (43):446–453
4. Dreesmann H (1886) Über Knochenplombirung. Zentralbl Chir (20):55–56
5. Espehaug B, Engesaeter LB, Vollset SE et al (1997). Antibiotic prophylaxis in total hip arthroplasty. Review of 10,905 primary cemented total hip replacements reported to the Norwegian arthroplasty register, 1987 to 1995. J Bone Joint Surg (Br) 79(4):590–595
6. Greene N, Holtom PD, Warren CA et al (1988) In vitro elution of tobramycin and vancomycin polymethylmethacrylate beads and spacers from Simplex and Palacos. Am J Orthop 27(3):201–205
7. Joseph TN, Chen AL, Di Cesare PE (2003) Use of antibiotic-impregnated cement in total joint arthroplasty. J Am Acad Orthop Surg 11(1):38–47. Review
8. Löhr W (1934) Die Behandlung der akuten und der chronische Osteomyelitis der Röhrenknochen mit dem Lebertrangips. Arch Klin Chir (180):206–222
9. Penner MJ, Duncan CP, Masri BA. (1999) The in vitro elution characteristics of antibiotic-loaded CMW and Palacos-R bone cements. J Arthroplasty 14(2):209–214
10. Schurman DJ, Trindade C, Hirshman HP et al (1978) Antibiotic-acrylic bone cement composites. Studies of gentamicin and Palacos. J Bone Joint Surg (Am) 60(7):978–984
11. Seeley SK, Seeley JV, Telehowski P et al (2004) Volume and surface area study of tobramycin-polymethylmethacrylate beads. Clin Orthop Relat Res (420):298–303
12. Simpson PM, Dall GF, Breusch SJ et al (2005) In vitro elution and mechanical properties of

antibiotic-loaded SmartSet HV and Palacos R acrylic bone cements. Orthopade 34(12): 1255–1262

13. Sorensen TS, Sorensen AI, Merser S (1990) Rapid release of gentamicin from collagen sponge. In vitro comparison with plastic beads. Acta Orthop Scand 61(4):353–356
14. Wahlig H, Dingeldein E (1980) Antibiotics and bone cements. Acta Orthop Scand 51(1):49–56
15. Wahlig H, Dingeldein E, Bergmann R et al (1978) The release of gentamicin from polymethylmethacrylate beads. An experimental and pharmacokinetic study. J Bone Joint Surg (Br) 60(2):270–275
16. Wahlig H, Schliep HJ, Bergmann R et al (1972) Über die Freisetzung von Gentamycin aus Polmethylmethacrylat. II. Experimentelle Untersuchungen in vivo. Langenbecks Arch Chir 331(3):193–212
17. Walenkamp G (1989) Small PMMA beads improve gentamicin release. Acta Orthop Scand 60(6):668–669
18. Walenkamp GHIM (1983) Gentamicin PMMA beads. A clinical, pharmacokinetic and toxicological study. Thesis University Nijmegen. 164 pages. ISBN 90–9000470-X
19. Witso E, Persen L, Loseth K et al (1999) Adsorption and release of antibiotics from morselized cancellous bone. In vitro studies of 8 antibiotics. Acta Orthop Scand 70(3):298–304
20. Witso E, Persen L, Loseth K et al (2000) Cancellous bone as an antibiotic carrier. Acta Orthop Scand 71(1):80–84

Clinical Applications: Hip

The Management of Infection in THA: A Historical Perspective

W. Petty

University of Florida, Gainesville, Florida USA

Introduction

Except for death and major vascular or neural injury, infection is the most feared complication associated with total hip replacement. Today, infection is uncommon but it is nonetheless of major concern because of the high monetary and personal cost required to resolve the complication.

In Charnley's reports of complications of low friction arthroplasty (LFA) performed by him, he indicated that the only appropriate treatment for infection was converting these hips to pseudoarthrosis. Though Charnley was opposed to replacement of previously infected hip arthroplasty prostheses, he reported good results when treating ancient septic arthritis with LFA and in patients who had infection in their opposite hip [7, 12].

Incidence and Prevention of Infection

In the early history of total hip replacement, without antibiotics or environmental control, the infection rate was disturbingly high, up to 11 percent (Table 1) [33]. When antibiotics began to be administered shortly before and for a brief time after surgery, the average infection rate for several series was reduced to 1.3 percent (Table 2) [33]. In contemporary series, the infection rate was 0.7 percent with the use of "clean" rooms when antibiotics were not added and 0.6 percent when antibiotics were added (Tables 3 and 4) [33]. The combination of an operating room with ultraviolet light and antibiotic administration resulted in an infection rate of 1.0 percent (Table 5) [33]. The difference in infection rates with the regular operating room and no antibiotics versus all other groups was highly statistically significant ($p < 0.001$). The incidence of infection in groups in which operations were performed in a "clean" room, whether or not antibiotics were given, was significantly less than the incidence in other groups ($p < 0.01$) [33].

The efficacy of unidirectional airflow operating rooms in reducing infection rates for total hip replacement was confirmed by Lidwell and associates, and the efficacy of antibiotics has been validated in many studies [21–23, 34]. Infection rates have been especially low in large series of total hip replacements in which both unidirectional airflow and antibiotics were employed. In one series of 659 arthroplasties, the combined early and late infection incidence in procedures performed without structural

Investigators	N° of Cases/Infections	Percent (%)
Charnley	190/13	6.8
Màller	683/27	4.0
Wilson et al	100/11	11.0
Patterson and Brown	368/30	8.2
Benson and Hughes	321/17	5.3
Murray	126/5	4.0
Ritter et al	96/6	6.5
Total	1880/109	5.8

Table 1. Deep infection in regular operating room and without antibiotics

Investigators	N° of Cases/Infections	Percent (%)
Eftakhar et al	800/4	0.5
Fitzgerald	3215/42	1.3
Murray	622/7	1.1
Lowell and Kundsen	621/19	3.1
Leinbach and Barlow	275/4	1.5
Welch et al	150/0	0
Collis and Steinhaus	298/0	0
Irvine et al	167/4	2.4
Bentley and Simmonds	117/2	1.7
Salvati	526/8	1.5
Total	6791/90	1.3

Table 2. Deep infection in regular operating room and with antibiotics

Investigators	N° of Cases/Infections	Percent (%)
Bradley	300/3	0.8
Charnley	2152/12	0.6
Ritter et al	278/3	1.1
Total	2730/18	0.7

Table 3. Deep infections in clean room operating room and without antibiotics

Investigators	N° of Cases/Infections	Percent (%)
Nelson	243/0	0
Irvine et al	107/1	0.9
Welch et al	600/0	0
Leinbach and Barlow	425/3	0.7
Bentley and Simmonds	130/1	0.8
Salvati	1249/12	1.0
Total	2754/17	0.6

Table 4. Deep infections in clean room operating room with antibiotics

Investigators	N° of Cases/Infections	Percent (%)
Lowell and Kundsen	665/5	0.8
Goldner et al	700/8	1.1
Total	1365/13	1.0

Table 5. Deep infections in ultraviolet light operating room and with antibiotics

bone grafts was 0.38 percent in primary operations. No infections were observed in 104 revisions. Infections were much more common when structural grafts were necessary, occurring in 6.8 percent of primary procedures and 3.0 percent of revision operations [42]. In another series of 1007 hip replacements, only 0.2 percent were associated with infections [31]. Another report revealed infections in 0.42 percent of primary arthroplasties and 0.47 percent of revision arthroplasties, for an overall incidence of 0.43 percent in 932 hip replacements [14].

In most series, the incidence of infection has been lower in patients who had primary hip arthroplasties than in patients who had previous surgery, whether total hip arthroplasty or other procedures, such as internal fixation. In one series of 711 hip replacements, the incidence of infection with primary surgery was 1.6 percent, whereas that with secondary surgery was 3.5 percent [34]. Some investigators have reported a relatively high infection rate in patients with rheumatoid arthritis. In one large series of total hip replacement, the overall infection incidence was 0.89 percent, but 1.2 percent of patients with rheumatoid arthritis developed infections [38]. Other risk factors for infection include presence of remote infections at the time of operation, immunosuppression, operative or postoperative complications, and positive culture findings of bacteria from postoperative wound discharge [45].

In the early development of total hip arthroplasty, previous infection in the hip, even if many years before, was considered a contraindication to this procedure [6]. Numerous reports now document that total hip arthroplasty can be performed successfully after previous sepsis, whether associated with hip replacement, another implant, or some other factor. The prognosis is worse if sepsis is active at the time of hip replacement surgery and for certain bacteria, especially Gram-negative organisms [1, 4, 8, 17, 18, 20, 26, 30, 40, 47].

Staphylococci are the bacteria most commonly isolated from infected total hip replacements. In most series, *Staphylococcus epidermidis* is more common than *Staphylococcus aureus*. Gram-negative organisms occur much less commonly but may be more difficult to treat and eradicate, in part because of their antibiotic sensitivity profile. Anaerobes may be the causative infectious agents in total hip arthroplasty, and careful culture techniques for these organisms are essential (Tables 6 and 7) [4, 9, 28]. Less commonly, infections may be associated with atypical mycobacteria and fungi [10, 15]. *Mycobacterium tuberculosis* may cause infection of total joint prosthesis, usually in a patient with previous infection of the hip associated with the

Table 6. Microorganisms isolated from specimens taken at the time of resection arthroplasty

McDonald DJ, Fitzgerald RH Jr., Ilstrup DM (1989) J Bone Joint Surg (Am) 71(6): 828–34
By permission.

Organism	N° of Isolates
Staphylococcus epidermidis	37
Staphylococcus aureus	19
Streptococcus viridans	10
Group-D *Streptococcus*	7
Escherichia coli	4
Proteus mirabilis	3
Pseudomonas aeruginosa	6
Enterobacter	4
Acinetobacter	1
Peptococcus	5
Bacillus ssp.	3
Corynebacterium ssp.	6
Bacteroides ssp.	2
β-hemolytic Streptococcus	2
Propionibacterium acnes	1
No organism isolated	2

Diagnosis	N° of Cases
Staphylococcus epidermidis	17*
Staphylococcus aureus	5*
Pseudomonas aeruginosa	2
Enterobacter	2
Microaerophilic Streptococcus	2
Escherichia coli	1
Propionibacterium acnes	1
Bacteroides fragilis	1*
Staphylococcus epidermidis and enterococcus	1

Table 7. Organisms cultured

* Recurrence
Callaghan JJ, Salvati EA, Brause BD et al (1985) Reimplantation for salvage of the infected hip: rationale for the use of gentamicin-impregnated cement and beads. The Hip. Edited by Robert H. Fitzgerald, Jr. St. Louis, C. V. Mosby Company, 1985. By permission

same organism. Recurrence of infection is reduced by appropriate chemotherapy at the time of and after the hip replacement [19, 41].

Most infections associated with total hip arthroplasty occur when bacteria gain access to the wound at the time of surgery. Infections resulting from hematogenous spread of organisms from remote sites have also been documented [24, 25, 27, 43, 44, 46]. These infections are usually associated with active infection elsewhere in the body. Bacteria from uninfected areas, such as those released during dental work or genitourinary manipulation, are much less common causes of infection in hip replacemtns [43, 46]. Lindquist and Slatis [25] reported three total hip replacements infected with microaerophilic *Streptococcus viridans* following dental procedures. Strazzeria and Anzel [44] reported a hip infection and *Actinomyces israelii*, an organism associated with dental caries and believed to exist almost exclusively in the mouth. This patient had not received antibiotics at the time of a tooth extraction.

These problems emphasize the importance of vigorous antibiotic treatment of any infection and a short course of antibiotic treatment for major dental procedures, genitourinary and bowel manipulations, and similar procedures that are known to cause significant bacteremia in patients who have total joint prostheses. Antibiotic selection is based on the organisms commonly present in the area of manipulation. The medication should be given about 1 hour before the procedure, if taken orally, and closer to the time of the procedure if administered parenterally. An additional oral antibiotic does 4 to 6 hours after the procedure may be wise.

Revision Total Hip Arthroplasty for Septic Failure

When infection occurs, treatment of infection in association with total hip arthroplasty may include 1) suppression of infection with antibiotic therapy, 2) early debridement with retention of the prosthesis, 3) one-stage revision, 4) two-stage revision, 5) resection arthroplasty, and 6) arthrodesis. Suppression with antibiotics is not curative and in many cases these patients eventually have treatment by one of the surgical options. The advantages and disadvantages of resection arthroplasty are well known. This excision arthroplasty often provides a significant reduction in pain but poor and often disabling functional results. Patients are easily fatigued because of weakness of the lower extremity and the increased energy required by the use of external support [2, 16, 29, 35].

One-Stage Exchange Arthroplasty for Septic Total Hip Replacement

Buchholz [3], a pioneer of one-stage exchange, has recommended this procedure as the treatment of choice for most deep infections involving a total hip replacement. The procedure requires excision of soft tissue and removal of the implant and cement. A new prosthesis is implanted immediately, using bone cement that contains antibiotics. Antibiotics are administered intravenously as well. Buchholz reported a 77 percent success rate in 583 patients and a 90 percent success rate when subsequent exchange procedures were performed after failure of the original revision.

Wroblewski [48] recorded a 75-percent success rate with one-stage revision without antibiotics in the cement. He later reported that the addition of gentamicin to the cement in revision surgery for deep infection increased the success rate from 75 to 91 percent [49].

In 1982, Miley, Scheller, and Turner [30] reviewed the results of one-stage reimplantations of 101 infected total hip arthroplasties. An antibiotic cement was used. After a minimum follow-up of 32 months, the infection had resolved in 87 hips.

Harris [13] reported the results of one-stage exchange arthroplasty in 18 patients followed for an average of 42 months. Treatment included antibiotic cement, intravenous antibiotics for 6 weeks, and oral antibiotics for several additional months. The success rate, as measured by the absence of sepsis and excellent functional results, was 78 percent.

Nasser, Lee, and Amstutz [32] reported the results of direct exchange arthroplasty for 30 septic total hip replacements after an average follow-up of 4 years. These direct exchanges were performed in patients who had antibiotic-sensitive organisms and viable soft tissues. Meticulous debridement was carried out to remove all infected implant, including all cement. Appropriate antibiotics, based on preoperative culture results, were placed in the cement in 28 of the 30 cases. On follow-up, all patients demonstrated good pain relief and improvement in function. No evidence of recurrent sepsis was observed. Two reoperations were necessary, both for aseptic loosening. These investigators concluded that direct exchange is an effective method for treatment of sepsis due to Gram-positive organisms.

Balderston and colleagues [1] reported a success rate of 83 percent for revision of infected total hip arthroplasties. Statistically significant negative prognosticators included the number of previous operations, elevated sedimentation rates, and gross infections at the time of surgery. Every conversion to total hip arthroplasty due to infection associated with other hip implants, such as sliding hip screws and other fracture fixation devices, was successful.

Two-Stage Revision of Septic Total Hip Replacement

In the United States, two-stage revision is a more popular treatment for infected total hip arthroplasty than one-stage revision. Reported success rates vary from 60 to 95 percent. Many of the earliest two stage revisions were initiated as resection arthroplasty or pseudoarthrosis as the definitive treatment. Because of poor function often accompanied by pain, courageous surgeons and equally courageous patients decided to attempt conversion of the pseudoarthrosis to another arthroplasty. Because many of these pseudoarthroses had been performed months to years previously, these conversions were difficult. Charnley stated that conversion of pseudoarthrosis to total hip was perhaps the most difficult of all hip arthroplasties that were secondary to previous hip operations.

Early in the history of revision hip arthroplasty for infection, the basic treatment between two stages was pseudoarthrosis. The patient was often placed in traction for at least a portion of the interval between stages. Some surgeons used continuous or intermittent flow of fluid, usually containing antibiotics. However, it was learned that this technique carried the risk of wound contamination with bacteria that were often resistant to antibiotics so the technique was abandoned.

None of the 82 two-stage revisions for infection reported by McDonald and colleagues [28] in 1989 incorporated antibiotics in the cement. Infection recurred in 13 percent of the cases, with an average follow-up of 5.5 years. Three of the seven patients in whom some cement had been left experienced a recurrence of infection. Seven recurrent infections occurred among the 26 patients who had surgery within a year, whereas only four occurred among the 56 patients who had reimplantations more than a year after resection arthroplasty. The conclusion of this study was that a two-stage reconstruction is an effective, safe technique, even when virulent organisms such as Gram-negative bacilli, Group D streptococci, or enterococci cause the infection.

Gustilo and Tsukayama [11] treated 18 patients with removal of the infected implant and thorough surgical debridement, followed by insertion of antibiotic-bone cement beads. Parenteral antibiotics were administered, and cementless revision with autogenous bone graft was performed 6 weeks later. During follow-up, which averaged 19 months, infection recurred in two hips. These preliminary results suggested that a cementless revision is a reasonable alternative to a cemented revision.

Pinto and coworkers [37] evaluated the results of two-stage revision with cementless components in 17 patients managed with resection arthroplasty followed by 4 weeks of parenteral antibiotics. The interval between the first and second stage was 3 months for Gram-positive infections and 12 months for Gram-negative infections. The average Harris hip score was 86 after an average follow-up of 32.1 months. No recurrent infections occurred, and none of the patients required further surgery.

Salvati and colleagues [39] evaluated antibiotic-impregnated cement in both one-stage and two-stage reimplantations. A total of 21 revision arthroplasties were performed in one stage, and eighteen were performed in two stages. The conditions of 32 hips was assessed after 4 years, at which time 22 hips had excellent results, 8 had good results, and 2 had fair results. Three recurrences of infection were reported. Progressive radiolucencies were seen about the acetabulum in 13 percent of the cases, and femoral radiolucencies were seen in 16 percent.

Carlsson and associates [5] described early results in 59 patients who underwent one-stage reimplantations and 18 who under-went two-stage revisions. The interval between the resection and reimplantation in the latter group varied from 2 to 4 months. After follow-up of 6 months to 3 – 1/2 [2] years, five hips that had been treated with one-stage reimplantation were infected and eight were doubtful. Three recurrent infections and one doubtful after the two-stage procedure were noted. The difference between the two groups was not statistically significant.

Local Delivery of Antimicrobial Agents

Systemic administration of antibiotics will deliver bactericidal levels of the agent to the wound, but higher levels may be achieved locally while keeping systemic levels low. This may be especially advantageous with antibiotics with a high potential for toxicity. Antibiotics may be delivered locally to wounds by 1) an irrigation system, 2) an implantable port or infusion pump, or 3) placement in a material, such as bone cement, that is left in the wound. Depot administration of antibiotics released from other materials, including absorbable polymers, is under investigation.

Because prolonged use of closed suction-irrigation systems is generally to be avoided, this is not a suitable method for local delivery of antibiotics. When this technique was used extensively, local levels of antibiotic higher than those achieved with systemic administration could not be maintained without increasing the systemic levels to the toxic range, because of systemic absorption from the wound. The effectiveness of the second option, use of implantable ports and pumps for local administration of antibiotics, has not yet been established.

Experimental studies in animals indicate that antibiotic-bone cement combination is highly effective in preventing infection of implants in wounds contaminated with bacteria [16]. The use of bone cement, both in bulk form and as beads, has been studied extensively for depot administration of antibiotics. All bone cements release most antibiotics studied. Aminoglycosides are preferred for depot administration in bone cement because of their broad spectrum and bactericidal activity, low potential for allergic reactions (none have been reported), thermal stability, and solubility in water. Although usually used for treatment of infections caused by Gram-negative bacteria, aminoglycosides are highly effective against staphylococci and moderately effective against streptococci [4].

Extensive European studies of cement containing an antibiotic, usually an aminoglycoside, for revision of infected total hip arthroplasty (often one-stage revision), yield a success rate ranging from 60 to 90 percent cure of infection [3, 5]. Chains of beads for antibiotic delivery in the wound are placed extensively throughout the wound, including inside the femoral canal. The wound must be closed and suction drainage discontinued as early as feasible to maintain a high concentration of the antibiotic in the wound. Most of the antibiotic is released in the first several days. If the beads are left in the wound for longer than 2 to 3 weeks, they may be difficult to remove because extensive scar tissue forms around them [4].

Surgeons have used hand-made spacers in the operating room, either free form or from molds, for many years in an attempt to maintain space for the subsequent placement of a revision prosthesis. Some have suggested that the spacers made from molds may allow improved function but these spacers are prone to failure when stressed because of their low structural integrity. In addition, because antibiotic is added in the operating room, its distribution in the cement may be irregular leading to inconsistent antibiotic release.

The technique of sterilizing the failed prosthesis and replacing it in the hip joint with cement containing antibiotics has been used by some in an attempt to provide improved function during the interval between stages. Though it does allow for more function between stages, this technique has the disadvantage of high time consumption during the operation and the placement of a foreign body that, though sterile, may include a proteinaceous biofilm that might provide an environment for bacterial growth.

More recent developments for treating hip arthroplasty infections in two stages include preformed antibiotic loaded spacers. These preformed spacers are especially advantageous because of their convenience, structural integrity, and their consistent release of antibiotic.

References

1. Balderston, RA, Hiller WD, Iannotti JP et al (1987) Treatment of the septic hip with total hip arthroplasty. Clin Orthop Relat Res (221):231–237
2. Bourne RB, Hunter GA, Rorabeck CH et al (1984) A six-year follow-up of infected total hip replacements managed by Girdlestone's arthroplasty. J Bone Joint Surg (Br) 66(3):340–343
3. Buchholz HW, Elson RA, Englebrecht E et al (1981) Management of deep infection of total hip replacement. J Bone Joint Surg (Br) 63(3):342–353
4. Callaghan JJ, Salvati EA, Brause BD et al (1985) Reimplantation for salvage of the infected hip: rationale for the use of gentamicin-impregnated cement and beads. the hip. Edited by Robert H. Fitzgerald, Jr. St. Louis, CV Mosby Company, 1985
5. Carlsson AS, Josefsson G, Lindberg L (1978) Revision with gentamicin-impregnated cement for deep infections in total hip arthroplasties. J Bone Joint Surg (Am) 60(8):1059–1064
6. Charnley J (1970) Acrylic Cement in Orthopaedic Surgery. Baltimore, Williams & Wilkins, 1970
7. Charnley J (1972) The long-term results of low-friction arthroplasty of the hip performed as a primary intervention. J Bone Joint Surg (Br) 54(1):61–76
8. Cherney DL, Amstutz HC (1983) Total hip replacement in the previously septic hip. J Bone Joint Surg (Am) 65(9):1256–1265
9. Furno P, Loubert G, Lambin Y et al (1982) Acute primary infection due to slow-growing anaerobes after total hip arthroplasty. Nouv Presse Med. 11(26):1991–3, 1982. (Published in French. Author's transl.)
10. Goodman JS, Seibert DG, Reahl GE Jr et al (1983) Fungal infection of prosthetic joints: a report of two cases. J Rheumatol 10(3):494–495
11. Gustilo RB, Tsukayama D (1998) Treatment of infected cemented total hip arthroplasty with tobramycin beads and delayed revision with the cementless prosthesis and bone grafting. Orthop Trans 12(3):739
12. Hardinge K, Cleary J, Charnley J (1979) Low-friction arthroplasty for healed septic and tuberculous arthritis. J Bone Joint Surg (Br) 61(2):144–147
13. Harris WH (1986) One-stage exchange arthroplasty for septic total hip replacement. Instructional Course Lectures Edited by L. Anderson, St. Louis, CV Mosby, 1986
14. Hill GE, Droller DG (1989) Acute and subacute deep infection after uncemented total hip replacement using antibacterial prophylaxis. Orthop Rev 18(5):617–623
15. Horadam VW, Smilack JD, Smith EC (1982) Mycobacterium fortuitum infection after total hip replacement. South Med J 75(2):244–246
16. Hunter G, Dandy D (1977) The natural history of the patient with an infected total hip replacement. J Bone Joint Surg (Br) 59(3):293–297
17. James ET, Hunter GA, Cameron HU (1982) Total hip revision arthroplasty: Does sepsis influence the results? Clin Orthop Relat Res (170):88–94
18. Jupiter JB, Karchmer AW, Lowell JD et al (1981) Total hip arthroplasty in the treatment of adult hips with current or quiescent sepsis. J Bone Joint Surg (Am) 63(2):194–200

19. Kim YY, Ko CU, Ahn JY et al (1988) Charnley low friction arthroplasty in tuberculosis of the hip. An eight to 13-year follow-up. J Bone Joint Surg (Br) 70(5):756–760
20. Laforgia R, Murphy JC, Redfern TR (1988) Low fiction arthroplasty for old quiescent infection of the hip. J Bone Joint Surg (Br) 70(3):373–376
21. Lidwell OM (181) Airborne bacteria and surgical infection. Am J Med 70(3):693–697
22. Lidwell OM (1982) Infection following orthopaedic surgery in conventional and unidirectional airflow operating theatres: the results of a prospective randomized study. Proceedings of 49th AAOS Meeting, New Orleans, LA
23. Lidwell OM, Lowbury EJ, Whyte W et al (1984) Infection and sepsis after operations for total hip or knee-joint replacement: influence of ultraclean air, prophylactic antibiotics and other factors. J Hyg (Lond) 93(3):505–529
24. Limbird TJ (1985) Hemophilus influenzae infection of a total hip arthroplasty. Clin Orthop Relat Res (199):182–184
25. Lindquist C, Slatis P (1985) Dental bacteremia-a neglected cause of arthroplasty infections? Three hip cases. Acta Orthop Scand 56(6):506–508
26. Lynch M, Esser MP, Shelley P et al (1987) Deep infection in Charnley low-friction arthroplasty. Comparison of plain and gentamicin-loaded cement. J Bone Joint Surg (Br) 69(3):355–360
27. Maniloff G, Greenwald R, Laskin R (1987) Delayed postbacteremic prosthetic joint infection. Clin Orthop Relat Res (223):194–197
28. McDonald DJ, Fitzgerald RH Jr, Ilstrup DM (1989) Two-stage reconstruction of a total hip arthroplasty because of infection. J Bone Joint Surg (Am) 71(6):828–834
29. McElwaine JP, Colville J (1984) Excision arthroplasty for infected total hip replacements. J Bone Joint Surg (Br) 66(2):168–171
30. Miley GB, Scheller AD Jr, Turner RH (1982) Medical and surgical treatment of the septic hip with one-stage revision arthroplasty. Clin Orthop Relat Res (170):76–82
31. Mulier JC, Vandepitte J, Stuyck J et al (1987) Long-term study of the preoperative infection rate in 1007 total hip replacements using prophylactic cefamandole and other precautions. Arch Orthop Trauma Surg 106(3):135–139
32. Nasser S, Lee YF, Amtutz HC (1989) Direct exchange arthroplasty in 30 septic total hip replacements without recurrent infection. Orthop Trans 13(3):519
33. Nelson JP (1977) The operating environment and its influence on deep wound infection. The hip. St. Louis, CV Mosby Company, 1977
34. Nelson JP, Glassburn AR Jr, Talbott RD et al (1980) The effect of previous surgery, operating room environment, and preventive antibiotics on postoperative infection following total hip arthroplasty. Clin Orthop Relat Res (147):167–169
35. Petty W, Goldsmith S (1980) Resection arthroplasty following infected total hip arthroplasty. J Bone Joint Surg 62(6):889–896
36. Petty W, Spanier S, Shuster JJ (1988) Prevention of infection after total joint replacement. Experiments with a canine model. J Bone Joint Surg (Am) 70(4):536–539
37. Pinto MR, Racette JW, Fitzgerald RH (1989) Staged hip reconstruction following infected cemented total hip arthroplasty. Orthop Trans 13(3):612
38. Poss R, Maloney JP, Ewald FC et al (1984) Six- to 11-year results of total hip arthroplasty in rheumatoid arthritis. Clin Orthop Relat Res (182):109–116
39. Salvati EA, Callaghan JJ, Brause BD (1986) Prosthetic reimplantation for salvage of infected hip. Instructional Course Lectures. Edited by L. Anderson. St. Louis, CV Mosby, 1986
40. Salvati EA., Chekofsky KM, Brause BD et al (1982) Reimplantation in infection: a 12-year experience. Clin Orthop Relat Res (170):62–75
41. Santavirta S, Eskola A, Konttinen YT et al (1988) Total hip replacement in old tuberculosis. A report of 14 cases. Acta Orthop Scand 59(4):391–395
42. Schutzer SF, Harris WH (1988) Deep-wound infection after total hip replacement under contemporary aseptic conditions. J Bone Joint Surg (Am) 70(5):724–727
43. Stinchfield FE, Bigliani LU, Neu HC et al (1980) Late hematogenous infection of total joint replacement. J Bone Joint Surg (Am) 62(8):1345–1350
44. Strazzeri JC, Anzel S (1986) Infected total hip arthroplasty due to Actinomyces israelii after dental extraction. A case report. Clin Orthop Relat Res (210):128–131
45. Surin VV, Sundholm K, Backman L (1983) Infection after total hip replacement. With special reference to a discharge from the wound. J Bone Joint Surg (Br) 65(4):412–418

46. Thomas BJ, Moreland JR, Amstutz, H. C (1983) Infection after total joint arthroplasty from distal extremity sepsis. Clin Orthop Relat Res (181):121 – 125
47. Vidal J, Salvan J, Orst G et al (1988) Total hip arthroplasty in the presence of sepsis. Rev Chir Orthop 74(3):223 – 231. (Published in French.)
48. Wroblewski BM (1983) Revision of infected hip arthroplasty. J Bone Joint Surg (Br) 65:224
49. Wroblewski BM (1986) One-stage revision of infected cemented total hip arthroplasty. Clin Orthop Relat Res (211):103 – 107

Girdlestone Arthroplasty after Hip Prosthesis Infection – A Two-stage Revision

S. Tohtz

Department of Orthopaedics, Charité-Standort Mitte, Berlin, Germany

Introduction

The most common complication of joint replacement is an aseptic loosening followed by prosthetic joint infection. The infrequent complication of prosthetic joint infection occurs with a frequency ranging from 0 % to 15 % [11]. The mortality rate associated with a deep prosthetic infection is estimated to be 2.7 % – 18 % [1, 9].

The principle treatment can be divided into four procedures [4]. 1) Antibiotic therapy without any surgical intervention: there is a low rate of success with this treatment combined with the necessity of prolonged antibiotic administration. This treatment should be reserved for patients which are not candidates for surgical removal of the implant. 2) Definitive resection arthroplasty (girdlestone situation) combined with an antibiotic treatment: the results are acceptable for treating the infection but the patients are limited in their function. This procedure is recommended in cases of recurrent infections, and in patients who are not considered ambulators. 3) Surgical debridement with retention of the prosthesis and long-term antibiotic therapy: this procedure can be chosen in the early postoperative infections (2 – 3 weeks) with an organism that is non-virulent. 4) Surgical revision with an exchange of the hip prosthesis in combination with systemic and/or local antibiotic therapy. The most common procedure is a single- or two-stage revision, both with acceptable results [6, 12].

Diagnosing the infection preoperatively requires the use of clinical, radiologic and hematologic assessment as well as an aspiration biopsy from the involved joint. An intraoperative biopsy of the periprothetic interface membrane for microbiological and histopathological analysis is taken to determine the organism and determine the antibiotic treatment prior to the second stage of reimplantation.

Material and Methods

From 01/2005 to 12/2005 we performed a revision hip surgery secondary to a periprosthetic joint infection in 22 patients (14 female, 8 male). Joint fluid was aspirated from all patients before revision and investigated for organisms by bacteriologic culture (duration of 14 days). In 15 hips a periprosthetic joint infection was present with a loose implant, in 7 joints a removal of a well fixed implant was necessary. During the first revision (removal of the septic prosthesis, osseous and soft tissue debridement)

Type	Infectious grading
I	Periprosthetic membrane of the wear particle induced type
II	Periprosthetic membrane of the infectious type
III	Periprosthetic membrane of the combined type (I/II)
IV	Periprosthetic membrane of the indeterminate type

Table 1. Histopathological consensus classification of the periprosthetic interface membrane [6]

tissue samples from the neocapsule and interface membrane were retrieved and bacteriological cultures and histopathological grading performed (Table 1).

Depending on the status of the infection, the bacterial identification and histological data as well as the patient's clinical evaluation, a two-stage revision or a definitive girdlestone operation was performed. A second aspiration culture of joint fluid was performed in patients with a planned reimplantation and was completed one week after the end of antibiotic treatment (culture duration: two weeks). Reconstruction was only considered if aspiration material from the joint was microbiologically sterile, radiographs showed normal findings and the laboratory parameters C-reactive protein (CRP), leukocytes blood count and erythrocyte sedimentation rate (ESR) were normal. Cemented, cementless or augments were utilized based on the amount of bone stock that remained at the time of reimplantation of a revision prosthesis.

Results

Aspiration performed preoperatively gave true positive results in 72.7 % (n = 16) and false negative in 27.3 % (n = 6), in soft tissue culture the true positive values reached 81.8 % (n = 18), the false negative values 18.2 % (n = 4). A high corresponding level of histopathological findings could be registered.

In 2005 a two stage revision was performed in 13 patients. In one case a preformed spacer was used, but because of a persistent infection a second revision was necessary and a definitive solution was not realized yet. In eight patients a girdlestone procedure was done. In two cases of them a two-stage revision was possible and completed in the following year, in six patients a definitive girdlestone hip was preferred (Table 2).

Recurrence of infection was observed in three patients (two girdlestone hips, one patient with a cement spacer).

Antibiotic treatment after revision surgery lasted 4 to 12 weeks.

Mean follow-up from reimplantation/definitive girdlestone up to clinical and radiological evaluation was 12 months (6–18).

The evaluation of the plain radiographs of the 13 patients who had a revision arthroplasty revealed periarticular ossification according to Brooker [2] in 4 cases: grade I in 2 (15.4 %) and grade II in 2 (15.4 %) patients. No cases of grade III or IV were observed. Loosening due to progressive migration of the implants was not seen in the short follow-up.

In these 13 patients, the remaining difference in leg length on the affected side was –0.8 cm (range –4.5 to +2.5). The Merle d'Aubigné score improved from 6.2 (range 3–15; median 6) points at the time of the girdlestone situation to 9.9 (range 6–17; median 10) points at the control after reconstruction. The HHS increased from 28.9 (range 4.7–74.1) to 46.9 points (range 13.9–81.7; median 48).

Table 2. Cumulative data of revision arhroplasty

No.	Diagnosis (N° of previous operations)	Joint fluid aspiration	Soft tissue culture	Histo-pathol. grading	Antibiotics	Surgical procedure
1	periprosthetic joint infection [PJI] (2)	Negative	β-haem. strept. (B) S.capitis S.haemoliticus	II	amp/sulbact ciproflox	two-stage-revision
2	PJI (4)	Negative	S. epidermidis S. aureus	II	clindamycin	two-stage-revision
3	PJI (1)	Negative	S. aureus	II	clindamycin	two-stage-revision
4	PJI (1)	Negative	S. epidermidis	IV	clindamycin	two-stage-revision
5	PJI (2)	S. epidermidis	Negative	I	amp/sulbact	two-stage-revision
6	PJI (1)	S. epidermidis	S. epidermidis	II	clindamycin linezolid	two-stage-revision
7	PJI (2)	Gram(+) cocci	Negative	IV	amp/sulbact	two-stage-revision
8	PJI (3)	Gram(+) cocci	E. coli	IV	ciproflox ampicillin	two-stage-revision
9	PJI (2)	Negative	S. aureus	IV	clindamycin	two-stage-revision
10	PJI (1)	S. epidermidis	S. epid.	IV	vancomycin rifampicin	two-stage-revision
11	PJI (1)	S. aureus	S. aureus	II	vancomycin rifampicin	two-stage-revision
12	Girdlestone (2)	S. aureus[a]	S. aureus[a]	II	vancomycin rifampicin	two-stage-revision
13	Girdlestone (2)	S. aureus[a]	S. aureus[a]	II	vancomycin rifampicin	two-stage-revision
14	PJI (12)	P. aeruginosa	P. aeruginosa	II	ciproflox gentamicin	spacer (Cemex®)
15	PJI (2)	E. coli	Negative	I	amp/sulbact	girdlestone[b]
16	PJI (2)	E. faecalis	E. faecalis	II, IV	moxifloxacin clindamycin	girdlestone
17	PJI (2)	KNS E. faecalis	KNS E. faecalis	II	clindamycin	girdlestone[b]
18	PJI (6)	P. mirabilis S. aureus E. coli	P. mirabilis S. aureus E. coli P. aeruginosa K. pneumoniae	III	vancomycin rifampicin	girdlestone[d]
19	PJI (1)	S. aureus	S. aureus	II	vancomycin rifampicin	girdlestone[d]
20	PJI (5)	β-haem. strept. (B) MRSA	β-haem. strept. (B) MRSA	II, IV	vancomycin rifampicin	girdlestone[b,d]
21	PJI (1)	S. aureus	Negative	II	clindamycin	girdlestone
22	PJI (3)	Negative	E. faecalis	II	amp/sulbact	girdlestone[c]

[a] bacterial species before/during explantation and debridement
[b] final solution because of general diseases
[c] final solution because of neoplasm/metastasis
[d] final solution because of multi-resistant bacterial spectrum

The use of walking aids was necessary in all cases of girdlestone situation and in one patient using a preformed spacer (9) and in 10 patients after two-stage-revision, 3 patients were able to walk without any walking aid.

Discussion

Revision of septic hip prosthesis with implant removal in one- or two-stage is the most common solution adpoted for the treatment of chronic infection. One-staged revision may be considered for patients without additional chronic disease, good vascularization of soft tissue and bones and bacteria susceptible to antibiotics [10]. Two-stage revision offers the advantage to postpone in a delayed stage, once infection has been eradicated, the choice of the type of reimplantation [12]. Over the last ten years, two-stage revision together with the use of antibiotic-loaded cement spacers has been increasingly used with infection eradication rate exceeding 90 % [5].

The present study shows that a periprosthetic joint infection can be revised without local application of antibiotics to the infected area using a two stage procedure.

The lack of of negative microbiological results due to aspiration or soft tissue culture is often caused by antibiotic treatment in the beginning of clinical symptoms. The higher sensitivity of soft tissue culture of the interface membrane and the histopathological grading gives a sufficient support to decide about the therapeutical management in a two-stage revision.

The reinfection rate can be minimized using an algorithm consist of microbiological and histopathological assessment combined with a surgical and well defined antibiotic treatment. We are using this procedure since more than two years with demontrated satisfying early results.

The usage of allogene bone material is only applicable in an infectionless stage. With a two stage procedure we are able to avoid revision implants in some cases of bone stock deficiency performing an allogene bone grafting of the acetabulum or using a structured bone graft for reconstruction of the proximal femur. It has been described that a successful bone augmentation in a postinfected stage is possible [6].

Our first results demonstrate the minor relevance of local application of antibiotic loaded spacers or beads in two-stage revision of septic THA and underline the significance of radical surgical debridement for successful therapy. Other techniques like the usage of a custom-made or a preformed spacer are possible [7, 8] but the presented technique is simple, cost-efficient and shows comparable efficacy to the current standard.

References

1. Berbari EF, Hanssen AD, Duffy MC (1998) Risk factors for prosthetic joint infection: case-control study. Clin Infect (5):1247–1254
2. Brooker AF, Bowerman JW, Robinson RA et al (1973) Ectopic ossification following total hip replacement. Incidence and a method of classification. J Bone Joint Surg Am 55(8):1629–1632
3. D'Angelo F, Negri L, Zatti G et al (2005) Two-stage revision surgery to treat an infected hip implant. A comparison between a custom-made spacer and a preformed one. Chir Organi Mov 90(3):271–279
4. Frommelt L (2006) Principles of systemic antimicrobial therapy in foreign material associated infection in bone tissue, with special focus on periprosthetic infection. Injury 37(Suppl 2):87–94
5. Hsieh PH, Shih CH, Chang YH et al (2004) Two stage revision hip arthroplasty for infection: comparison between the interim use of antibiotic-loaded cement beads and a spacer prosthesis. J Bone Joint Surg (Am) 86(9):1989–1997

6. Kordelle J, Frommelt L, Kluber D, Seemann K (2000) Results of one-stage endoprosthesis revision in periprosthetic infection cause by methicillin-resistant Staphylococcus aureus. Z Orthop 138(3):240–244
7. Morawietz L, Classen RA, Schroder JH et al (2006) Proposal for a histopathological consensus classification of the periprosthetic interface membrane. J Clin Pathol 59(6):591–597
8. Nusem I, Morgan DA (2006) Structural allografts for bone stock recontruction in Two-stage revision for infected total hip arthroplasty: good outcome in 16 of 18 patients followed for 5–14 years. Acta Orthop 77(1):92–97
9. Powers KA, Terpenning MS, Voice RA et al (1990) Prosthetic joint infections in the elderly. AM J Med 88(5N):9N-13N.
10. Sofer D, Regenbrecht B, Pfeil J (2005) Early results of one-stage septic revision arthroplasties with antibiotic-laden cement. A clinical and statistical analysis. Orthopade 34(6):592–602
11. Steckelberg JM, Osmon DR (2000) Prosthetic joint infection. In Bisno A, Waldvogel F, eds. Infections associated with indwelling devices. Washington, DC: American Society for Mikrobiology, 2000:173–209
12. Volin SJ, Hinrichs SH, Garvin KL (2004) Two-stage reimplantation of total joint infections: a comparison of resistant and non-resistant organisms. Clin Orthop Relat Res (427):94–100

22 One-stage Non-cemented Revision of Septic Hip Prosthesis Using Antibiotic-loaded Bone Graft

H. Winkler, A. Stoiber

Osteitis Center Privatklinik Döbling, Wien, Austria
Orthopaedic Department, Weinviertel Klinikum, Schwerpunktkrankenhaus Mistelbach, Austria

Introduction

Total hip replacement (THR) has revolutionized orthopaedic surgery. Each year millions of traumatic, inflammatory or degenerative hip joint lesions favourably are treated with THR worldwide. Although meanwhile a routine procedure, infections inevitably occur in a certain percentage of interventions, depending from a variety of accompanying circumstances. Today, the risk of infection for primary THR is estimated around 1 %, in revision cases it may rise up to 20 %. It may be expected that the real number is even higher since detection of infection not always is feasible [4, 11, 13]. The absolute number of patients with infection continuously increases as the number of patients requiring THR and revisions grows.

Treatment of infected THR most frequently includes removal of the implant and long-term antimicrobial treatment with re-implantation after all signs of infection have ceased. Such cases still are considered a disaster, both for the patient and for the treating team. Reasons for the difficulties in treatment include the specific adherence of bacteria to foreign material [8] and the poor penetration of antibiotics into infected osseous sites. After removal of necrotic bone the remaining defects must be filled. Leaving the dead space would result in early re-infection and diminished mechanical stability.

Dead space management therefore represents one critical point of septic surgery. For filling the defects bone grafts would be most advisable, since they may restore bone stock and grant immediate mechanical support. However, usual grafts can only be applied several weeks after debridement when all signs of infection have ceased. Otherwise the non-vital grafts immediately would become re-colonised with remaining bacteria.

To overcome the inferior performance of systemic application in bone infections local administration of antibiotics has been in use since long. Major concern of studies investigating locally applied antibiotics has been efficacy against bacteria as well as compatibility with surrounding tissue. Among all tested antibiotics vancomycin has been suggested as most suitable, since it provides bactericidal activity against the most relevant germs and shows the least cytotoxic effect against growing osteoblasts [5, 10]. As another excellent option for local application aminoglycosides are in clinical use since several years and have proven efficacy and good compatibility with vital tissue [9]. For local application of the antibiotics a carrier with good storage capacity is needed.

Bone cement (Polymethylmetacrylate, PMMA) is most widely evaluated as an antibiotic carrier. It provides dead space management as well as prolonged release of antibiotics and therefore is in use in one stage procedures since more than 30 years [1]. However, several possible disadvantages must be taken into account: 1. there is no restoration of bone stock, 2. sclerotic bone, which is present in most revision cases, does not interconnect properly with PMMA, 3. in case of failure the consecutive revision is rather difficult since the cement must be removed again, 4. the "empty" carrier may act as bed for new colonization with surviving selected bacteria [12]. These concerns certainly are some of the reasons, why this approach did not gain widespread popularity.

To overcome the disadvantages of cement uncemented implants and biological carriers have been suggested as an alternative. Cancellous bone shows a large surface after purification on which antibiotics can adhere. Witso et al. have shown, that several antibiotics may be stored and released by allograft bone [18, 19]. The same group has used netilmicin in combination with allografts for reconstruction in revision hip arthroplasty and found no adverse effects [17]. Buttaro at al. favorably used vancomycin impregnated grafts for reconstruction after infected THR [3]. Although concentration in the postoperative drainage fluid was extremely high they did not observe any adverse effects, neither systemically nor in graft incorporation [2]. However, both groups have used the grafts only in the second stage of a two stage revision after resolution of clinical, laboratory and radiological evidence of sepsis.

Our own *in vitro* studies, using a proprietary impregnation technique, revealed high initial concentrations of antibiotics in areas adjacent to antibiotic impregnated grafts with a prolonged release for several weeks [16]. The aim of our study was to investigate the performance of these compounds under the conditions of florid infection together with uncemented implants.

Material and Methods

Between 1998 and 2004, 37 patients with culture proven deep infection of a THR were treated using a standardized protocol. Loose implants were removed and meticulous excision of all PMMA, granulation, necrotic and infected tissue was performed. Cleaning was finalized using intensive pulsed lavage with saline. The cleaned sites were evaluated for bone deficiencies and consecutively filled with antibiotic impregnated bone graft.

The grafts originated from cadaveric donors, procured following the protocols of the European Association of Tissue Banks [6]. The retrieved cancellous parts were morsellized to granules with a diameter between 2 and 6 mm and cleaned thoroughly from marrow and adhering soft tissue leaving intact structures of bone matrix and mineral content. The bone was impregnated with high loads of antibiotic, using a specific incubation technique [16].

There were two options of antibiotic impregnation: vancomycin or tobramycin, the choice being dependent on the causative pathogen isolated. Vancomycin was used in all cases, combinations with tobramycin in cases of mixed infections. The impregnation procedure produced an antibiotic-bone compound (ABC) with high levels of antibiotic inside the graft: For vancomycin levels were in the range of 100 mg per 1 cc

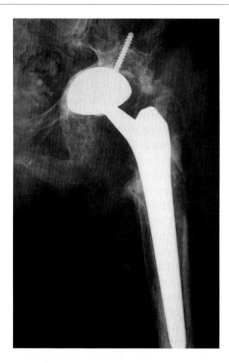

Fig. 1. Antibiotic bone compound (ABC) ventrally and dorsally of a Zwey-mueller stem and in the acetabulum

of bone, for tobramycin in the range of 75 mg per 1 cc. On average an amount of 80 cc of ABC was used per case (range: 30 to 150 cc). After gross preparation ABC was filled into cavities using a modified technique of impaction grafting [7, 14] followed by preparation of the bone for the insertion of chosen implants. All prosthetic implants were anchored following the principles of press-fit fixation without additional use of cement.

The choice of the respective implants was dependent from the amount of accompanying bone defects, in uncomplicated cases a hemispheric cup was preferred in combination with a rectangular diameter stem. Fixation intraoperatively was qualified as stable in all cases. After insertion of the implant ABC was placed around eventually uncovered parts, in special ventrally and dorsally of the proximal parts of the stem (Fig. 1). Wounds were drained for three days and closed immediately. Perioperative antibiotic treatment consisted of second generation cephalosporines intravenously for two weeks. Postoperatively levels of vancomycin were monitored both in the drainage fluid and in serum.

Cultures taken intraoperatively revealed growth of coagulase-negative staphylococci (18x), *Staphylococcus aureus* (11x), methicillin-resistant *S. aureus* (MRSA) (4x), enterococci (9x) and other Gram-positive pathogens (3x), respectively. In 6 hips Gram-negative germs were found additionally. All of them were susceptible for either vancomycin or tobramycin or both. Postoperative mobilisation did not differ from non-septic surgery. Patients were evaluated clinically and radiographically 2 weeks, 6 weeks, 3 months, 6 months and one year after surgery and then annually. Laboratory data were collected the same time and included CRP, ESR, blood count, urea and creatinine.

Results

Postoperative serum levels of vancomycin were between 0 and 3.9 µg/ml with a median of 0.2 µg/ml. Vancomycin level in the drainage fluid were between 8 and 2243 µg/ml with a median of 345 µg/ml. Wound healing was uneventful in all cases. No adverse side effects could be observed during the whole follow up period, in special renal function did not show any difference compared to preoperative values. Mean hospital stay was 16 days (10 – 32 days). Rehabilitation was in the range of uncomplicated primary surgery in cases with short history of infection (up to 3 months) and prolonged in relation to duration of infection and amount of preceding surgery.

All patients could be followed with a minimum of 2 years and a maximum of 8 years (mean 4,1 years). 35 patients showed no sign of infection until the last follow up. In two hips there was recurrence of infection, diagnosed 6 and 12 weeks after surgery respectively. In one of them the well fixed stem had not been exchanged, in another one a technical error during impregnation of the bone graft could be evaluated. Both could be successfully re-operated using the same technique with complete removal of implants and appropriately impregnated bone graft.

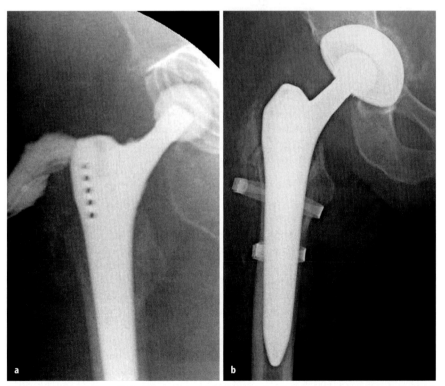

Fig. 2. a Infection of a well fixed uncemented THR (Fistulography). **b** Postoperative radiograph showing ABC at the medial aspect of the acetabular component and the proximal part of the femoral component

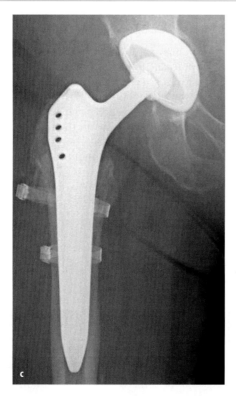

Fig. 2c. 6 years later partial resorption in unloaded areas is visible, remaining parts of the allograft are well incorporated. Lucent lines in Gruen zone 2 and 3 but no dislocation and no clinical sign of loosening or infection

Radiologically we could observe partial resorption of allograft bone in non-weight-bearing areas and intramedullarily (Figs. 2a – c). Incorporation of the allografts appeared normal compared to conventional grafting. There was no sign of loosening in any of the implants or dislocation of bone fragments.

Discussion

To our knowledge this is the first report on the use of antibiotic impregnated bone grafts in the treatment of infected THR in a single stage procedure. It must be emphasized that ABC can only be considered as one tool in a complex treatment protocol consisting of 1. complete removal of all foreign material, 2. meticulous debridement of the infected site, 3. complete dead space management with allograft bone, 4. stable fixation of new implants and 5. adequate wound coverage. However, to our opinion only sufficient impregnation of the graft with antibiotics makes such a protocol feasible.

So far impregnated bone grafts have been used clinically only as a more or less prophylactic tool since it has been used in patients with high risk but without any sign of florid infection. Buttaro's group added 500 mg of vancomycin powder to one morsel-lized femoral head, which may be estimated to represent a volume of roughly 50 cc cancellous bone. Similar techniques and concentrations were used by Witso et al. Both groups found similar levels of antibiotic in the drainage fluid as we did in our series. However, we could show that with our technique an amount of 5 g vancomycin may be incorporated in the same amount of bone graft, which represents about the ten-fold concentration. The reason for the comparable concentration in drainage fluids and serum in our opinion is, that drainage fluid can be monitored only for a few days until drainage is discontinued. During that time vancomycin is released in the same pattern, independent from the impregnation technique.

We believe that this "burst release" is finished after several days. This pattern of release seems to be sufficient in cases where no florid infection or only a low bioburden is present. Florid infections in our opinion require a more prolonged release that should maintain antibiotic levels above the MIC for several weeks. This requirement seems to be fulfilled with our impregnation technique, which provides a double pattern release: the same amount of antibiotic seems to be released immediately, as in the other series, however, this amount represents only about 10 % of the total implanted dosage. An additional 9-fold amount shall be released slowly within a period between 2 and 8 weeks after surgery. These consistent levels protect both the graft and the implant against recolonisation even in highly contaminated areas during the time of release and at the same time may help in eradicating remaining bacterial colonies. Only under these circumstances one stage revision seems to be justified.

Although very high concentrations of antibiotic were present at the operative site we did not see any adverse effects. Systemic effects seem to be avoided by the poor penetration of vancomycin between blood stream and tissue. This property always has been considered a disadvantage when vancomycin was administered intravenously. In our application the disadvantage turns into an advantage, because vice versa there is also poor penetration from the tissue into the vascular system which avoids quick removal of the antibiotic from the implant site, keeping serum levels low and tissue levels high. Local wound healing and remodeling of the graft seem not to be impaired due to the low cytotoxic property of vancomycin and tobramycin respectively.

Some authors criticize local application of antibiotics since they fear induction of resistencies. We believe this fear is not justified in our application. Moreover the opposite seems to be true: resistencies are created by sub-inhibitory concentrations of antibiotics as they are common in infected bone during systemic antibiotic therapy. The extremely high concentrations after local application leave no chance for bacteria to survive or even develop resistance. Development of small colony variants or similar phenotypes as created by antibiotic loaded cement [12] is unlikely since in contrast to PMMA the grafts release all the incorporated antibiotic load within several weeks while about 90 % of antibiotics inside PMMA stay there forever and are only released in subinhibitory amounts whenever cracks appear in the aging cement.

Although there are not yet significant numbers of cases and a rather short follow up period, it seems, that one stage non-cemented revision in combination with ABC provides an excellent tool in the treatment of infected THR. However, several principles need to be observed. In addition to the described protocol we now recommend removing even well fixed prostheses and taking care, that at least 50 cc of well impregnated bone graft is implanted.

Since we have found that intraoperatively taken cultures sometimes reveal growth of bacteria that have not been found in the preoperative aspirate, we now always use vancomycin and tobramycin in combination, such covering also potentially undetected Gram-negative germs and taking advantage of the synergistic effect of the two antibiotics [15].

Following the described principles eradication of pathogens, grafting of bony defects and re-insertion of an uncemented implant may be accomplished in a one stage procedure. Since the graft gradually is replaced by healthy own bone, improved conditions may be expected for the long term performance and especially in the case of another revision.

References

1. Buchholz HW, Elson RA, Engelbrecht E et al (1981) Management of deep infection of total hip replacement. J Bone Joint Surg (Br) 63(3):342–353
2. Buttaro MA, Gimenez MI, Greco G et al (2005) High active local levels of vancomycin without nephrotoxicity released from impacted bone allografts in 20 revision hip arthroplasties. Acta Orthop 76(3):336–340
3. Buttaro MA, Pusso R, Piccaluga F (2005) Vancomycin-supplemented impacted bone allografts in infected hip arthroplasty. Two-stage revision results. J Bone Joint Surg (Br) 87(3):314–319
4. Costerton W (2005) Biofilm theory can guide the treatment of device-related orthopaedic infections. Clin Orthop Relat Res (437):7–11. Review
5. Edin ML, Miclau T, Lester GE et al (1996) Effect of cefazolin and vancomycin on osteoblasts in vitro. Clin Orthop Relat Res (333):245–251
6. European Association of Tissue Banks, European Association of Muskulosceletal Transplantation (1999) Common Standards for Musculo Skeletal Tissue Banking. Vienna: Oebig Transplant
7. Gie GA, Linder L, Ling RS et al (1993) Contained morselized allograft in revision total hip arthroplasty. Surgical technique. Orthop Clin North Am 24(4):717–725
8. Gristina AG (1987) Biomaterial-centered infection: microbial adhesion versus tissue integration. Science 237(4822):1588–1595
9. Miclau T, Edin ML, Lester GE et al (1995) Bone toxicity of locally applied aminoglycosides. J Orthop Trauma 9(5):401–406
10. Miclau T, Edin ML, Lester GE et al (1998) Effect of ciprofloxacin on the proliferation of osteoblast-like MG-63 human osteosarcoma cells in vitro. J Orthop Res 16(4):509–512
11. Nelson CL, McLaren AC, McLaren SG et al (2005) Is aseptic loosening truly aseptic? Clin Orthop Relat Res (437):25–30
12. Neut D, van de Belt H, Stokroos I et al (2001) Biomaterial-associated infection of gentamicin-loaded PMMA beads in orthopaedic revision surgery. J Antimicrob Chemother 47(6):885–891
13. Neut D, van Horn JR, van Kooten TG et al (2003) Detection of biomaterial-associated infections in orthopaedic joint implants. Clin Orthop Relat Res (413):261–268
14. Schimmel J, Buma P, Versleyen D et al (1998) Acetabular reconstruction with impacted morselized cancellous allografts in cemented hip arthroplasty: a histological and biomechanical study on the goat. J Arthroplasty 13(4):438–448
15. Watanakunakorn C, Tisone JC (1982) Synergism between vancomycin and gentamicin or tobramycin for methicillin-susceptible and methicillin-resistant Staphylococcus aureus strains. Antimicrob Agents Chemother 22(5):903–905
16. Winkler H, Janata O, Berger C et al (2000) In vitro release of vancomycin and tobramycin from impregnated human and bovine bone grafts. J Antimicrob Chemother 46(3):423–428
17. Witso E, Persen L, Benum P et al (2004) High local concentrations without systemic adverse effects after impaction of netilmicin-impregnated bone. Acta Orthop Scand 75(3):339–346
18. Witso E, Persen L, Loseth K et al (1999) Adsorption and release of antibiotics from morselized cancellous bone. In vitro studies of 8 antibiotics. Acta Orthop Scand 70(3):298–304
19. Witso E, Persen L, Loseth K et al (2000) Cancellous bone as an antibiotic carrier. Acta Orthop Scand 71(1):80–84

Two-stage Revision of Infected Total Hip Arthroplasty. Comparison Between a Custom-made and a Preformed Spacer

F.A. Grassi, F. D'Angelo, G. Zatti, P. Cherubino

Department of Orthopaedics and Traumatology "Mario Boni", University of Insubria, Varese, Italy

Introduction

Infection is one of the most severe complications of joint replacement. The main goals of treatment are eradication of infection and restoration of joint function [9].

Many surgical solutions have been proposed, all relying on components removal and accurate debridement of pathologic tissue [14].

At present, there is not yet a unanimous consent on the best way to treat infection, nonetheless many surgeons prefer to perform two-stage revisions because of the encouraging results reported in literature, with success rates ranging from 87 % to 100 % [6, 7, 9, 12, 13].

Two-stage revision foresees the temporary use of a PMMA spacer impregnated with one or more antibiotics. The spacer exerts a mechanical and a biological function: it avoids the peri-articular soft tissue shortening, keeping the correct limb positioning and it sterilizes the infected areas by means of local antibiotic release [2, 8].

Aim of this study is to compare the results achieved in the treatment of infected total hip arthroplasties (THA) with a two-stage revision, using two different types of spacers: hand-made (Fig. 1) or preformed (Fig. 2).

Materials and Methods

Between 1995 and 2003, 20 patients (10 M, 10 F) underwent a two-stage revision procedure for the treatment of infected THA. The diagnosis of infection was based on clinical and bio-humoral parameters (ESR > 30 mm/h and CRP > 10 mg/l), integrated by imaging studies (X-rays and labelled leucocytes bone scan) and microbiological assays (cultures from draining fistulae) [10].

The mean age of the patients at the time of surgery was 68 years (range 53–74).

The infecting pathogen was *Staphylococcus aureus* (3), *Staphylococcus epidermidis* (2), *Staphylococcus* spp. (2), *Streptococcus pneumoniae* (1), *Streptococcus agalactiae* (1) and *Escherichia coli* (1). Polymicrobial infection was diagnosed in 4 cases: *S. aureus* + *Enterococcus faecalis* (1), *S. aureus* + *Staphylococcus* spp. (3). In the remaining patients the pathogen was not detected.

The therapeutic protocol included a first procedure to remove the components, bone cement and all infected tissues, followed by implantation of the antibiotic-loaded acrylic cement (ALAC) spacer. Systemic antibiotics were administered in

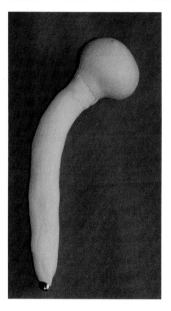 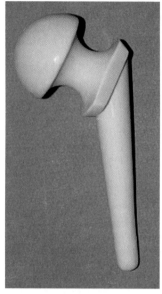

◁◁
Fig. 1. Custom-made spacer: a blade-plate is used to provide mechanical strength

◁
Fig. 2. Preformed spacer (Spacer-G)

accordance to the results of microbiological assays on intraoperative biopsies; therapy lasted a minimum of 4 weeks (range, 4 to 8 weeks).

Patients were evaluated on a monthly basis; normalisation of biohumoral parameters was the condition required for performing the second stage procedure. At this time the spacer was removed and a definitive prosthesis was implanted.

Patient were divided into two groups according to the type of spacer used:

Group A: 8 patients with a custom-made spacer, prepared in the operating room with antibiotic loaded bone cement (Cemex Genta – Tecres Spa, Italy) coating a metal stem so to reproduce an hip prosthesis

Group B: 12 patients with a preformed, industrially manufactured spacer (Spacer-G – Tecres, Italy)

At follow-up, all the patients were evaluated both clinically, using the Harris Hip Score (HHS), and radiographically. A statistical analysis was performed in order to highlight differences between the two groups in terms of duration of operative time, hospitalisation, intra-operative blood loss and clinical results. The level of significance was set at $p < 0.05$.

Results

19 patients were evaluated at an average follow-up of 5 years (range 3 – 10).

The spacer implantation time was on average 6.3 months (2 – 11) for group A and 5.3 months (3 – 13) in Group B.

Table 1

	Group A	Group B
Operatory time 1st st.	164 min (140–210)	127 min (60–180)
Blood loss 1st st.	2112 ml (500–3200)	1618 ml (500–3000)
Operatory time 2nd st.	149 min (105–190)	109 min (55–210)
Blood loss 2nd st.	1416 ml (800–2000)	1587 ml (500–4000)
Hospital stay	20 days (7–44)	13 days (7–28)

No significant differences were observed between the two groups in term of operative time, hospitalisation and blood loss (Table 1). One recurrence of infection was observed in both groups: in Group A, a septic mobilization occurred after 2 months from revision surgery; in Group B, two weeks after spacer implantation, complete slough of the wound along with purulent secretion occurred. Resection-arthroplasty was performed in both cases along with systemic antibiotic treatment.

The observed mechanical complications were as follows:

- in Group A, one dislocation and one breakage of the spacer, one aseptic loosening of the revision stem;
- in Group B, one dislocation of the spacer.

At the latest follow-up, mean Harris Hip Score (HHS) increased from 35 (pre-op) to 76 in Group A and from 43 (pre-op) to 76 in Group B. The differences between pre-op and post-op scores were statistically significant (Student's "t" test for paired data) in both groups.

Discussion

Orthopaedic infection is a costly complication both in human and economic terms. Systemic antibiotic therapy alone is generally not able to eradicate infection, as the concentration required in the infected site is not always achieved due to soft tissue and vascular compromise, and the mechanisms of self-defense of the pathogens [4].

That is why the removal of the infected implant is a mandatory step for the success of the procedure. Revision may be performed in one or two stages. A higher success rate is reported for two-stage revision with the use of a temporary spacer made of antibiotic loaded bone cement associated to systemic antibiotic therapy [6, 8, 12, 13]. Two-stage revision allows the preservation of some joint function, facilitates reimplantation and accelerates rehabilitation after revision surgery [6, 8].

This study compared the results achieved with two different type of spacers in infected THA.

The use of a preformed spacer [8] does not allow the surgeon to choose the antiobiotic-cement mixture according to microbiological data. However, local concentrations of the antibiotic eluted from the spacer are 50 to 100 times higher than those reached after systemic administration: thus an antimicrobial activity, even on resistant germs, can be exerted [5].

The chemical and physical properties of the ALAC spacer should be well defined and reproducible. The standardisation of the manufacturing process reduces the risk of mechanical problems [1] and insufficient drug release, which can derive from mistakes in the preparation of the device. Custom-made spacers are burdened by a higher incidence of mechanical complications [10]. In our series, breakage of one device occurred because the supporting hardware was too thin.

A satisfactory matching between the spacer head and the acetabulum is desirable, in order to provide sufficient joint function, avoid dislocation and preserve bone stock between the two surgical stages. Any incongruence can lead to eccentric loads on contact surfaces, increasing the risk of bone wear and resorption. In our experience, the less satisfying adaptability of custom-made spacers influenced the choice of the acetabular component at revision: an oblong cup was used in 57 % of patients of Group A and only in 18 % of Group B patients.

In conclusion, a two-stage revision procedure with temporary implantation of an ALAC spacer allowed us to achieve a high rate of successful results in the treatment of infected THA. The use of a preformed spacer offers some advantages with respect to custom-made devices: more reproducible mechanical and chemical behaviours, easier implantation, preservation of bone stock [3]. These advantages resulted in a lower incidence of local complications and better functional results.

References

1. Baleani M, Traina F, Toni A (2003) The mechanical behaviour of a preformed hip spacer. Hip International 13(3):159–162
2. Bertazzoni Minelli E, Benini A, Magnan B et al (2004) Release of gentamicin and vancomycin from temporary human hip spacers in two-stage revision of infected arthroplasty. J Antimicrob Chemother 53(2):329–334
3. D'Angelo F, Negri L, Zatti G et al (2005) Two-stage revision surgery to treat an infected hip implant. A comparison between a custom-made spacer and a pre-formed one. Chir Organi Mov 90(3):271–279
4. Ghisellini F, Ceffa R (1997) Manuale atlante di trattamento delle infezioni di protesi articolari e di utilizzo delle miscele di cemento co antibiotici. Roma Ed. Mediprint, 1997
5. Kyung-Hoi Koo, Jin-Won Yang, Se-Hyun Cho et al (2001) Impregnation of vancomycin, gentamicin and cefotaxime in a cement spacer for two-stage cementless reconstruction in infected total hip arthroplasty. J Arthroplasty 16(7):882–892
6. Leunig M, Chosa E, Speck M et al (1998) A cement spacer for two-stage revision of infected implants of the hip joint. Int Orthop 22(4):209–214
7. Lieberman JR, Callaway GH, Salvati EA et al (1994) Treatment of the infected total hip arthroplasty with a two-stage reimplantation protocol. Clin Orthop Relat Res (301):205–212
8. Magnan B, Regis D, Biscaglia R et al (2001) Preformed acrylic bone cement spacer loaded with antibiotics. Use of two-stage procedure in 10 patients because of infected hip after total replacement. Acta Orthop Scand 72(6):591–594
9. McDonald DJ, Fitzgerald RH Jr, Ilstrup DM (1989) Two-stage reconstruction of a total hip arthroplasty because of infection. J Bone Joint Surg (Am) 71(6):828–834
10. Schoellner C, Fuerderer S, Rompe JD et al (2003) Individual bone cement spacer (IBCS) for septic hip revision – preliminary report. Arch Orthop Trauma Surg 123(5):254–259
11. Spangehl MJ, Younger AS, Masri BA et al (1997) Diagnosis of infection following total hip arthroplasty. J Bone Joint Surg (Am) 79(10):1578–1588
12. Younger AS, Duncan CP, Masri BA (1998) Treatment of infection associated with segmental bone loss in the proximal part of the femur in two stages with use of an antibiotic-loaded interval prosthesis. J Bone Joint Surg (Am) 80(1):60–69
13. Younger AS, Duncan CP, Masri BA, McGraw RW. (1997) The outcome of two-stage arthroplasty using a custom-made interval spacer to treat the infected hip. J Arthroplasty 12(6):615–623
14. Zimmerli W, Ochsner PE (2003) Management of infection associated with prosthetic joints. Infection 31(2):99–108

Two-stage Revision of Infected Total Hip Replacement Using a Preformed, Antibiotic-loaded Acrylic Cement Spacer

B. Magnan, D. Regis, A. Costa, P. Bartolozzi

Department of Orthopaedics, University of Verona, Policlinico "GB Rossi", Verona, Italy

Introduction

Infection is one of the most serious local complications of total hip replacement [16, 19, 23, 39, 42]

The observation of meticulous standards of asepsis in operating theatres [11, 37] and the routine application of systemic and topic antibiotic treatments with cemented implants [22, 26, 27] had a significant role in reducing infection rates in recent decades: current case series indicate an incidence of less than 1 % [2, 31, 40].

Nevertheless, the widespread practice of total hip replacement and the subsequent increase in revision surgery mean that infection is still a significant clinical problem, affecting the patient with dramatic consequences [20].

Chronic infection of joint prosthesis requires surgical removal of the implant, in order to eradicate the infective process [13, 42].

Reimplantation of the prosthesis may take place at the same time as surgical removal of the infected device – one-stage revision technique [7, 8, 9, 10, 35], or be delayed – two-stage revision procedure [12, 20, 25, 24, 27, 43, 46]. This option depends on the personal treatment approach, which is often determined by microbiological evaluations.

Two-stage revision technique means reimplantation after a variable interval, 4 up to 8 weeks, during which a temporary antibiotic (AB)-loaded polymethylmethacrylate (PMMA) spacer is usually positioned into the original prosthetic site.

The insertion of such a spacer fulfils two different aims: first a mechanical function, as it can avoid the periarticular soft tissue shortening, keeping correct limb positioning; moreover, a biological function, as it sterilizes the infected areas by means of a local antibiotic release [3, 4, 5, 17, 32, 41, 44].

The extemporary preparation of a spacer in the operating room is not easy because of some difficulties in the realization of an optimal mix of the components and the need of a metal reinforcement which is able to prevent the mechanical failure of the device.

Moreover, it is hard to obtain a shape which can correctly fit into the host bone and achieve a good limb positioning.

The skill of surgeons and the variable morphology of bony segments following removal of pre-existing implant have variously influenced the final shape of the spacer [1, 15, 25, 30, 46]. The shape of the spacer, indeed, has been demonstrated to affect the surgical outcome in two ways: first, it interferes with the antibiotic release, that depends on the correct mix with the cement and on the total surface of the spacer. Moreover, it is correlated to the incidence of complications such as pain, dislocation and limb malposition as they may be subsequent to the possible incongruity of the spacer with the bone and to its mechanical stability.

We evaluated the advantages of a preformed PMMA spacer in different sizes which allows some degree of joint motion and weight-bearing in selected cases, as well as a defined, sustained antibiotic release fitting into the residual bony segments of the infected implant.

Material and Method

The device we employed is called "Spacer-G" and it is manufactured on an industrial scale (Tecres SpA, Italy). The spacer has a central load-bearing structure comprising a hollow cylindrical rod in AISI 316L stainless steel, with a 10 mm maximum diameter, which is fully covered with antibiotic-loaded "Cemex" bone cement (Fig. 1).

In the first 10 cases the spacer was available only in one size: 54 mm head, 180 g in weight, 165 cm^2 in surface. Then additional sizes were added. Currently the spacer is available with head diameters of 46, 54 and 60 mm, with short or long stem.

29 patients with an infected total hip arthroplasty were treated from September 1996 to February 2006. There were 15 males and 14 females, whose age ranged from 58 and 84 years (average 70). The previous prostheses had been implanted minimum 2 and maximum 166 months before (average 54). Intra-operative detection of the

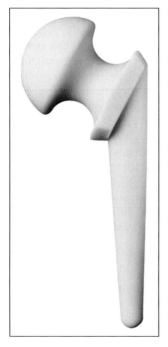

Fig. 1. Spacer-G. The device is manufactured with a central weight-bearing hollow cylindrical rod entirely covered by antibiotic-loaded PMMA

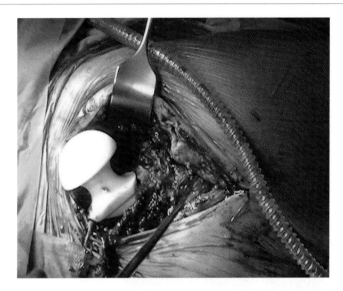

Fig. 2. Spacers were applied in all cases by a lateral approach, requiring an extended trochanteric osteotomy in some selected cases for the removal of an infected long stem

infecting germ was only possible in 8 cases: *Staphylococcus epidermidis* (2), *Staphylococcus aureus* (2), Group-B β-haemolytic *Streptococcus* (1), *Pseudomonas aeruginosa* (1), *Escherichia coli* (1), *Mycobacterium tuberculosis* (1).

Removal of the prosthesis and debridement of the infected periprosthetic tissues were followed by the implantation of an antibiotic-loaded preformed PMMA spacer during the same surgical procedure.

In the first 5 patients, the device was loaded just with gentamicin, widely used in association with bone cement [2, 45], in the overall quantity of 1.9 g.

In the following 24 patients, the PMMA constituting the spacer was supplemented with a 2.5 % concentration of gentamicin and a 2.5 % concentration of vancomycin.

The effective release of these antibiotics from the spacer according to reproducible release kinetics was demonstrated by means of in vitro pharmacological tests [2, 3, 5, 28, 34, 37, 45].

Surgery was performed using a direct lateral approach: removal of all implanted devices and meticulous debridement of the periprosthetic infected tissue was followed by insertion of the spacer in the femoral canal, achieving an easy reduction in all patients (Fig. 2).

Clinical outcome conditioned an early rehabilitation programme, including active and passive joint mobilization and muscle strengthening exercises. Assisted weight-bearing was allowed in selected cases when the spacer demonstrated adequate mechanical stability and depending on the residual bone quality (Fig. 3).

Serological trend following the first stage of the procedure was monitored through parameters widely used as markers of phlogosis – Erythrocyte-Sedimentation Rate (ESR) and C-Reactive Protein (CRP); normalization or substantial reduction of these values were discriminant in the planning of the subsequent revision [39].

Infection-healed patients underwent the final prosthetic reimplantation using different implants, both cemented (Fig. 4) and uncemented. Acrylic cement supplemented with a 2.5 % concentration of Gentamicin (Cemex Genta – Tecres SpA, Italy)

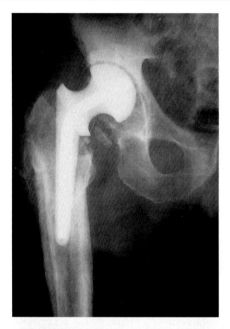

Fig. 3. Post-operative X-ray of the hip spacer: the residual bone quality is determining in the rehabilitation programme. Weight-bearing is allowed in selected cases when an adequate mechanical stability of the spacer and a good residual bone quality are present (Fig. 3)

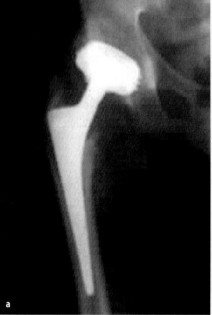

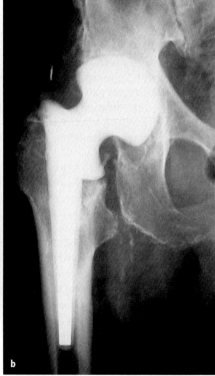

Fig. 4. Clinical case: 55 year-old man affected by a chronic infected uncemented THR (**a**). In a two-stage revision procedure a Spacer-G is applied after the removal of all infected implants (**b**)

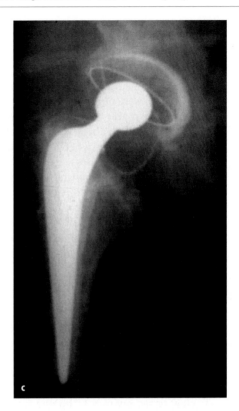

Fig. 4. (*cont.*) Final reimplantation of a antibiotic-loaded cemented THR is performed after 4 months from the first stage (**c**). The patients is infection-free at a 8 years follow-up

was used for fixation of acetabular component for cemented devices, 18 cups and 14 femoral components, while uncemented component were implanted in the remaining patients.

Multiple samples of periprosthetic tissues were routinely obtained during second-stage surgery for bacteriological assessment.

All patients were treated with 4 weeks of 400 mg/daily intravenous administration of Teicoplanin followed by a 4-weeks of oral treatment with 1.5 g/daily Ciprofloxacin.

Patients then underwent quarterly controls including clinical examination, conventional X-rays and laboratory parameters.

Results

The spacer remained *in situ* for an average time of 155 days (minimum 70 – maximum 272).

25 patients achieved a substantial decrease of the serological markers of infection.

In 4 cases such decrease did not occur, and this was considered to be a contraindication to prosthetic reimplantation: the surgical procedure therefore consisted in removal of the spacer. In two cases the infective germs were *M. tuberculosis* and multi-resistant *S. aureus* (MRSA). In the other 2 cases the pathogen agent was not detected.

In 1 patient a normalization of the biohumoral parameters was obtained, but acute recurrence of infection occurred, requiring a resection-arthroplasty.

In all reimplanted patients samples for bacteriological examination taken in the operating room were negative.

In 4 cases the spacer dislocated, because the head diameter was too small to adequately fit the acetabular bone. The dislocation was treated by non-surgical reduction and immobilization using a pelvi-condylar plaster cast for 1 month.

The 24 patients were assessed after the prosthetic reimplantation procedure with a mean 52 months follow-up (minimum 36 – maximum 100) showing no clinical or biohumoral signs of infection recurrence.

A definitive healing of infection was obtained in 27/29 cases (93.1 %).

Joint motion was possible up to 90° – 110° of hip flexion.

Radiographs demonstrated no radiolucent lines or focal osteolysis; no prosthetic component migration was observed.

Discussion

Better results as regards definitive resolution of infection with delayed reimplantation technique (91 %) compared with the one-stage revision (82 %) [20] are reported in literature: moreover, the latter requires the supply of an experienced microbiological assessment even in presence of small amounts of material, as can be sampled with a preoperative aspiration [29].

The two-stage revision technique was conventionally limited to removal of the infected prosthesis with local administration of antibiotics by means of continuous irrigation. This procedure is today better performed by temporary variously-shaped spacers [1, 15, 30, 46, 47]; these devices are usually prepared in the operating theatre consisting of a mixture of bone cement and antibiotics.

In spite of increased results with the two-stage technique, it should be emphasised that patients undergo a period never less than two months during which functional autonomy and thus the quality of life are significantly restricted; this condition may involve lengthy hospitalization [20] and a prolonged rehabilitation.

The mechanical features of the ideal spacer are currently well-defined: its femoral stem must be long enough and its neck and head should be adequately dimensioned in order to ensure the stability of the implant. Moreover, a metal "core" as a reinforcement, which must be completely covered by PMMA, is recommended.

A well-shaped spacer creates the local conditions for the second-stage reimplantation and promotes sitting and standing, thereby allowing some range of motion.

Patients treated with a temporary spacer could be encouraged to undertake weight-bearing with crutches, but the risk of mechanical failure or overloading of the acetabulum should not be neglected.

However, the condition mainly affecting the possibility of weight-bearing is not the mechanical resistance of the spacer, but the bone stock after the first implant. This factor should suggest to the surgeon the adequate rehabilitation programme in order to prevent bone lysis or even acetabular protrusion of the spacer.

In a first phase of clinical application, attention was focused on an aminoglycosidantibiotic, gentamicin, presenting a wide spectrum of activity (especially effective versus Gram-negative pathogens); a sustained release of this antibiotic into biological fluids and the attainment of prolonged local concentrations have already been demonstrated [2, 3, 4, 5, 10, 20, 38, 45].

This behaviour has been confirmed in studies with the preformed spacer by measuring elution of the antibiotic over time [3, 4]. In these studies, a release level of 6 – 14 % of the initial concentration of antibiotic was still found 6 months after surgical implant: these values proved to be effective versus the main microbial agents responsible for infection around prostheses.

The chemical-physical characteristics of gentamicin ensure optimal dispersion when mixed with PMMA, as well as high-temperature resistance which prevents structural modifications during the exothermic polymerization.

Actually it has been developed a PMMA spacer supplemented with gentamicin but also with vancomycin.

While gentamicin has been an effective treatment for most of the pathogens causing periprosthetic infection, recent selection of Gram-positive cocci resistant to aminoglycosides suggests that alternative drugs, active against methicillin-resistant bacteria, should also be considered [5, 16].

The release of vancomycin, is now well documented [3, 4, 5, 28, 34].

The routine use of vancomycin-loaded acrylic cement should be considered when epidemiologic data demonstrate a high rate (> 50 %) of methicillin-resistant [6], suggesting the supplementation of antibiotics provided with a tested efficacy versus most frequently involved pathogens.

In our experience, the "Spacer-G" used in the two-stage revision of infected total hip replacements shows to fulfil the theoretical mechanical and biological requirements which stimulated its initial development.

This device maintained a correct gap between the two bone segments allowing a partial range of motion, which improved the quality of life of the patients during postoperative period, and enabled their functional recovery following prosthetic reimplantation.

Dislocation of the preformed spacer is the only observed complication, and this is caused by a marked incongruency between the head of the device and the residual acetabular cavity, by an insufficient offset of the device or by a rotational instability of the stem on the femur, especially in the infected long stem revision: this aspect was also described by Leunig et al.[30], emphasizing the need of multi-sized models.

Sustained and effective release of antibiotics mixed with acrylic bone cement ensures the availability of high concentrations at the site of infection in the treatment of septic process, as part of the two-stage procedure [3, 4, 5, 12, 24, 26, 34, 46].

In conclusion, according to similar recent experiences [1, 25, 30, 46, 47], we can state that the spacer employed in this study proved to be able to ensure a good joint stability and length restoration during the time of insertion, thus allowing early rehabilitation.

This device also provides a system for a sustained release of the antibiotics which were supplemented to PMMA prior to surgery.

References

1. Abendschein W (1992) Salvage of infected total hip replacement: use of antibiotic/PMMA spacer. Orthopaedics 15(2):288–289
2. Baker AS, Greenham LW (1998) Release of gentamicin from acrylic bone cement. Elution and diffusion studies. J Bone Joint Surg (Am) 70(10):1551–1557
3. Bertazzoni Minelli E, Benini A, Biscaglia R et al (1999) Antibiotic release from removed temporary hip spacers. Proceedings of 9th European Congress of Clinical Microbiology and Infectious Diseases, Berlin Germany, March 21–24, 1999
4. Bertazzoni Minelli E, Benini A, Biscaglia R et al (1999) Release of gentamicin and vancomicin alone and in combination from polymethylmethacrylate (PMMA) cement. Proceedings of 21th International Congress of Chemoterapy, Birmingham, UK, July 4–7, 1999
5. Bertazzoni Minelli E, Benini A, Magnan B et al (2004) Release of gentamicin and vancomycin from temporary human hip spacers in two-stage revision of infected arthroplasty. J Antimicrob Chemother 53(2):329–334
6. Borrè S, Ricciardello PT et al (1992) Eziopatogenesi delle infezioni in artroprotesi e relative profilassi perioperatoria. Lo Scalpello (6):399–403
7. Buchholz HW, Elson RA et al (1981) Management of deep infection of total hip replacement. J Bone Joint Surg (Br) 63(3):342–353
8. Buchholz HW, Elson RA, Heinert K (1984) Antibiotic-loaded acrylic cement: current concepts. Clin Orthop Relat Res (190):96–108
9. Callaghan JJ, Katz RP, Jhonston RC (1999) One stage revision surgery of the infected hip. A minimum 10 year follow-up study. Clin Orthop Relat Res (369):139–143
10. Carlsson AS, Josefsson G, Lindberg L (1978) Revision with gentamicin-impregnated cement for deep infections in total hip arthroplasties J Bone Joint Surg (Am) 60(8):1059–1064
11. Charnley J (1972) Postoperative infection after total hip replacement with special references to air contamination in the operating room Clin Orthop Relat Res (87):167–187
12. Colier RA, Capello WN (1994) Surgical treatment of the infected hip implant. Two stage reimplantation with a one month interval Clin Orthop Relat Res (298):75–79
13. Coventry MB (1975) Treatment of infections occurring in total hip surgery. Orthop Clin North Am 6 (4):991–1003
14. Diefenbeck M, Mucley TH, O Hoffmann (2006) Prophylaxis and treatment of implant-related infection by local application of antibiotics Injury 37 Suppl 2:95-S104
15. Duncan CP, Beauchamp CP (1993) A temporary antibiotic-loaded joint replacement system for management of complex infections involving the hip. Orthop Clin North Am 24(4):751–759
16. Duncan CP, Masri BA (1994) The role of antibiotic-loaded cement in the treatment of an infection after a hip replacement. J Bone Joint Surg (Am) 76(11):1742–1751
17. Elson RA, Jephcott AE, McGechie DB et al (1997) Antibiotic loaded acrylic cement J Bone Joint Surg (Br) 59(2):200–205
18. Espehaug B, Engesaeter LB, Vollset SE et al (1997) Antibiotic prophylaxis in total hip arthroplasty. Review of 100.905 primary cemented total hip replacements reported to the Norwegian arthroplasty register, 1987 to 1995. J Bone Joint Surg (Br) 79(4):590–595
19. Fitzgerald RH Jr (1995) Infected total hip arthroplasty: diagnosis and treatment. J Am Acad Orthop Surg 3(5):294–262
20. Garvin KL, Evans BG et al (1994) Palacos gentamicin for the treatment of deep periprosthetic hip infection. Clin Orthop Relat Res (298):97–105
21. Haddad FS, Masri BA et al (1999) The treatment of infected hip replacement. The complex case. Clin Orthop Relat Res (369):144–156
22. Hanssen AD, Osmon DR, Nelson CL (1996) Prevention of deep periprosthetic joint infection. J Bone Joint Surg (Am) 78 (3):458–471
23. Hanssen AD, Rand JA (1998) Evaluation and treatment of infection at the site of total hip or knee arthroplasty. J Bone Joint Surg (Am) 80(6):910–922
24. Hsieh PH, Shih CH, Cheng YH et al (2004) Two stage revision hip arthroplasty for infection: comparison between the interim use of antibiotic-loaded cement beads and a spacer prosthesis. J Bone Joint Surg (Am) 86(9):1989–1997
25. Ivarsson I, Wahlstrom O et al (1994) Revision of infected hip replacement. Two stage procedure with a temporary gentamicin spacer. Acta Orthop Scand 65(1):7–8

26. Josefsson G, Lindberg L, Wiklander B (1981) Systemic antibiotics and Gentamicin-containing bone cement in tha prophylaxis of postoperative infections in total hip arthroplasty. Clin Orthop Relar Res (159):194–200
27. Joseph TN, Chen AL, Di Cesare PE (2003) Use of antibiotic-impregnated cement in total joint arthroplasty. J Am Acad Orthop Surg 11(1):38–47
28. Kuechle DK, Landon GC, Musher DM et al (1991) Elution of Vancomycin, Daptomycin and Amikacin from acrylic bone cement Clin Orthop Relat Res (264):302–308
29. Lachiewicz PF, Rogers GD, Thomason HC (1996) Aspiration of the hip joint before revision total hip arthroplasty. Clinical and laboratory factors influencing attainment of positive culture. J Bone Joint Surg (Am) 78(59):749–754
30. Leunig M, Chosa E et al (1998) A cement for two-stage revison infected implants of the hip joint. Int Orthop 22(4):209–214
31. Malchau H, Herberts P (1996) Prognosis of total hip replacement. Surgical and cementing technique in THR: A revision-risk study of 134,056 primary operation. 63rd AAOS Ann Meeting, Atlanta, USA, Febr 1996
32. Marks KE, Nelson CL, Lautenschlager EP (1976) Antibiotic-impregnated acrylic bone cement. J Bone Joint Surg (Am) 58(3):358–364
33. Martini C, Vedovi E, Corno M et al (1997) Trattamento riabilitativo in pazienti portatori di spaziatore temporaneo in polimetacrilato addizionato con antibiotico per mobilizzazione settica di protesi d'anca. Acts to: Argomenti di riabilitazione, Venezia, Italy, Nov 15th 1997
34. Penner MJ, Masri BA, Duncan CP (1996) Elution characteristics of Vancomycin and Toabramycin combined in acrylic bone cement. J Arthroplasty 11(8):939–944
35. Raut vv, Siney PD, Wroblewski BM (1995) One-stage revision of total hip arthroplasty for deep infection.Long term follow-up. Clin Orthop Relat Res (321):202–207
36. Ritter MA (1999) Operating room environment. Clin Orthop Relat Res (369):103–109
37. Salvati EA, Callaghan JJ, Brause BD et al (1986) Reimplantation in infection. Elution of gentamicin from cement and beads. Clin Orthop Relat Res (207):83–93
38. Salvati EA, Chekofsky KM et al (1982) Reimplantaion in infection. A 12-year experience. Clin Orthop Relat Res (170):62–75
39. Sanzen L, Carlsson AS (1989) The diagnostic value of C-reactive protein in infected protein in infected total hip arthroplasties J Bone Joint Surg (Br) 71(4):638–641
40. Schutzer Sf, Harris WH (1988) Deep wound infection after total hip replacement under contemporary aseptic conditions. J Bone Joint Surg (Am) 70(5):724–727
41. Steinbrink K (1990) The case for revision arthroplasty using antibiotic-loaded acrylic cement. Clin Orthop Relat Res (261):19–22
42. Tsukayama DT, Estrada R, Gustilo RB (1996) Infection after total hip arthroplasty. A study of the treatment of one hundred and six infections. J Bone Joint Surg (Am) 78(4):512–523
43. Ure KJ, Amstutz HC, Nasser S et al (1998) Direct-exchange arthroplasty for the treatment of infection after THR. An average ten-year follow-up. J Bone Joint Surg (Am) 80(7):961–968
44. Wahlig H, Dingeldein E (1980) Antibiotics and bone cements. Experimental and clinical long-term observations Acta Orthop Scand 51(1):49–56
45. Wahlig H, Dingeldein E, Buchholtz HW et al (1984) Pharmacokinetic study of gentamicin-loaded cement in total hip replacements. Comparative effects of varying dosage. J Bone Joint Surg (Br) 66(2):175–179
46. Younger ASE, Duncan CP, Masri BA (1998) Treatment of infection associated with segmental bone loss in the proximal part of the femur in two stages with use of an antibiotic-loaded interval prosthesis. J Bone Joint Surg (Am) 80(1):60–69
47. Zilkens KW, Casser HR, Ohnsorge J (1990) Treatment of an old infection in a total hip replacement with an interim spacer prosthesis. Arch Orthop Trauma Surg 109(2):94–96

Two-stage Revision of Septic Hip Prosthesis with Uncemented Implants

X. Flores Sánchez, E. Guerra Farfan, J. Nardi Vilardaga

Department of Orthopaedics, Vall d'Hebron University Hospital, Barcelona, Spain

Introduction

We expose the experience of the Musculo-Skeletal Septic Pathology Unit (UPSAL) of the Vall d'Hebron University Hospital (HUVH) in the treatment of infection associated with total hip arthroplasty, using the two-stage procedure with uncemented implants [6, 14, 23, 34, 51, 61].

Material and Methods

Between August 1972 and September 2002 the UPSAL treated 205 infections associated with total hip arthroplasty (periprosthetic joint infection); 161 cases were primary THA and 44 cases revisions.

These infected arthroplasties led to, until the end of 2002, 299 treatment options (Fig. 1) which included:

- Suppressive antibiotic treatment [5, 78, 110]   n: 19
- Debridement and cleaning of implants [16, 82]   n: 36
- 1-stage revision [6, 8, 39, 82, 83, 101]   n: 22
- 2-stage revision [7, 34, 61, 112]   n: 57
- Girdlestone resection arthroplasty [12, 33]   n: 129
- Debridement of resection arthroplasty due to persistent infection   n: 36

As can be observed in Fig. 1, in the early years the most frequent option was resection arthroplasty, this being justified by the type of patients treated: chronic stages which had been subject to multiple surgical procedures in the centres where the problem had originally arisen.

In more recent years, as a centre of reference, the predominant option was the two-stage revision arthroplasty. The case series reported and analysis of our previous results made it advisory. Until 1994 in UPSAL, with the one and two-stage revision techniques, using Buchholz cemented implants [6, 34, 99], one third of patients showed persistent infection, two thirds were resolved of their septic process, but 30 % showed an aseptic loosening in the follow-up within 6 years (average follow up 117.4 months).

In 1996 we started a two-stage treatment [14, 112] protocol using uncemented implants [22, 32, 67, 68, 86] in those cases with chronic infection, unknown or multi-

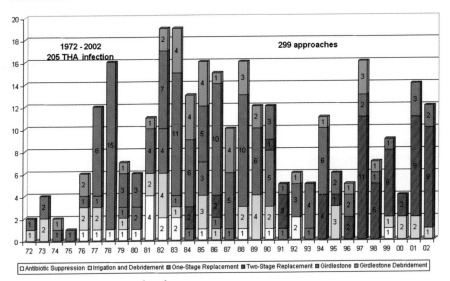

Fig. 1. Treatment options employed

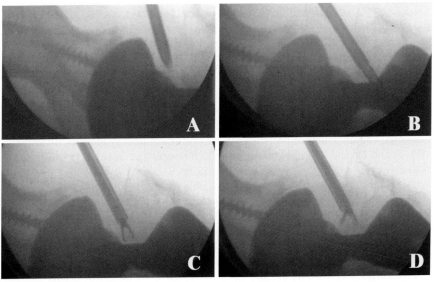

Fig. 2. Sampling for anatomopathological and microbiological study on bone-implant or bone-cement interface level

resistant bacteria, loss of bone stock and failure of one-stage revision [15, 38, 51, 54, 63].

We utilized arthrocenthesis as well as bone-implant or bone-cement interface biopsy to improve the successful bacterial identification. This interface biopsy was carried out in the operating room as the first procedure, before the first-stage, with a percutaneous trocar guided with radiographic C-arm.

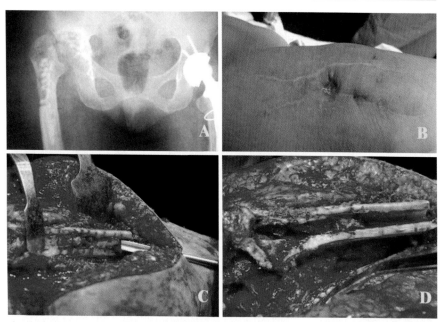

Fig. 3. (A) Right hip X-ray in a patient with recurrent septic activity following THR. Unremoved bone cement is visible. **(B)** Clinical aspect of the patient subject to several previous operations. **(C)** Clinical aspect of the femoral osteotomy done to remove the remains of the cement mantle. **(D)** Clinical aspect after removal of the cement mantle

After bacterial identification, the first open surgical procedure must include an extensive debridement of both soft and bone tissue and foreign material. In both cemented and uncemented prosthesis the debridement usually requires osteotomies (Fig. 3) and or drill holes possibly leading to fractures and false tracts which makes the subsequent cementing challenging [29, 35, 86, 94]. The osteomized or perforated bone makes pressurizing the cement impossible within the medullary canal already weakened by revision arthroplasty. Acrylic cement often escapes on to soft tissue which can lead to future complications (Fig. 4) [94].

Once the debridement is achieved antibiotic spacers, [53, 65] custom made in both form and antibiotic content [31, 73, 76] will release high concentrations of antibiotics "*in situ*". This spacer avoid the retraction of the periarticular tissues and allows walking with crutches [9, 20, 48, 49, 50, 84, 97, 98, 104, 106]. We have little experience with preformed spacers for both technical and economic reasons [84], and have proceeded from after the first stage to the preparation of custom made "personalised" spacers in relation to antibiotic content (secondary to the previous identification of the bacteria). Once the PMMA cement and corresponding antibiotics are added (up to 4 g of antibiotic for every 40 g unit of acrylic cement) it is wrapped in a sheet of latex and place it into the residual cavity and pressing it so that it takes up all the defects, and finally with the proximal part of the femur correctly lined up with the limb (Fig. 5). When the cement begins to harden we use Moore's corkscrew in the centre of the spacer approaching through the rear of the hip: this technical detail eases the placing

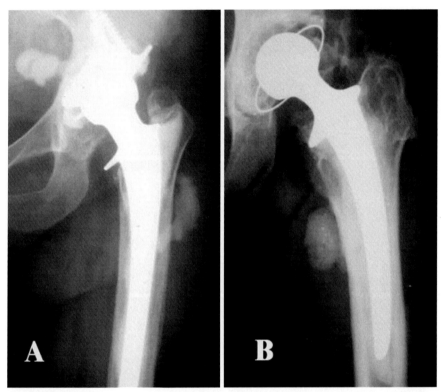

Fig. 4. (A, B) X-ray of cement leakage to soft tissues due to the presence of bone defects at a acetabular (**A**) or femoral (**B**) level

and extraction of the spacer (Fig. 6). Once the plastic properties of the cement have disappeared and before the exothermic reaction happens, we remove the spacer until it cools and then reinsert it.

During the intermediate period between the first and second stage, approximately three months, the patient continues on antibiotic treatment. According to the literature the duration of the treatment varies between 2 and 3 months [5, 23, 27, 58, 73, 78, 110]. We adopted the 3-month period (orally, if possible), as it is the length of treatment advised for chronic osteomyelitis [14, 34, 63, 91, 112, 113].

Fifteen days after of intermediate period, if the patient is stable clinically and laboratory values are normal, analytical nor nuclear imagines, we proceed to the second stage revision [1, 8, 35, 53]. Frozen sections are sent for analysis [2] to confirm there is no acute inflammation. If present a second debridement is carried out, tissue samples taken and a new antibiotic-spacer inserted. If the frozen section is negative for acute inflammation we continue with revision arthroplasty using uncemented implants [26]. Published evidence suggests that these uncemented implants have better long-term survival in revision surgery [26]. Moreover, the use of cement can inhibit the cellular response mechanisms due to heat from polymethylmetacrylate, by depressing the quimiotaxis and fagocytosis of the polimorphonuclear leukocytes, as

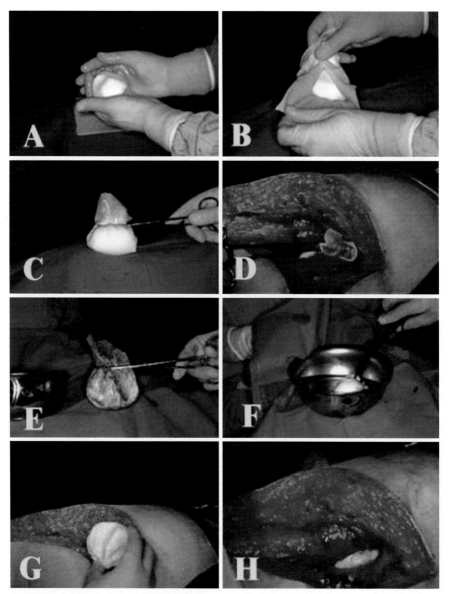

Fig. 5. Different phases in custom made "personalized" spacer
A "Ball" shaping of acrylic cement with antibiotics
B Fitting cement wrapped in a latex sheet
C Closing of latex "sheet"
D Fitting in to the residual space and shaping with fingers
E Once the acrylic cement begins to harder it is removed without being deformed
F The exothermic reaction (temperature around 90 °C) is carried out outside the patient using a coolant
G Once cool and completely hardened it is fitted into the residual space
H Clinical aspect of spacer "*in situ*"

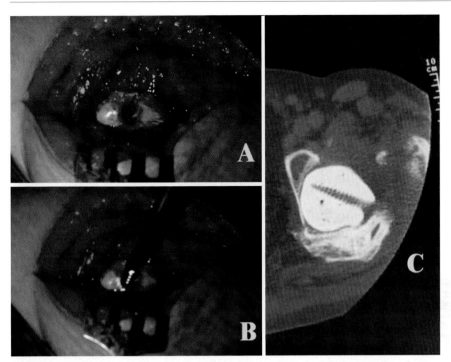

Fig. 6. Technical detail, the screwed orifice achieved by inserting the tip of a Moore's corkscrew, before the cement hardens completely. The use of Moore's corkscrew in the second stage aids spacer removal. X-ray of spacer "in situ" taking up all of the residual space. The profile of the screwed hole that will aid its extraction is also visible

demonstrated by Petty [30, 74, 75], and others. The use of cemented arthroplasties can explain the growth of resistant organisms secondary to using antibiotic cement.

Methods

Since 1996 we have used this method of treatment in 44 hip arthroplasties associated with a chronic infected hip arthroplasty, and this series constitutes the basis of our study. There were 25 men and 19 women, with an average age of 64.2 years, ranging from 20 to 88. Forty-seven percent of patients presented with comorbidities (23 patients were classified as physiological type A, 18 as type B and 3 type C). Fifteen patients (34.1 %) had previous surgery before presenting to our institution.

The THA involved were 37 primary prosthesis (25 cemented, 5 uncemented and 7 hybrids) and 7 revision hip arthroplasties (5 cemented, 1 uncemented and 1 hybrid).

The type of infection was: in 5 cases type II (2 early and 3 haematogenous), the others type IV (37 late and 2 haematogenous).

The bacteria responsible was gram positive in 54.6 % of cases, gram negative in 31.8 %, polymicrobian infections were present in 6.8 % of cases, other bacteria and the absence of a positive culture made up the remaining 7 %.

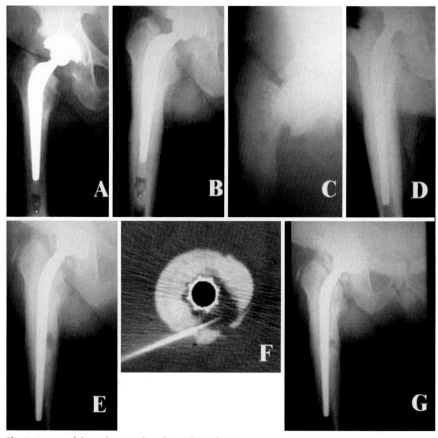

Fig. 7. X-rays of the only case that showed reinfection

A Primary total hip arthroplasty

B Periprosthetic infection, chronic stage, a reactive hyperostosis is noted

C Spacer "*in situ*" after first stage of revision

D X-ray of the uncemented stem used in the second stage of revision total hip arthroplasty

E After 10 months, thigh pain, alteration of specific analytic parameters and "endostic osteolytic" and periostitis signs occurrence

F Biopsy of the osteolytic cavity using a trocar guided by computerized axial tomography. *S. epidermidis* is isolated, with the same resistance profile as in the original germ

G After six months antibiogram-based antibiotic treatment disappearance of clinical signs and normalisation of the endostic osteolytic image is achieved

Results

Results for the first 25 cases treated with two stage revision with a cementless prosthesis, from 1996 to 2002 are reported. Two patients have died for reasons unrelated to the septic process, and their implants revealed no evidence of infection. The remaining 23 patients had an average age of 61.2 years (ranging between 20 and 88), 13 women and 10 men.

An average follow up of 74.5 months (ranging between 47.5 and 125 months), 22 of 23 patients were free of infection (95.7 %). One patient (4.3 %) had a reactivation of the periprosthetic infection in the form of thigh pain, increased ESR and CRP. He had a positive bone scan 10 months after the second stage (Fig. 7). The bacteria identified from biopsy with trocar aided revealed the same characteristics as the bacteria responsible for the original infection (*Staphylococcus epidermidis*). After obtaining the corresponding sensitivity the patient received oral antibiotic treatment for a period of 6 months, resolving the clinical signs, serum parameters and radiographic and nuclear imagines. The success of the therapy is attributed to the antibiotic treatment and an uncemented implant with an absence of a second interface as would be in the case with a cemented implant.

With an average follow up of 6 years (74.5 months) [47], all patients still have their implants and no loosening has been observed.

The functional result according to the Merle – d'Aubigue – Postel scale [18, 19] was completely satisfactory with pain scoring 5.86 (ranging between 5 and 6), mobility 4.93 (ranging between 2 and 6) and aided walking 4.86 (ranging between 2 and 6).

Discussion

Appropriate treatment of periprosthetic infection needs to identify the bacteria and obtain its sensitivity to different antibiotics before performing any surgery. The correct and systematic use of specific antibiotics after radical debridement surgery is fundamental in treating any residual bacterias which may exist in the surgical field. Obtaining this information is also important in two stage revision, if antibiotic spacers are used [13, 40, 56], whether prefabricated [24, 25, 41] or personalised [37]. That is why in the periprosthetic infection treatment protocol we systematically include a first operation in our unit, aimed at obtaining tissue samples from bone-cement or prosthesis-bone interface, the area where the infectious process develops [107], with a percutaneous trocar and biopsy tweezers guided by radiographic C-arm. In this way we try to get better sensitivity and specificity than that obtained through joint aspiration, whose sensitivity ranged 55 % and 86 %, placing the specificity between 94 % and 96 % [3, 95]. Clearly this elementary action will be more important in the near future, when new microbiological techniques will allow us to more easily and systematically isolated and cultivated bacteria in the stationary phase of growth cycle container in the slime [100]. Our treatment is aime at those germs and hill not is limited to planktonic forms. The differing sensitivity profile of the bacteria contained in the biofilms is responsable for the majority of failures [77, 102], as the coagulase-negative *Staphylococcus* is implicated in nearly all of them.

Two-stage replacement is the most frequently used method in THA infections, it must be considered the first choice procedure in acute cases with serious sepsis and which endanger the life of the patient. However, periprosthetic infection is often late to show itself in chronic form. Two-stage revision is indicated when: the bacteria responsable is unknown; we deal with virulent bacterias; there is insufficient bone stock; the patient presents associated systemic pathologies or has failed with one-stage revision. For some authors [93] the existence of sinus tracks is a reason to indicate two-stage revision but we believe that their existence is a manifestation of the chronic nature does not in itself require this response. A correct debridement which includes the sinus tracks is totally compatible with one-stage revision, if all the conditions for this technique are fulfilled.

For some authors [93] the existence of precarious host immunity and medical conditions and insufficient bone stock are contraindications of a two-stage revision and in such cases recommend the one-stage revision with cemented implants. In our opinion precisely such cases should be treated with two-stage revision as it offers a higher guarantee of success in patients with a relative immunosuppression. It is also in situations of insufficient bone stock when associated surgery is needed, use of bone grafts and special implants, which are not indicated in one-stage revision. The use of cemented implants gives rise to precarious cementing due to a smooth implantation surface. Poor bone quality with cortical deficiencies and endostic sclerosis make long-term stability and implant survival less likely with cemented techniques. They are also associated with potential false ways and frequent femoral osteotomies carried out during debridement surgery. The use of cemented implants makes it impossible to repair the problem biologically, which may have a deleterious effect on the immune system and which may also become an inhibiting factor upon local defence mechanisms as we will mention later. A correct joint reconstruction should only be considered when the septic process has been eradicated [108]. However it is clear that the overall treatment strategy must be guided by the patient's ability to tolerate surgical procedures and their projected longevity [93]. Two- stage approach entails the morbidity associated with multiple surgeries and prolonged immobilization, and may be unacceptable for frail older patients [27]. In these cases long-term suppressive oral antimicrobial therapy alone or definitive resection arthroplasty may be an acceptable option. With this latter procedure, successful eradication of infection can be achieved in 60 % to 100 % of cases [4, 10, 12].

Published evidence gathered recently in the literature by Sia and Colbs [93] is very demonstrative. Out of a total of 601 periprosthetic hip infections [26, 28, 34, 44, 55, 61, 69, 70, 72, 88, 92, 99, 105, 109, 112], two-stage revision provided 88 % of good results, 530 cases were free of infection whereas one-stage revision carried out in other 914 cases only obtained 77 % of good results freeing 701 patients from infection [6, 8, 11, 42, 43, 90, 101, 111].

The results published upon total prosthetic hip replacement surgery showed higher medium-term survival rates, when cementless implants were used. In his article, Fehring [26] checks implant survival in non-septic replacement surgery. Out of a total of 283 cases using cemented implants, 92 needed a second revision within 7 years, whereas in further 468 cases of revision for aseptic weakening those that used uncemented implants noted a 1.28 % (6 of 468) re-revision rate with the same follow-up as the previous group.

The success of the cemented techniques lies in the micro-interdigitation of cement within the cancellous structure of the femur, after a failed femoral arthroplasty leaves a sclerotic tube incapable of allowing such interdigitation. In replacement surgery a good femoral fixation using cemented techniques is not possible. For that reason uncemented distal fixation implants are used. Not using cement at a proximal level favours spontaneous biological repair and allows the use of bone grafts to restore its precarious stock.

Surgical debridement carried out in the first stage, it is origin of solutions of continuity at level of proximal femur, in form of extended trocanteric osteotomies, to withdraw the femoral implants or the cement used in its fixation, false tracts related to accidental perforations or even intraoperative fractures. None of these situations favours a correct cementation but are compatible with the use of cementless implants associated with reconstruction techniques with bone grafts.

The use of uncemented distal support implants associated with transosseous approaches and proximal femoral fractures allows the spontaneous reconstruction of the weakened proximal bone.

Published evidence suggests that these uncemented implants have better long-term survival in revision surgery [26]. Also, the use of cement can inhibit the cellular response mechanism due to heat from polymethylmetacrylate, by depressing the quimiotaxis and fagocytosis of the polimorphonuclear leukocytes, as demonstrated by Petty [30, 74, 75], and others. The use of cemented arthroplasties can explain the growth of resistance organisms secondary to using antibiotic cement. Not using antibiotic cement as an implant fixation method is, for some authors [96], a disadvantage as it means they can not use high doses of antibiotic "*in situ*" during the second stage of replacement. We believe that the use of antibiotic cement is unnecessary as the septic process is clinically controlled and its use in the pathology which concerns us is still a potential problem since after some weeks the doses of antibiotic released have sub-therapeutic quantities and even favour the appearance of resistance. Thornes in its study of experimental infection [98] demonstrates that antibiotic-loaded bone cement offers an optimal surface for the colonization, and a prolonged exposure to antibiotics facilitates the appearance of resistance by mutation. Another negative aspect of polymethylmetacrylate as shown by Petty [74, 75] is the inhibition of local cellular defences, by depressing the quimiotaxis and fagocytosis of the polimorphonuclear leukocytes.

Conclusion

To correctly treat periprosthetic infection it is crucial to **identify the bacteria** and obtain its sensitivity to different antibiotics. The correct and systematic use of specific antibiotics after radical debridement surgery is fundamental in treating any residual bacteria which may exist in the surgical field. Obtaining this information is also very useful, if antibiotic spacers [13, 40, 56] are used, whether prefabricated [24, 25, 41] or personalised [37] in the intermediary period between stages in two-stage prosthetic revision surgery in the septic prosthesis hip as it allows us to adapt the type of antibiotics mixed with the acrylic cement to the specific needs of each case.

The inclusion of a previous operation in our protocol, the biopsy of tissue samples from bone-cement or prosthesis-bone interface improves upon the traditional diagnostic method, joint aspiration, in identifying the bacteria responsible for the septic process. The bacteria was not identified in less than 7 % of cases, substantially improving sensitivity and specificity of joint aspiration, whose scores ranged between 55 % – 86 %, and 94 % – 96 % respectively [3, 95]. This is possible because bacteria investigation is carried out in the area where the process is most active, the bone-cement or prosthesis-bone interface [107]. Also, the solid specimens obtained in this way allow for microbiological and anatomopathological investigation. Clearly this elementary action will be more important in the near future, when new microbiological techniques will allow us to more easily and systematically isolate and cultivate bacteria contained in the slime 100], ultrasounding the prosthetic components already forms part of normal practice in some centres, such as the Mayo Clinic. Our treatment will be aimed at these bacteria and will not be limited to their planktonic forms. Our only failure was related to the presence of a coagulase-negative *Staphylococcus* which is responsible for most failures in other series [77, 102].

For us **two-stage replacement** can be considered the gold standard. It is the most frequently used method in treatment of THA infections [26, 28, 34, 44, 55, 61, 69, 70, 72, 88, 92, 99, 105, 109, 112], and is also the procedure of choice in acute cases which show serious and systemic sepsis and endanger the patient's life. However, periprosthetic infection is often late to show itself in chronic form. Two-stage revision is indicated when: the bacteria responsable is unknown; we deal with virulent bacteria; there is insufficient bone stock; the patient presents associated systemic pathologies or has failed with one-stage revision. The published literature shows clearly that out of a total of 601 periprosthetic hip infections [26, 28, 34, 44, 55, 61, 69, 70, 72, 88, 92, 93, 99, 105, 109, 112], two-stage revision provided 88 % of good results, 530 cases were free of infection, whereas one-stage revision carried out in another 914 cases only obtained 77 % of good results freeing 701 patients from infection [6, 8, 11, 42, 43, 90, 93, 101, 111].

Two-stage replacement is also especially indicated in those cases with precarious host immunity and medical conditions, since this method offers a higher guarantee of success in patients with a relative immunosuppression. It is also a safe procedure in situations of insufficient bone stock where associated reconstructive surgery is needed, use of bone grafts and special implants, none of which are indicated in one-stage revision.

We obtained excellent results in terms of infection resolution, with an average follow up of 74.5 months; with 95.7 % of patients (22 of 23 cases) showing no relapse.

The advantages of **uncemented implants** are that they have the potential long-term fixation in a revision situation; the longer duration of uncemented implants justifies their use.

The results published in total prosthetic hip replacement surgery show higher medium-term survival rates when cementless implants are used. In his article, Fehring [26] checks implant survival in non-septic replacement surgery. Out of a total of 283 cases using cemented implants, 92 needed a second revision within 7 years whereas in another 468 cases of revision for aseptic weakening those that used uncemented implants noted a 1.3 % (6 of 468) re-revision rate with the same follow-up as the previous group.

The success of the cemented techniques lies in the micro-interdigitation of cement within the cancellous structure of the femur. In replacement surgery a good femoral fixation using cemented techniques is not possible. Poor bone quality with cortical deficiencies and endostic sclerosis make long-term stability and implant survival less likely with cemented techniques. For that reason uncemented distal fixation implants are used.

Other circumstances may be responsible for precarious cemented fixation. Surgical debridement carried out in the first stage can create disruptions at level of proximal femur, in form of extended trocanteric osteotomy, to withdraw the femoral implants or the cement used in its fixation, false tracts related to accidental perforations or even intraoperative fractures. None of these situations favours a correct cementation but are compatible with the use of cementless implants associated with reconstruction techniques with bone grafts. The use of cemented implants makes a biological repair impossible; the use of uncemented diaphyseal fixation implants [38, 42, 55] associated with transosseous approaches allows the spontaneous reconstruction of the weakened proximal bone. The method proposed is useful in conditions of bad cementing techniques [15, 22]. On some occasions the loss of bone stock is so extensive that a correct spontaneous repair cannot be expected and in these cases the two-stage revision using cementless implants allows us to use bone grafts to restore precarious bone stock in a biological way. Obviously a correct joint reconstruction that includes the use of bone grafts can only be considered when the septic process has been eradicated [108]. The advantages of cementless revision for infection are that they have the potential long-term fixation in a revision situation. Authors, such as Fehring [26], among others, arrive at the same conclusion.

None of our 23 patients showed signs of prosthetic dysfunction, with a follow up of 74.5 months. It is a useful method which avoids cementing in those cases where that would be precarious for the coexistence of fractures, false tracts, windows or osteotomies created during the debridement stage.

Cement with antibiotics is not essential for the treatment of infection associated with arthroplasties using this technique. Our eradication rate infection of 95.7 % (22 of 23 cases) certainly is superior in comparison with other series using antibiotic-impregnated cement. The advantages of cementless revision for infection are that they have the potential long-term fixation in a revision situation, and they lack the inhibitory effect on polymorphonuclear leukocytes arising from the presence of polymethylmetacrylate, which may have a deleterious effect on the immune system [74, 75]. Another effect negative originated by antibiotic-cement, it is derived from the potential risk of appearance of antibiotic-resistant bacteria by mutation. Some weeks after the use of the antibiotic-cement, the antibiotic liberation from the cement takes place to sub-therapeutic doses [45, 98].

Finally, eliminating the bone-cement interface allowed for healing with a simple antibiotic treatment retaining the implant. If the infection relapses, the elimination of the bone-cement interface allows healing with a simple antibiotic treatment, retaining the implant. In this series, the only case relapsed, we believe was due to the close relationship of the implant with the endostic vascular bed, a single prosthesis-bone interface where the humoral and cellular immune systems of the patient could act. It is possible that had there been a bone-cement interface, the result would not have been the same and the infection would have been spread by this interface due to a deleterious effect on the immune system caused by the polymethylmetacrylate and the avascular character of the prosthesis-cement interface. Elimination of one of the interfaces, the cement–prosthesis, which could never receive an antibiotic treatment, uncemented components and distal support, intimate contact between the circulatory system and the implant lets antibiotics reach the implant surface in the event of persistent infection.

References

1. Aalto K, Osterman K, Peltola H, Rasanen J (1984) Changes in erythrocyte sedimentation rate and C-reactive protein after total hip arthroplasty. Clin Orthop Relat Res (184):118–120
2. Athanasou NA, Pandey P, de Steiger R et al (1995) Diagnosis of infection by frozen section during revision arthroplasty. J Bone Joint Surg (Br) 77(1):28–33
3. Atkins BL, Athanasou N, Deeks JJ et al (1998) Prospective evaluation of criteria for microbiological diagnosis of prosthetic-joint infection at revision arthroplasty. The OSIRIS Collaborative Study Group. J Clin Michrobiol 36(10):2932–2939
4. Bittar ES, Petty W (1982) Girdlestone arthroplasty for infected total hip arthroplasty. Clin Orthop Relat Res (170):83–87
5. Borden LS, Geraen PF (1987) Infected total knee arthroplasty. A protocol for management. J Artrhoplasty 2(1):27–36
6. Buchholz HW, Elson RA, Engelbercht E et al (1981) Management of deep infection of total hip replacement. J Bone Joint Surg (Br) 63(3):342–353
7. Buttaro MA, Pusso R, Piccaluga F (2005) Vancomycin-supplemented impacted bone allografts in infected hip arthroplasty. Two-stage revision results. J Bone Joint Surg (Br) 87(3): 314–319
8. Callaghan JJ, Katz RP, Johnston RC (1999) One-stage revision surgery of the infected hip. A minimum 10-year followip study. Clin Orthop Relat Res (369):139–143
9. Calton TF, Fehring TK, Griffin WL (1997) Bone loss associated with the use of spacer blocks in infected total knee arthroplasty. Clin Orthop Relat Res (345):148–154
10. Canner GC, Steinberg ME, Heppenstall RB et al (1984) The infected hip after total hip arthroplasty. J Bone Joint Surg (Am) 66(9):1393–1399
11. Carlsson AS, Josefsson G, Lindberg L (1978) Revision with gentamicin-impregnated cement for deep infections in total hip arthroplasties. J Bone Joint Surg (Am) 60:1059–1064
12. Castellanos J, Flores X, Llusa M et al (1998) The Girdlestone pseudoarthrosis in the treatment of infected hip replacements. Int Orthop 22(3):178–181
13. Chimento GF, Finger S, Barrack RL (1996) Gram stain detection of infection during revision arthroplasty. J Bone Joint Surg (Br) 78(5):838–839
14. Christel P, Djian P (1994) Recent advances in adult hip joint surgery. Curr Opin Rheumatol 6(2):161–171
15. Cierny G, DiPasquale D (2002) Periprosthetic total joint infections. Staging, treatment and outcomes. Clin Orthop Relat Res (403):23–28
16. Crockarell JR, Hanssen AD, Osmon DR et al (1998) Treatment of infection with debridement and retention of the components following hip arthroplasty. 80(9):1306–1313
17. Cuckler JM, Star AM, Alavi A et al (1991) Diagnosis and management of the infected total joint arthroplasty. Orthop Clin North Am 22(3):523–530
18. D'Aubigne M (1954) Functional results of hip arthroplasty. J Bone Joint Surg (Am) 36: 451–475
19. D'Aubigne M (1970) Cotation chifrée de la function de la manche. Rev Clin Orthop 56: 481–486
20. David A Wininger, Robert J Fass (1996) Antibiotic-impregnated cement and beads for orthopedic infections. Antimicrob Agents Chemother 40(12):2675–2679
21. Della Valle CJ, Bogner E, Desai P et al (1999) Analysis of frozen sections of intraoperative specimens obtained at the time of reoperation after hip or knee resection arthroplasty for the treatment of infection. J Bone Joint Surg (Am) 81(5):684–689
22. Duffy GP, Berry DJ, Rand JA (1998) Cement versus cementless fixation in total knee arthroplasty. Clin Orthop Relat Res (356):66–72
23. Duggan JM, Georgiadis GM, Kleshinski JF (2001) Management of prosthetic joint infections. Infect Med 18(12):534–541
24. Duncan CP, Beauchamp C (1993) A temporary antibiotic-loaded joint replacement system for management of complex infections involving the hip. Orthop Clin North Am 24(4): 751–759
25. Duncan CP, Masri B (1993) Antibiotic depots. J Bone Joint Surg (Br) 75(3):349–350
26. Fehring TK, Calton TF, Griffin WL (1999) Cementless fixation in 2-stage reimplantation for periprosthetic sepsis. J Arthroplasty 14(2):175–181

27. Fisman D, Reilly DT, Karchmer AW et al (2001) Clinical effectiveness and cost-effectiveness of 2 management strategies for infected total hip arthroplasty in the elderly. Management of Infected Arthroplasty 32(3):419–430
28. Fitzgerald RH Jr (1995) Infected total hip arthroplasty: diagnosis and treatment. J Am Acad Orthop Surg 3(5):249–262
29. Fitzgerald RH, Jones DR (1985) Hip implant infection: treatment with resection arthroplasty and late total hip arthroplasty. Am J Med 78(6B):225–228
30. Garvin KL, Hinrichs SH, Urban JA (1999) Emerging antibiotic-resistant bacteria. their treatment in total joint arthroplasty. Clin Orthop Relat Res (369):110–123
31. Garvin KL, Salvati EA, Brause BD (1998) Role of gentamicin-impregnated cement in total joint arthroplasty. Orthop Clin North Am 19(3):605–610
32. Gorab RS, Covino BM, Borden LS (1993) The rationale for cementless revision total hip replacement with contemporary technology. Orthop Clin North Am 24(4):627–633
33. Grauer JD, Amstutz HC, O'Carroll PF et al (1989) Resection arthroplasty of the hip. J Bone Joint Surg 71(5):669–678
34. Haddad FS, Masri BA, Garbuz DS, Duncan CP (1999) The treatment of the infected hip replacement. The complex case. Clin Orthop Relat Res (369):144–156
35. Haddad FS, Muirhead-Allwood SK, Manktelow AR et al (2000) Two stage uncemented revision hip arthroplasty for infection. J Bone Joint Surg (Br) 82(5):689–694
36. Hanssen AD, Rand JA, Osmon DR (1994) Treatment of the infected total knee arthroplasty with insertion of another prosthesis: the effect of antibiotic-impregnated bone cement. Clin Orthop Relat Res (309):44–55
37. Hanssen AD, Osmon DR (2002) Evaluation of a staging system for infected hip arthroplasty. Clin Orthop Relat Res (403):16–22
38. Hanssen AD, Rand JA (1999) Evaluation and treatment of infection at the site of a total hip or knee arthroplasty. Instr Course Lect (48):111–122.Review
39. Harris WH (1986) One staged exchange arthroplasty for septic total hip replacement. AAOS Instr Course Lect (35):226–228
40. Heck D, Rosenberg A, Schink-Ascani M et al (1995) Use of antibiotic-impregnated cement during hip and knee arthroplasty in the United States. J Arthroplasty 10(4):470–475
41. Hofmann AA, Kane KR, Tkach TK et al (1995) Treatment of infected total knee arthroplasty using an articulating spacer. Clin Orthop Relat Res (321):45–54
42. Hope PG, Kristinsson KG, Norman P et al (1989) Deep infection of cemented total hip arthroplasties caused by coagulase-negative staphylococci. J Bone Joint Surg (Br) 71(5):851–855
43. Hughes P.W., Salvati E.A., Wilson P.D., et al. (1979) Treatment of subacute sepsis of the hip by antibiotics and joint replacement criteria for diagnosis with evaluation of twenty-six cases. Clin Orthop Relat Res (141):143–157
44. Ivarsson I, Wahlstrom O, Djerf K et al (1994) Revision of infected hip replacement: two-stage procedure with a temporary gentamicin spacer. Acta Orthop Scand 65(1):7–8
45. Joseph TN, Chen AL, Di Cesare PE (2003) Use of antibiotic-impregnated cement in total joint arthroplasty. J Am Acad Orthop Surg 11(1):38–47. Review
46. Kantor GS, Osterkamp JA, Dorr LD et al (1986) Resection arthroplasty following infected total hip replacement arthroplasty. J Arthroplasty 1(2):83–89
47. Katz RP, Callaghan JJ, Sullivan PM et al (1997) Long-term results of revision total hip arthroplasty with improved cementing technique. J Bone Joint Surg (Br) 79(2):322–326
48. Klekamp J, Dawson JM, Haas DW, Deboer D, Christie M (1999) The use of vancomycin and tobramycin in acrylic bone cement. J Arthroplasty 14(3):339–346
49. Kuechle DK, Landon GC, Musher DM, Noble PC (1991) Elution of vancomycin, daptomycin and amikacin from acrylic bone cement. Clin Orthop Relat Res (264):302–308
50. Kyung-Hi Koo, Jin-Won Yang, Se-Hyun Cho et al (2001) Impregnation of vancomycin, gentamicin, and cefotaxime in a cement spacer for two-stage cementless. reconstruction in infected total hip arthroplasty. J Arthroplasty 16(7):882–892
51. LaPorte DM, Waldman BJ, Mont MA, Hungerford DS (1999) Infections associated with dental procedures in total hip arthroplasty. J Bone Joint Surg (Br) 81(1):56–59
52. Lecuire F, Collodel M, Basso M et al (1999) Revision of infected total hip prosthesis by ablation reimplantation of an uncemented prosthesis. 57 case reports. Rev Chir Orthop Reparatrice Appar Mot 85(4):337–348

53. Leunig M, Chosa E, Speck M et al (1998) A cement spacer for two-stage revision of infected implants of the hip joint. Int Orthop 22(4):209–214
54. Levin JS, Rodriguez AA, Luong K (1997) Fistula between the Hip and the Sigmoid Colon after Total Hip Arthroplasty. A case report. J Bone Joint Surg (Am) 7(8):1240–1242
55. Lieberman JR, Callaway GH, Salvati EA et al (1994) Treatment of the infected total hip replacement with a two-stage reimplantation protocol. Clin Orthop Relat Res (301):205–212
56. Love C, Marwin SE, Tomas MB et al (2004) Diagnosing infection in the failed joint replacement: a comparison of coincidence detection 18F-FDG and 111In-labeled leukocyte/99mTc-sulfur colloid marrow imaging. J Nucl Med 45(11):1864–1871
57. Mackowiak PA, Jones SR, Smith JW (1978) Diagnostic value of sinus-tract cultures in chronic osteomyelitis. JAMA 239(26):2772–2775
58. Mader JT, Wang J, Calhoun JH (2001) Antibiotic therapy for musculoeskeletal infections. Instr Course Lect J Bone Joint Surg (Am) 83(12):1878–1890
59. Malkani AL, Lewallen DG, Cabanela ME et al (1996) Femoral component revision using an uncemented, proximally coated, long-stem prosthesis. J Artroplasty 11(4):311–318
60. Masterson EL, Masri BA, Duncan CP (1998) Treatment of infection at the site of total hip replacement. Instr Course Lect 47(2):297–306
61. McDonald DJ, Fitzgerald RH, Ilstrup DM (1989) Two-stage reconstruction of a total hip arthroplasty because of infection. J Bone Joint Surg (Am) 71(6):828–834
62. McElwaine JP, Colville J (1984) Excision arthroplasty for infected total hip replacements. J Bone Joint Surg (Br) 66():168–171
63. McPherson EJ, Woodson C, Holtom P et al (2002) Periprosthetic total hip infection. outcomes using a staging system. Clin Orthop Relat Res (403):8–15
64. Michelinakis E, Papapolychronlou T, Vafiadis J (1996) The use a cementless femoral component for the management of bone loss in revision hip arthroplasty. Bull Hosp Jt Dis 55(1): 28–32
65. Migaud H, Chantelot C, Besson A et al (1997) Temporary antibiotic-loaded cemented prosthesis for two-stage septic hip arthroplasty. Rev Chir Orthop Reparatrice Appar Mot 84(5): 466–468
66. Miley G.B., Scheller A.D., Turner R.H. (1982) Medical and surgical treatment of the septic hip with one-stage revision arthroplasty. Clin Orthop Relat Res (170):76–82
67. Morscher E (1983) Cementless total hip arthroplasty. Clin Orthop Relat Res (181):76–91
68. Morscher E, Babst R, Jenny H (1990) Treatment of infected joint arthroplasty. Int Orthop 14(2):161–165
69. Nelson CL, Evans RP, Blaha JD et al (1993) A comparison of gentamicin-impregnated polymethylmethacrylate bead implantation to conventional parenteral antibiotic therapy in infected total hip and knee arthroplasty.Clin Orthop Relat Res (295):96–101
70. Nestor BJ, Hanssen AD, Ferrer-Gonzalez R et al (1994) The use of porous prostheses in delayed reconstruction of total hip replacements that have failed because of infection. J Bone Joint Surg (Am) 76(3):349–359
71. Osmon DR (2001) Antimicrobial resistance: guidelines for the practicing orthopaedic surgeon. Instr Course Lect J Bone Joint Surg (Am) 83(12):1891–1901
72. Pagnano MW, Trousdale RT, Hanssen AD (1997) Outcome after reinfection following reimplantation hip arthroplasty. Clin Orthop Relat Res (338):192–204
73. Pang-Hsin Hsieh, Chun-Hsiung Shih, YU-Han Chang et al (2004) Two-stage revision hip arthroplasty for infection: Comparison between the interim use of antibiotic-loasded cement beads and a spacer prothesis. J Bone Joint Surg (Am) 86(9):1989–1997
74. Petty W (1978) The effect of methylmethacrylate on bacterial phagocytosis and killing by human polymorphonuclear leukocytes. J Bone Joint Surg (Am) 60(6):752–757
75. Petty W (1978) The effect of methylmethacrylate on chemotaxis of polymorphonuclear leukocites. J Bone Joint Surg (Am) 60(4):492–498
76. Powles JW, Spencer RF, Lovering AM (1998) Gentamicin release from old cement during revision hip arthroplasty. J Bone Joint Surg (Br) 80(4):607–610
77. Proctor RA, van Langevelde P, Kristjansson M et al (1995) Persistent and relapsing infections associated with small-colony variants of Staphylococcus aureus. Clin Infect Dis 20(1): 95–102
78. Rand JA, Bryan RS, Morrey BF et al (1986) Management of infected total knee arthroplasty.Clin Orthop Relat Res (205):75–85

79. Raut VV, Orth MS, Orth MC et al (1996) One stage revision arthroplasty of the hip for deep gram negative infection. Int Orthop 20(1):12–14
80. Raut VV, Siney PD, Wroblewski BM (1994) One-stage revision of infected total hip replacements with discharging sinuses. J Bone Joint Surg (Br) 76(5):721–724
81. Raut VV, Siney PD, Wroblewski BM (1995) One-stage revision of total hip arthroplasty for deep infection: long-term followup. Clin Orthop Relat Res (321):202–207
82. Raut VV, Siney PD, Wroblewsky BM (1986) One-stage revision of infected cemented total hip arthroplasty. Clin Orthop Relat Res (211):103–107
83. Raut VV, Siney PD, Wroblewsky BM (1995) Cemented Charnley revision arthroplasty for severe femoral osteolysis. J Bone Joint Surg (Br) 77(3):362–365
84. Ries MD, Jergesen H (1999) An inexpensive molding method for antibiotic-impregnated cement spacers in infected total hip arthroplasty. J Arthroplasty 14(6):764–765
85. Romanò C, Romanò D, Meani E (2002) Two-stage non-cemented revision of infected total hip prosthesis. Proceedings of ISTA Oxford (UK)
86. Rothman RH, Cohn JC (1990) Cemented versus cementless total hip arthroplasty. A critical review. Clin Orthop Relat Res (254):153–169
87. Sakalkale SP, Eng K, Hozack WJ et al (1999) Minimum 10-Year Results of a Tapered Cementless Hip Replacement. Clin Orthop Relat Res (362):138–144
88. Salvati EA, Chekofsky KM, Brause BD et al (1982) Reimplantation in infection: a 12-year experience. Clin Orthop Relat Res (170):62–75
89. Sanzen L, Sundberg M (1997) Periprosthetic low-grade hip infections. Erythrocyte sedimentation rate and C-reactive protein in 23 cases. Acta Orthop Scand 68(5):461–465
90. Sanzen L, Carlsson AS, Josefsson G et al (1988) Revision operations on infected total hip arthroplasties: two- to nine-year follow-up study. Clin Orthop Relat Res (229):165–172
91. Schroeder HM, Kristensen PW, Petersen MB et al (1998) Patient survival after total knee arthroplasty. 5-year data in 926 patients. Acta Orthop Scand 69(1):35–38
92. Segawa H, Tsukayama DT, Kyle RF et al (1999) Infection after total knee arthroplasty: a retrospective study of the treatment of eighty-one infections. J Bone Joint Surg (Am) 81(10):1434–1445
93. Sia IG, Berbari EF, Karchmer AW (2005) Prosthetic Joint IndectionsInfect Dis Clin N Am 19():885–914
94. Smith PN, Eyres KS (1999) Safe removal of massive intrapelvic cement using ultrasonic instruments. J Arthroplasty 14(2):235–238
95. Spangehl MJ, Masri BA, O'Connell JX et al (1999) Prospective analysis of preoperative and intraoperative investigations for the diagnosis of infection at the sites of two hundred and two revision total hip arthroplasties. J Bone Joint Surg (Am) 81(5):672–683
96. Spangehl MJ, Younger AS, Masri BA et al (1998) Diagnosis of infection following total hip arthroplasty. Instr Course Lect (47):285–295
97. Taggart T, Kerry RM, Norman P et al (2002) The use of vancomycin-impregnated cement beads in the management of infection of prosthetic joints. J Bone Joint Surg (Br) 84(1):70–72
98. Thornes B, Murray P, Bouchier-Hayes D (2002) Development of resistant strains of staphylococcus epidermidis on gentamicin-loaded cement in vivo. J Bone Joint Surg (Br) 84(5):757–760
99. Tsukayama DT, Estrada R, Gustilo RB (1996) Infection after total hip arthroplasty. A study of the treatment of one hundred and six infections. J Bone Joint Surg (Am) 78(4):512–523
100. Tunney MM, Patrick S, Gorman SP et al (1998) Improved detection of infection in hip replacements: a currently underestimated problem. J Bone Joint Surg (Br) 80(4):568–572
101. Ure KJ, Amstutz HC, Nasser S et al (1998) Direct-exchange arthroplasty for the treatment of infection after total hip replacemnet. An average ten-year follow-up. J Bone Joint Surg (Am) 80(7):961–968
102. Von Eiff C, Proctor RA, Peters G (2000) Small colony variants of staphylococci: a link to persistent infections. Berl Munch Tierarztl Wochenschr 113(9):321–325.Review
103. Von Eiff C, Proctor RA, Peters G (2000) Staphylococcus aureus small colony variants: formation and clinical impact. Int J Clin Pract Suppl (115):44–49
104. Walker PS, Culligan SG, Hua J et al (2000) Stability abd bone preservation in custom designed revision hip stems. Clin Orthop Relat Res (373):164–173

105. Wang JS, Franzén H, Lidgren L (1999) Interface gap after implantation of a cemented femoral stem in pigs. Acta Orthop Scand 70(3):234–239
106. Wang JW, Chen CE (1997) Reimplantation of infected hip arthroplasties using bone allografts. Clin Orthop Relat Res (335):202–210
107. Widmer AF (2001) New developments in diagnosis and treatment of infection in orthopedic implants. Clin Infect Dis 33(Suppl 2):94–106
108. Wilde AH (1994) Management of infected knee and hip prostheses. Curr Opin Rheumatol 6(2):172–176
109. Wilson MG, Dorr LD (1989) Reimplantation of infected total hip arthroplasties in the absence of antibiotic cement. J Arthroplasty 4(3):263–269
110. Windsor RE (1990) Two-stage reimplantation for the salvage of total knee arthroplasty complicated by infection. Further follow-up and refinement of indications. J Bone Joint Surg (Am) 72(2):272–278
111. Wroblewski B.M. (1986) One-stage revision of infected cemented total hip arthroplasty. Clin Orthop Relat Res (211):103–107
112. Younger AS, Duncan CP, Masri BA (1998) Treatment of infection associated with segmental bone loss in the proximal part of the femur in two stages with use of an antibiotic-loaded interval prosthesis. J Bone Joint Surg (Am) 80(1):60–69
113. Younger AS, Duncan CP, Masri BA et al (1997) The outcome of two-stage arthroplasty using custom-made onterval spacer to treat the infected hip. J Arthroplasty 12(6):615–623

Long-stem Preformed Spacers Followed by Uncemented Implants: A Solution for Wide Femoral Opening or Bone Loss in Two-stage Revision

C. Romanò, E. Meani

Department for Treatment of Osteoarticular Septic Complications (COS) –
Director: Prof. Enzo Meani
Operative Unit for Septic Prosthesis – Responsible: Prof. Carlo L. Romanò
"G.Pini" Orthopaedic Istitute, Milan, Italy

Introduction

Infection after total hip arthroplasty is a serious complication, and several treatment strategies have been proposed [5, 7, 10, 29, 35].

Two-stage reimplantation using an interval spacer of antibiotic-impregnated bone cement has been investigated previously as a method to eradicate infection and prevent limb shortening [12, 15, 20, 21, 41].

Revision surgery of infected hip prosthesis is often associated with femoral bone loss, due to the septic process in itself, associated mechanical loosening of the prosthesis, surgical debridement, cement and/or well fixed prosthesis removal. Preformed antibiotic-loaded spacers (Spacer-G – Tecres Spa, Italy) offer known mechanical resistance [1, 3], predictable antibiotic release [4] and reduced surgical time [26]. Additionally the long-stem versions allow to overcome proximal femoral bone loss, providing immediate primary stability and allowing partial weight bearing [38] (Fig. 1).

Medium-term results of a consecutive series of patients with chronically infected total hip arthroplasty, treated according to the same protocol are reported. The protocol included a two-stage revision using preformed antibiotic-loaded cement spacers and cementless modular long stem revision prosthesis together with prolonged systemic antibiotic therapy after first and second stage

Materials and Methods

From year 2000 to 2006 103 patients, affected by chronic septic hip prosthesis, underwent two stage hip revision in our Department. For the purpose of this study we have considered the first 48 consecutive patients, at a follow-up ranging from 2 to 6 years from revision. Two patients were lost to follow-up.

In all the cases the infected prosthesis was removed and a preformed antibiotic-loaded spacer (Spacer-G – Tecres Spa, Italy) was implanted. Spacer-G is an off-the-shelf preformed antibiotic-loaded cement hip spacer. It is available in three in different head sizes and two stem lengths, short (110 mm) and long (210 mm), that may be intra-operatively chosen. The inner part of the spacer features a stainless still rod that provides mechanical resistance. The cement is pre-loaded by the manufacturer with gentamicin at a concentration of 1.9 % (w/w).

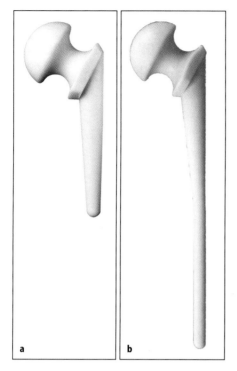

Fig. 1. Preformed antibiotic-loaded spacers (Spacer-G – Tecres Spa, Italy); **a** short (110 mm) and **b** long (210 mm) stemmed spacers come in three different head sizes (not shown)

8 to 12 weeks (mean 10.7 +- 2.1) after implantation, the spacer was removed and the patients underwent reconstruction using cementless modular prosthesis and non-cemented cups.

All the patients received systemic antibiotic treatment with two antibiotics for six weeks after the first and the second stage, on the basis of the antibiogram.

There were 18 men and 30 women. Mean age at the time of the operation was 56.8 years (range, 18–79). 29 patients were Type B hosts according to the Cierny-Mader classification system [8].

20 of the initial prosthetic components were cemented, 22 uncemented and 6 hybrid (femoral stem cemented, cup uncemented). Pre-operative limb shortening ranged from 0 to 60 mm.

The interval between the previous index operation and the revision ranged from 1 to 8 years. 17 patients underwent a previous revision operation and in the remaining patients all but 6 had at least one previous failed debridement.

Specimens for culture were obtained from wound drainage in 25 patients, from hip aspirate in 19 patients, only intra-operatively in 3 patients.

All the hips in this series were treated through a lateral approach, with the patient laying in supine position. In 32 cases the bone loss was Grade 3 or 4 according to Paprowsky classification and/or a large window femoral opening or a trans-femoral approach was necessary to remove a solidly fixed cemented or cementless femoral component or cement mantle.

After prosthesis removal and accurate bone and soft tissues debridement, Spacer-

G was inserted. In all the cases the spacer was fixed in the proximal part (Fig. 2), to prevent implant rotation, with one pack of antibiotic-loaded cement (Cemex Genta – Tecres Spa, Italy – gentamicin 2.5 %) to which vancomycin (5 %) was also intra-operatively added. The vancomycin powder was thoroughly mixed with the cement powder before the addition of liquid monomer. In the presence of gentamicin-resistant strains, vancomycin was also added to the spacer with the drilling technique, as described by Bertazzoni Minelli [4].

After spacer implantation and reduction, the osteotomy eventually performed was re-approximated around the antibiotic cement spacer with resorbable suture and no metallic cerclages or plates were used for further synthesis. No bone grafts were used

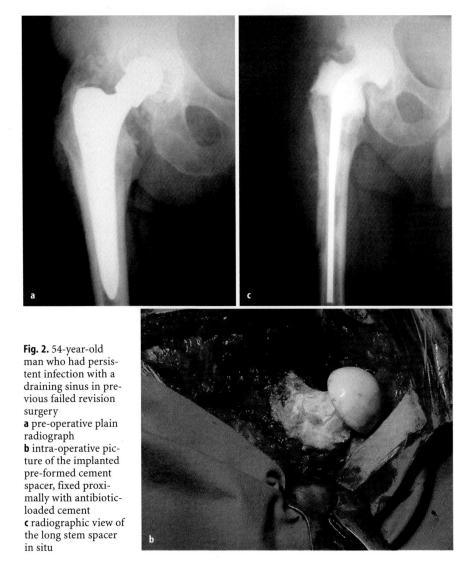

Fig. 2. 54-year-old man who had persistent infection with a draining sinus in previous failed revision surgery
a pre-operative plain radiograph
b intra-operative picture of the implanted pre-formed cement spacer, fixed proximally with antibiotic-loaded cement
c radiographic view of the long stem spacer in situ

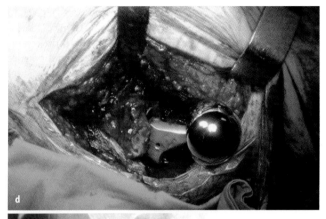

Fig. 2d. Revision with modular cementless implant and large (38 mm) metal-on-metal ball and socket, at 76 days after spacer implant

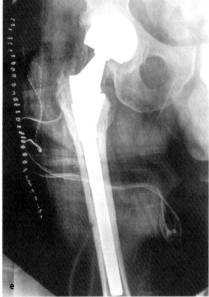

◁
Fig. 2e. Early post-operative X-ray

at the time of spacer implantation. 32 patients had severe proximal femoral bone loss, that required the use of a long-stem cement spacer and, 9 patients received autologous (three) or homologous (six) bone grafts with autologous platelet-rich-plasma.

Postoperatively, patients were allowed touch-down weight bearing for one month and then partial weight bearing on the operated extremity with two crutches until re-implantation.

All the patients received a minimum of 6 weeks of organism-specific antibiotics postoperatively and returned for clinical follow-up at the completion of their antibiotic course.

Routine laboratory studies were obtained including complete blood count with differential, erythrocyte sedimentation rate (ESR), and C-reactive protein (CRP). Patients were scheduled for removal of the spacer and revision arthroplasty 2 to 4 weeks after completion of intravenous antibiotics or 8 to 12 weeks after spacer implantation. Patients with successful eradication of their infection, as evidenced by complete blood count with differential and C-reactive protein within the normal ranges underwent the second stage of their reconstruction. If clinical suspicion of persistent infection remained, despite negative laboratory studies, joint aspiration before reimplantation was performed for cultural examination and white blood cells count. In all cases, intraoperative cultures were obtained at the time of the second stage procedure.

At revision the hip was exposed through the same lateral incision, and all the spacers were removed without difficulty.

All the hips were treated with modular titanium cementless femoral components (Profemur, Wright, or S-ROM Johnson&Johnson DePuy). Unconstrained cementless acetabular components were used in all cases. Touch-down weight bearing was allowed for 6 weeks followed by 50 % weight bearing for 6 weeks. Full weight-bearing and abductor strengthening were permitted 12 weeks after surgery. After operation, parenteral antibiotics were administered for 6 weeks. After each procedure closed suction drainage was inserted and removed after 48 hours.

All the patients underwent enoxaparin 0.4 ml/die for 30 days after surgery to prevent trombohaembolic complications and celecoxib 200 mg/die administration for 14 days after revision surgery, to prevent heterotopic ossifications [37].

Our primary outcomes included eradication of infection, spacer stability and integrity and implant stability.

Failure of treatment was a recurrence of infection, defined as the occurrence of clinical signs of infection (redness, swelling, pain, fistulae) whenever at follow-up.

Preoperative and post-operative hematologic studies included the determination of erythrocyte sedimentation rate, white blood cell count, and C-reactive protein level. Plain radiographs included anteroposterior and trans-lateral views of the hip joint.

Radiographic examination was performed at 2, 6 and 12 months postoperatively, followed by yearly intervals thereafter. These were compared to determine femoral component subsidence and signs of osteolysis.

Hip function was recorded using the method of Merle d'Aubigne et al [30]. In this scoring system, 6 points were awarded for the following: pain, walking ability, and movement range. This amounted to a total score of 18 for a normal hip. A rating of 17 to 18 was considered excellent; 15 to 16, good; 13 to 14, fair; and < 13, poor. Clinical failure was defined as a Merle d'Aubigne hip score of < 13.

Heterotopic ossification was quantified using the classification proposed by Brooker et al [6].

The spacer dislocation and use of allograft were also noted and included in the analysis. Complications including persistent infection, fractures, implant instability, subsidence or proximal migration, and revision were noted.

Results

The 48 patients included in this study were followed for an average of 48 months (range, 24 – 72). Two patients were lost to follow-up at 24 and 34 months post-operatively, respectively.

The average preoperative hip score by Merle d'Aubigne et al [30] was 4.9 points (range, 3 – 12). Before operation, erythrocyte sedimentation rate averaged 82 mm/h (range, 12–155), and C-reactive protein level averaged 72 mg/L (range, 5–258). Erythrocyte sedimentation rates, C-reactive protein levels, or both were high in 44 patients.

Identified organisms were the followings: *Staphylococcus aureus* in 21 patients and *Staphylococcus epidermidis* in 19 patients (methicillin-resistant staphylococcal strains: 22), *Pseudomonas aeruginosa* in 8 patients, *Escherichia coli* in 2 patients, *Enterobacter cloacae* in 1 patient, *Serratia marcescens* in 1 patient, no isolates in two patients. 6 patients showed a mixed flora.

The duration of the first stage of the operation averaged 165 minutes (range, 125–220). Blood transfusions averaged 4.5 units of blood.

The interval between the first-stage and second-stage operations ranged from 8 to 12 weeks (mean 10.7 ± 2.1).

During the interval, most patients had tolerable pain in the hip; 32 patients had no pain, 14 patients had mild pain and 2 patients had moderate pain.

36 patients were able to walk with partial weight bearing and 12 with touch-down weight bearing. 1 patient who had a femoral nerve palsy walked with a knee-brace.

A cementless femoral component was implanted in all the 48 revised hips (Profemur R modular long-stem, Wright-Cremascoli or S-ROM, Johnson&Johnson DePuy). Acetabular revisions were performed with uncemented components in all the cases.

The duration of the second-stage operations averaged 175 minutes (range, 130–250). Blood transfusions averaged 4.2 units (range, 3–12) of blood. The closed suction drain was removed at 2 days after the second-stage operation. The total drainage ranged from 210 to 650 mL (average, 470).

At the time of the latest follow-up one patient (2.2%) showed clinical evidence of infection recurrence. This was a Type B host, according to Cierny-Mader (rheumatoid arthritis and immunosuppressive treatments).

The hip score was improved to an average of 13.8 points (range, 10–16). 26 patients (55%) had excellent or good results, 14 patients had fair results, and 4 patients had poor results. The short operated limbs were lengthened a mean of 19 mm (range, 0–35).

At the latest follow-up all the acetabular components were stable and none of the femoral components were revised. In 42 hips, the femoral stems were fixed by bone ingrowth and good proximal bone remodeling was achieved (Fig. 3). The remaining 4 femoral stems subsided 2 to 5 mm, but they were stabilized by stable fibrous ingrowth. The 9 hips that received morcellized autologous (3 patients) or homologous (6 patients) bone grafts and platelet-rich-plasma had complete healing within 6 months with bone ingrowth.

Postoperative complications included nine spacer cranial dislocation, that required no treatment but prevented weight bearing, one femoral nerve palsy, partially recovered after 12 months, two revision prosthesis dislocations, that required open reduction and change of the modular neck offset. No Grade 3 or 4 heterotopic ossification occurred.

Four patients had side effects during antibiotic treatment, including gastrointestinal tract dysfunction in one patient, temporary liver dysfunction in two patients and bone marrow depression in one patient. These side effects were resolved after temporary withdrawal of antibiotics.

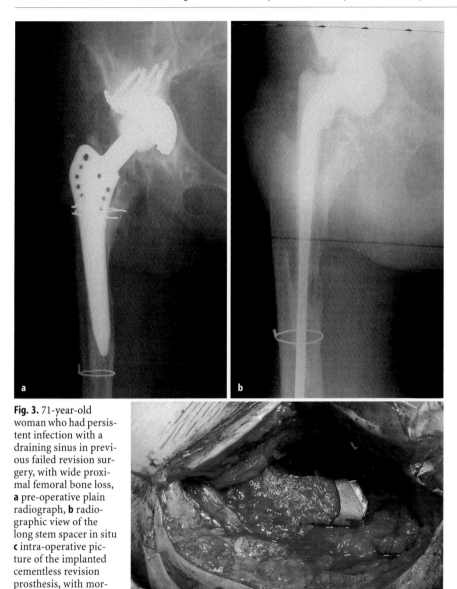

Fig. 3. 71-year-old woman who had persistent infection with a draining sinus in previous failed revision surgery, with wide proximal femoral bone loss, **a** pre-operative plain radiograph, **b** radiographic view of the long stem spacer in situ **c** intra-operative picture of the implanted cementless revision prosthesis, with morcellized homologous bone grafts and platelet-rich-plasma in the proximal third of the femoral component

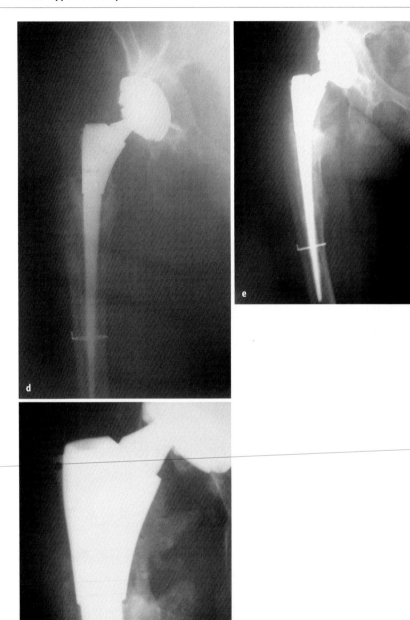

Fig. 3d. early post-operative X-ray, **e** at two years follow-up, **f** note the optimal new bone formation and osteointegration of the graft

Discussion

Duncan and Beauchamp [21] who introduced the concept of the interval spacer in a two-stage procedure for the treatment of infected THA, developed a refined interval spacer (prosthesis of antibiotic-loaded acrylic cement [PROSTALAC]) that has to be prepared intraoperatively by the surgeon. The eradication rate of infection was 93.5 %. The merits of PROSTALAC were a decrease in hip pain and the ability of patients to walk between the 2 stages. The Spacer-G preformed cement spacer allows early weight bearing and (protected) walking ability, pain-free hip mobility and predictable antibiotic local release, while it adds the following advantages: reduced operatory time and different sizes available, including long-stem spacers. Long-stem preformed spacers appear particularly useful in consideration of the frequent occurrence of proximal femoral bone loss in hip infection surgery either due to the loosening of the prosthesis, the septic process and/or to surgical debridement or intra-operative fractures [2, 9, 11, 17, 31, 36, 42]. Long-stem spacers provide also in these challenging cases, primary stability and mechanical resistance allowing partial weight bearing, while the range of movement and limb length is maintained [38].

Cranial dislocation of the spacer was the main complication in the present series (19 %) and, although it did not required any treatment, its occurrence did not allow to maintain limb length and prevented weight bearing. Concurrent acetabulum bone loss and/or muscle insufficiency and the fixed offset of the spacer are the main reasons for the relatively high rate of this complication. The patients should adequately be informed prior to spacer implant of the possible occurrence of this complication that does not seem to affect the final result, but significantly reduces walking ability during the interval between spacer and revision surgery. It should be noted that, even in the case of spacer dislocation, the presence of the spacers is helpful in preventing further limb shortening, in assuring local antibiotic delivery while filling the dead space caused by prosthesis removal.

Dislocation of the revision prosthesis occurred in two cases (4 %) both of whom required open reduction and change of modular neck offset. Although this rate of dislocation is relatively low, compared to other studies, in which revision prosthesis dislocation rate ranges from 10.2 % to 31 % [13, 14, 31], both cases in our series had spacer dislocation prior to revision surgery. In case of spacer dislocation we now recommend, whenever possible, earlier revision (6 to 8 weeks after spacer implant) and the use of larger (36-mm or more) metal on metal socket balls at reimplantation. This led us to observe no dislocation after revision in the most recent series of 44 patients operated in the last two years.

Cementless revision arthroplasty provided a higher success rate than the cemented revision in a similar follow-up in aseptic loosening in different studies [13, 14, 23, 32] and long-term survival of antibiotic-loaded cemented prosthesis has been shown to be rather low [7]. In the revision of the infected hip prosthesis, however, the cementless system may have a possible disadvantage because local antibiotics cannot be delivered without using the cement. On the other side one may argue that if the antibiotic in the cement spacer did not provide local antibiotic levels able to eradicate the infection during a two-three months period, this will not be achieved by the necessarily lower levels of antibiotics added to the cement used for fixation of a revision prosthesis.

Relatively few studies have reported the results of 2-stage reimplantation using cementless components in an infected hip. Nestor et al [35] reported an 18 % rate of recurrent infection in their study of 34 cementless revisions for the treatment of infected total hip prosthesis. They concluded that cementless revision does not improve the rate of resolution of infection. On the contrary Fehring et al [15] and Haddad et al [18] reported an 8 % infection recurrence in their studies.

Eradication of infection in our series was achieved in 45/48 cases, 2 patients were lost to follow-up and one (2.2 %) showed infection recurrence. With the protocol used (local and systemic antibiotic treatment), cementless revision appears safe and effective to eradicate infection and allow good stability on the medium term. Our results are better than the 80 % to 95 % eradication rates reported in the literature for chronic infection [7, 10, 16, 25]; we are now extending our series of patients and follow-up periods to verify these very encouraging preliminary data. Our results are also remarkable considering our patient population in whom 16 (28 %) had at least one failed previous revision procedure and 28 (55 %) were Cierny-Mader B–type host.

S. aureus and *S. epidermidis* are the predominant organisms of infection after joint arthroplasty. Methicillin-resistant *Staphylococci* (MRS) have been identified as an important pathogen in patients who have an infection at the site of a joint prosthesis and this also occurred in our series with a relative prevalence of 47 %. Vancomycin is the most potent agent against MRS. Gentamicin is potent against *Enterobacteriaceae* and *P. aeruginosa*, which are common pathogens of infection after joint arthroplasty. Nevertheless, many gram-positive and negative organisms are resistant to gentamicin. Therapeutic levels of vancomycin and gentamicin, have been found *in vitro* and in drainage fluid after they were used with cement [19, 22, 24, 27, 28, 33, 34]. In our series vancomycin was added in the cement used to fix the spacer implant and with a drilling technique in the spacer itself.

Levels of vancomycin in serum after the use of vancomycin-loaded cement have been shown to be negligible, and an association between the use of vancomycin in cement and the isolation of vancomycin-resistant *Enterococci* (VRE) have not been shown [12, 28].

It has been claimed that a drain should not be inserted to spare the antibiotic-rich periprosthetic fluid [40]. A drain should be inserted, however, to prevent a haematoma that could create a medium for organism growth. Drain insertion decreases the dead space after the haematoma formation. In the present study, a closed suction drain was inserted in all patients, and we found that drain insertion was not correlated with infection recurrence.

Systemic antibiotic administration has been performed for approximately six weeks after the first and second stage operation. The antibiotic choice has been made on the basis of cultural examination and antibiogram and two antibiotics have been administered parenterally and orally during the first 3 or 4 weeks and then only orally for the remaining 2 or 3 weeks in all the patients. In the lack of comparative studies it is not possible to drive any conclusion either if this prolonged systemic antibiotic treatment was an over-treatment or, on the contrary and as we suggest, if it may have played a role in the overall good success rate in this series of patients. Four of our patients (9 %) had side effects due to antibiotics, including temporary liver dysfunction and bone marrow depression. These side effects might be related to postoperative intravenous antibiotics or antibiotics used in the cement spacer (or both). However, the safety of the antibiotic delivery from the cement spacer has been previously established [12] and the side effects resolved after temporary withdrawal of intravenous antibiotics in all the patients.

We have observed no side effects due to the use of autologous or homologous morcellized bone graft at the time of revision and this is to our knowledge the first report on the use of platelet-rich-plasma in revision surgery in previously infected hip prosthesis. Platelet-rich-plasma has been shown in different studies [39] to provide locally growth factors able to promote and accelerate bone healing both in animal and in humans. Even if it was not the aim of this study to demonstrate a quicker or larger bone growth in patients treated with platelet-rich-plasma in two-stage cementless revision of septic hip prosthesis, our data point out the safety of this technology in this application and the need for further studies, given the frequent occurrence of bone loss in revision surgery in infections.

References

1. Affatato S, Mattarozzi A, Taddei P et al (2003) Investigations on the wear behaviour of the temporary PMMA-based hip Spacer-G Proc Inst Mech Eng 217(1):1–8
2. Aribindi R, Paprosky W, Nourbash P et al (1999) Extended proximal femoral osteotomy, AAOS Instr Course Lect (48):19–26
3. Baleani M, Traina F, Toni A (2003) The mechanical behaviour of a pre-formed hip spacer. Hip International 13(3):159–162
4. Bertazzoni Minelli E, Benini A, Magnan B et al (2004) Release of gentamicin and vancomycin from temporary human hip spacers in two-stage revision of infected arthroplasty. J Antimicrob Chemother 53(2):329–334
5. Bittar ES, Petty W (1982) Girdlestone arthroplasty for infected total hip arthroplasty. Clin Orthop Relat Res (170):83–87
6. Brooker A, Bowerman J, Robinson R (1973) Ectopic ossification following total hip replacement: incidence and a method of classification J Bone Joint Surg (Am) 55(8):1629–1632
7. Buchholz HW, Elson RA, Engelbrecht E et al (1981) Management of deep infection of total hip replacement. J Bone Joint Surg (Br) 63(3):342–353
8. Calhoun JH, Cierny G, Holtom P et al (1994) Symposium: current concepts in the management of osteomyelitis, Contemp Orthop 28(2):157–185
9. Cameron HU (1991) Use of a distal trochanteric osteotomy in hip revision, Contemp Orthop 23(3):235–238
10. Carlsson AS, Joseffson G, Lindberg LT (1978) Revision with gentamicin-impregnated cement for deep infections in total hip arthroplasties. J Bone Joint Surg (Am) 60(8):1059–1064
11. Chen W-M, McAuley JP, Engh CA et al (2000) Extended slide trochanteric osteotomy for revision total hip arthroplasty. J Bone Joint Surg (Am) 82(9):1215–1219
12. Duncan CP, Masri BA (1995) The role of antibiotic-loaded cement in the treatment of an infection after a hip replacement. Instr Course Lect (44):305–313. Review
13. Engelbrecht DJ, Weber FA, Sweet MB et al (1990) Long-term results of revision total hip arthroplasty. J Bone Joint Surg (Br) 72(1):41–45
14. Engh CA, Glassman AH, Griffin WL et al (1988) Results of cementless revision for failed cemented total hip arthroplasty. Clin Orthop Relat Res (235):91–110
15. Fehring TK, Calton TF, Griffin WL (1999) Cementless fixation in 2-stage reimplantation for periprosthetic sepsis. J Arthroplasty 14(2):175–181
16. Garvin KL, Evans BG, Salvati EA et al (1994) Palacos gentamicin for the treatment of deep periprosthetic hip infections. Clin. Orthop Relat Res (298):97–105
17. Glassman AH, Engh CA, Bobyn JD (1987) A technique of extensile exposure for total hip arthroplasty. J. Arthroplasty 2(1):11–21
18. Haddad FS, Muirhead-Allwood SK, Manktelow AR et al (2000) Two-stage uncemented revision hip arthroplasty for infection. J Bone Joint Surg (Br) 82(5):689–694

19. Hill L, Klenerman L, Trustey S, Blowers R (1975) Diffusion of antibiotics from acrylic bone-cement in vitro. J Bone Joint Surg (Br) 59(2):197–199
20. Ivarsson I, Wahlstrom O, Djerf K et al (1994) Revision of infected hip replacement: Two-stage procedure with a temporary gentamicin spacer. Acta Orthop Scand 65(1):7–8
21. Kendall RW, Masri BA, Duncan CP et al (1994) Temporary antibiotic loaded acrylic hip replacement: a novel method for management of the infected THA. Semin Arthroplasty 5(4):171–177
22. Kuechle DK, Landon GC, Musher DM et al (1975) Elution of vancomycin, daptomycin, and amikacin from acrylic bone cement. Clin Orthop Relat Res (264):302–308
23. Lawrence JM, Engh CA, Macalino GE et al (1994) Outcome of revision hip arthroplasty done without cement. J Bone Joint Surg (Am) 76(7):965–973
24. Levin PD (1975) The effectiveness of various antibiotics in methyl methacrylate. J Bone Joint Surg (Br) 57(2):234–237
25. Lieberman JR, Callaway GH, Salvati EA et al (1994) Treatment of the infected total hip arthroplasty with a two-stage reimplantation protocol. Clin. Orthop (301):205–212
26. Magnan B, Regis D, Biscaglia R et al (2001) Preformed acrylic bone cement spacer loaded with antibiotics. Use of two-stage procedure in 10 patients because of infected hips after total replacement. Acta Orthop Scand 72(6):591–594
27. Marks KH, Nelson CL, Lautenschlager EP (1976) Antibiotic-impregnated acrylic bone cement. J Bone Joint Surg (Am) 58(3):358–364
28. Masterson EL, Masri BA, Duncan CP (1998) Treatment of infection at the site of total hip replacement. Instr Course Lect (47):297–306
29. McDonald DJ, Fitzgerald RH Jr, Listrup DM et al (1989) Two-stage reconstruction of a total hip arthroplasty because of infection. J Bone Joint Surg (Am) 71(6):828–834
30. Merle d'Aubigne R, Postel M, Mazabraud A et al (1965) Idiopathic necrosis of the femoral head in adults. J Bone Joint Surg (Br) 47(4):612–633
31. Miner TM, Momberger NG, Chong D et al (2001) The extended trochanteric osteotomy in revision hip arthroplasty: a critical review of 166 at mean 3-year, 9-month follow-up. J Arthroplasty 16(8 Suppl 1):188–194
32. Moreland JR, Bernstein ML (1995) Femoral revision hip arthroplasty with uncemented, porous-coated stems. Clin Orthop Relat Res (319):141–150
33. Murray WR (1984) Use of antibiotic-containing bone cement. Clin Orthop Relat Res (190):89–95
34. Nelson CL, Evans RP, Blaba JD et al (1993) A comparison of gentamicin-impregnated poly-methylmethacrylate bead implantation to conventional parenteral antibiotic therapy in infected total hip and knee arthroplasty. Clin Orthop Relat Res (295):96–101
35. Nestor BJ, Hanssen AD, Ferrer-Gonzalez R, Fitzgerald RH Jr (1994) The use of porous prostheses in delayed reconstruction of total hip replacements that have failed because of infection. J Bone Joint Surg (Am) 76(3):349–359
36. Peters PC, Head WC, Emerson RH (1993) An extended trochanteric osteotomy for revision total hip replacement, J Bone Joint Surg (Br) 75(1):158–159
37. Romano CL, Duci D, Romano D et al (2004) Celecoxib versus indomethacin in the prevention of heterotopic ossification after total hip arthroplasty. J Arthroplasty 19(1):14–18
38. Romano CL, Meani E (2004) The use of pre-formed long stem antibiotic-loaded cement spacers for two-stage revisions of infected hip prosthesis. Multimedia Education Center American Academy of Orthopaedic Surgeons, San Francisco, CA – March 10–14, 2004
39. Tonelli P, Mannelli D, Brancato L et al (2005) Counting of platelet derived growth factor and transforming growth factor-beta in platelet-rich-plasma used in jaw bone regeneration. Minerva Stomatol 54(1–2):23–34
40. Younger AS, Duncan CP, Masri BA (1998) Treatment of infection associated with segmental bone loss in the proximal part of the femur in two stages with use of an antibiotic-loaded interval prosthesis. J Bone Joint Surg (Am) 80(1):60–69
41. Younger AS, Duncan CP, Masri BA et al (1997) The outcome of two-stage arthroplasty using a custom-made interval spacer to treat the infected hip. J Arthroplasty 12(6):615–623
42. Younger TI, Bradford MS, Magnus RE et al (1995) Extended proximal femoral osteotomy. A new technique for femoral revision arthroplasty. J Arthroplasty (10):329–338

Two-stage Revision Surgery in Septic Total Hip Arthroplasty

C.H. LOHMANN[1,2], M. FUERST[2], O. NIGGEMEYER[2], W. RUETHER[1,2]

Departments of Orthopaedics, [1]University of Hamburg-Eppendorf, Hamburg, Germany
[2] Rheumaklinik Bad Bramstedt, Germany

Introduction

Infections of total joint arthroplasties is one of the most debilitating situation for the patients that have received an artificial joint replacement. The infection rate of total joint arthroplasty varies between different reports (0.3 % [19], 1.0 – 1.7 % [3, 13, 26], 3 % [16], 7 % [17]. However, with today's modern surgical techniques, antibiotic prophylaxis and clean air surgical suits, the infection rate should not exceed 2 % [24].

The pathway of the infection consists of contamination with pathogens, their adhesion, colonization, invasion of tissues, and exacerbation of the infection. In normal tissue there is a balance between the pathogen and the humoral defence which depends on the rate of multiplication of the pathogens and the ability to eliminate them [8].

The specific situation in the periprosthetic infection is the ability of bacteria to form a biofilm on the implant surfaces with a high affinity to smooth surfaces and polyethylene. It is known for a long time that a foreign body material infection can be induced by a very low number of pathogens: 100 bacteria are considered to be a sufficient number to cause an infection of an implant [6, 22]. This then initiates a cascade of events that involves the competition for the implant surface between osteoblasts, fibroblasts, and bacteria [11].

This paper gives an overview of the treatment with two-stage revision surgery in periprosthetic infections. The clinical results of a high-risk cohort of patients with rheumatoid arthritis as their presenting underlying diagnosis. They were treated with total joint replacement and became infected. A two stage revision was performed and the results reported.

Our treatment protocol follows an algorithm that includes preclinical, analytical as well as clinical, therapeutical procedures. Patients with an exacerbated infection or early infection of their total joint are rather rare. Most often patients present with low-grade infection.

The patient with onset of pain in an artificial joint is screened with routine radiographs and blood tests. Isotope scans can be performed but are not highly specific [15, 23]. Fluoroscopy may be helpful to rule out impingement as well as CT scans may show malpositioning of the implant components. An aspiration is performed under sterile conditions, the sample is sent to a microbiology laboratory that ensures a culture time of more than 10 days to detect low-grade infections [1, 18]. If the results are not conclusive, an open or arthroscopic biopsy is performed and tissue from the inner joint capsule is analysed by microbiology and pathology [9].

The proof of a periprosthetic infection requires the removal of all prosthetic components, including well-fixed components [12, 14]. Aggressive debridement is performed in order to eliminated necrotic and infected tissues. In case of cemented implants, the parts of the cement mantles are very thoroughly removed from the implant bed. An antibiotic spacer formed from cement is inserted into the joint for two reasons: 1. Local release of antibiotics is desirable for a certain period of time. Therefore, specific antibiotics for the bacteria may be added to the cement. 2. The leg length can be maintained by the use of a spacer and mobilization of the patients is easier than with just only implant removal alone. Intravenous antibiotic treatment is given to the patient for 2 weeks, and 4 weeks orally.

6 weeks after removal of the prosthetic components, the spacer is removed, the implant site is again thoroughly debrided and the revision joint replacement is performed. The antibiotic treatment is continued for 2 additional weeks.

Materials and Methods

The septic revisions of patients with total hip, knee and elbow arthroplasties of the Rheumaklinik Bad Bramstedt from 1990 to 2000 were reviewed. Only total joint arthroplasties that were implanted in the Rheumaklinik Bad Bramstedt were included to this review. The infection rate in the cohort was 0.72 %.

Patient's Profile

There were 47 patients, 24 were females and 23 were males. Underlying disease was rheumatoid arthritis (RA) in 21 patients, 26 patients had joint replacement secondary to degenerative osteoarthritis (OA). The age ranged from 21 to 86 years with a mean age of 62 years. The total joint replacements were 15 total hips, 29 total knees, and 3 elbow prostheses. The follow-up time was 70 months (3 – 162 months). Endpoints of the review were septic recurrence, death, or last follow up contact with the patient (Table 1).

Clinical symptoms and diagnostics

All patients had obvious clinical symptoms with pain in their joints, reduced range of motion. The laboratory parameters for infection were elevated in 76.6 %. An aspiration was performed in all cases and bacteria could be detected in 85.1 %. Isotope scan was performed in 83.7 % of the cases and had a sensitivity of 100 %.

Radiological signs of loosening were seen only in 34 % of the cases.

Number of Patients	47 (24 male, 23 female)
Age	21 – 86 yrs.
Site	15 Hips, 29 Knees, 3 Elbows
Diagnosis	26 Arthritis, 21 RA
Follow up	70 mts. (3 – 162)

Table 1. Clinical profile of the patients

Results

At the time of the surgery, samples for bacteriology were taken. In 2 patients an infection could not be proven by intraoperative samples. However, in 95.8 % of the cases the preoperative diagnosis of periprosthetic infection was supported by intraoperative sampling. All patients were subjected to a two-stage revision. The patients received 6 weeks of antibiotic treatment during a period with a spacer in the infected site. The patients received cemented artificial joint replacements for revision implant.

In this cohort 36 patients (76.6 %) were free of infection at the time of their last follow up. 3 of the patients died not related to surgery without a recurrence of infection. 11 patients (23.4 %) had a recurrence of their infection. The underlying diagnoses of these patients were in 7 cases rheumatoid arthritis and only in 4 cases degenerative arthritis. The sites of the infection in the rheumatoid patients were 4 hips, 2 knees and 1 elbow. In the other group of the patients, there were only patients with infected endoprostheses of the knee.

The overall success rate to cure the periprosthetic infection was 83 % in the arthritis group and 71 % in the rheumatoid arthritis group (Table 2).

Table 2. The clinical outcome of the patients after two stage revision surgery

	No recurrence	Recurrence
Diagnosis	36 14 RA, 22 Arthritis	11 7 RA, 4 Arthritis

Discussion

This paper reveals the effectiveness of two stage revision surgery in cases of periprosthetic infections. The rate of infection in this cohort of patients was 0.72 %. This reflects the infection rates (0 % – 2 %) that are reported in the literature elsewhere [3, 13, 26]. 23.4 % of the patients had a recurrence. The predominant patients with a recurrence of infection were patients with rheumatoid arthritis as underlying arthropathy (63.4 %).

The importance for the success of the revision of a periprosthetic infection has several factors. The appropriate sampling and handling of the specimens. The specimen should be representative for the site of infection and free of contaminating bacteria. We consider joint fluid or biopsy tissue as representative. This may lead to an increased rate of successful diagnostic procedures. The identification of the pathogens is described between 60 % [7] up to 80 % [2] and 90 % [21]. Using our diagnostic algorithm, it was possible to identify the pathogen in more than 85 % of the cases.

The eradication of the implant associated infections without removing foreign body is not possible [10]. Thus, the removal of the implants is mandatory in late infection. However, other options that are in clinical use should be also discussed in the following paragraphs.

The retention of the prosthesis is only an option for early infection following 6 weeks after implantation of the artificial joint. This includes the revision, debridement, exchange of the mobile parts of the prosthesis and/or suction/irrigation which is followed by long-term systemic antibiotic therapy. However, this is a treatment that should only be applied to patients within 6 weeks after their joint replacement [5].

The most promising treatment is the exchange of the prosthesis in a one stage revision or a two stage revision procedure. One stage revision procedures require the exchange of the procedure with a debridement of the implant bed and the cemented re-implantation with the addition of specific antibiotics to the bone cement [10, 20, 24, 25]. The treatment with two stage revision surgery was described earlier.

The risk factors for implant infections are variable and several factors have been shown to be primary risks and other have been shown to be supportive [4].

The risk factors like previous joint replacement, postop wound infection, malignant disease, and increased NNIS score are associated with a increased of periprosthetic infection. Relative risk factors amongst others are rheumatoid arthritis and steroid therapy and also placement of the implant close to the skin. This is represented in our results: In the group of patients with degenerative arthritis, we observed infections only in patients with knee total replacements. Furthermore, the infection rate was clearly increased in patients with rheumatoid arthritis and long term steroid therapies.

The advantage of the two stage revision surgery includes a continuous local release of antibiotics. Those antibiotics must be able to infiltrate bony tissues, should have low tissue toxicity and high tissue compatibility. Additional systemic therapy is mandatory. [28].

Two stage revision surgery is treatment of choice in our algorithm. Only treating with systemic antibiotics is not effective in our opinion and should be considered only in a highly selective patients. This treatment alone can only be considered as suppression of the infection but not as eradicating the infection. We believe that the addition of antibiotics in the spacer cement for 6 weeks has advantages for the effective treatment in periprosthetic infections. Systemic therapy is mandatory, Rifampicin is one of the most valuable agents to treat infected implant. Usually, a combination therapy is favourable in systemic antibiotic therapy [27]. Our patient profile shows that patient with rheumatoid arthritis and steroid therapy do not only have a higher risk for implant infection but also for their recurrence.

References

1. Atkins BL, Athanasou N, Deeks JJ et al (1998) Prospective evaluation criteria for microbiological diagnosis of prosthetic joint infection at revision arthroplasty. J Clin Microbiol 36(10):2932–2939
2. Barrack RL, Harris WH (1993) The value of aspiration of the hip joint before revision total hip arthroplasty. J Bone Joint Surg (Am) 75(1):66–67
3. Bengston S, Knutson K, Lidgren L (1989) Treatment of infected knee arthroplasty. Clin Orthop Relat Res (245):173–178
4. Berbari EF, Hanssen AD, Duffy MC et al (1998) Risk factors for prostetic joint infections: case control-study. Clin Infect Dis 27(5):1247–1254
5. Crockarell JR, Hanssen AD, Osmon DR et al (1998) Treatment of infection with debridement and retention of the components following hip arthroplasty. J Bone Joint Surg (Am) 80(9):1306–1313
6. Elek SD, Conen PE (1957) The virulence of Staphylococcus pyogenes for man; a study of the problems of wound infection. Br J Exp Pathol 38(6):53–86

7. Fehring TK, Cohen B (1996) Aspiration as a guide to sepsis in revision total hip arthroplasty. J Arthroplasty 11(5):543–547
8. Frommelt L (2006) Principles of systemic antimicrobial therapy in foreign material associated infection in bone tissue, with special focus on periprosthetic infection. Injury 37(Suppl 2):S87–94
9. Fuerst M, Fink B, Rüther W (2005) The value of preoperative knee aspiration and arthroscopic biopsy in revision total knee arthroplasty. Z Orthop Ihre Grenzgeb 143(1):36–41
10. Garvin KL, Hanssen AD (1995) Infection after total hip arthroplasty. Past, present and future. J Bone Joint Surg (Am) 77(10):1576–1588. Review
11. Gristina AG (1994) Implant failure and immuno-incompetent fibro-inflammatory zone. Clin Orthop Relat Res (298):106–118
12. Haddad FS, Muirhead-Allwood SK, Manktelow AR et al (2000) Two-Stage uncemented revision hip arthroplasty for infection. J Bone Joint Surg (Br) 82(5):689–694
13. Hanssen AD, Osmon DR, Nelson CL (1997) Prevention of deep periprosthetic joint infection. Instr Course Lect (46):555–567
14. Hanssen AD, Rand JA (1999) Evaluation and treatment of infection at the site of a total hip or knee arthroplasty. Instr Course Lect (48):111–122
15. Johnson JA, Christie MJ, Sandler MP et al (1998) Detection of occult infection following total joint arthroplasty using sequential technetium-99m HDP bone scintigraphy and indium-111 WBC imaging. J Nucl Med 29(8):1347–1353
16. Knutson K, Tjornstrand B, Lindgren L (1985) Survival of knee arthroplasties for rheumatoid athritis. Acta Orthop Scand 56(5):422–425
17. Kristensen O, Nafei A, Kjaersgaard-Andersen P et al (1992) Long-term results of total condylar knee arthroplasty in rheumatoid arthritis. J Bone Joint Surg (Br) 74(6):803–806
18. Lachiewicz PF, Rogers GD, Thomason HC (1996) Aspiration of the hip joint before revision total hip arthroplasty. Clinical and laboratory factors influencing attainment of a positive culture. J Bone Joint Surg (Am) 78(5):749–754
19. Lidwell OM (1986) Clear air operation and subsequent sepsis in the joint. Clin Orthop Rel Res (211):91–102
20. Masterson EL, Masri BA, Duncan CP (1998) Treatment of infection at the site of total hip replacement. Instr Course Lect (47):297–306
21. Spangehl MJ, Masri BA, O'Connell JX et al (1999) Prospective analysis of preoperative and intraoperative investigations for the diagnosis of infection at the site of two hundred and two revision total hip arthroplasties. J Bone Joint Surg (Am) 81(5):672–683
22. Stoodley P, Kathju S, Hu FZ et al (2005) Molecular and imaging techniques for bacterial biofilms in joint arthroplasty infections. Clin Orthop Relat Res (437):31–40
23. Teller RE, Christie MJ, Martin W et al (2000) Sequential indium-lableled leucocyte and bone scans to diagnose prosthetic joint infections. Clin Orthop Relat Res (373):241–247
24. Toms AD, Davidson D, Masri BA et al (2006) The management of per-prosthetic infection in total joint arthroplasty. J Bone Joint Surg (Br) 88(2):149–155
25. Tsukayama DT, Goldberg VM, Kyle R et al (2003) Diagnosis and management of infection after total knee arthroplasty. J Bone Joint Surg (Am) 85(Suppl 1):75–80
26. Zimmerli W (1995) Role of antibiotics in the treatment of infected joint prosthesis. Orthopäde 24(4):308–313
27. Zimmerli W, Tampuz A, Ochsner PE (2004) Prosthetic-joint infections. N Engl J Med 351(16):1645–1654. Review
28. Zimmerli W, Widmer AF, Blatter M et al (1998) Role of rifampicin for treatment of orthopedic implant-related staphylococcal infections: a randomized controlled trial. Foreign-Body Infection (FBI) Study Group. JAMA. 279(19):1537–1541

28 One-stage, Two-stage or Multi-stage Revision: the Reason of a Choice

M. Diefenbeck[1], A. Tiemann[1], G.O. Hofmann[1,2]

[1] Klinik für Unfall- und Wiederherstellungschirurgie, Berufsgenossenschaftliche Kliniken Bergmannstrost, Halle / Saale, Germany
[2] Klinik für Unfall-, Hand- und Wiederherstellungschirurgie, Friedrich-Schiller-Universität Jena, Germany

Introduction

Infection remains a serious complication following arthroplasty. Despite the improvement in surgical technique and implant design, the overall rate of infection ranges from about 0.5 – 1.4 % in total hip arthroplasty [12, 25].

The exact infection rate varies depending on localization, technique (cemented vs. cementless), duration of follow-up and implant used (Table 1).

To understand the difficulties in treating periprosthetic infections, we have to focus on some microbiological concerns. Bacteria adherent to the surface of implants change their biological behaviour. They produce a biofilm, the so-called glycocalix [20], which creates a microenvironment protective against antibiotics and the host's immune system (Fig. 1) [20, 33, 42]. Moreover, they reduce their metabolic activity and thus increase their generation times [4]. Because antibiotics act on growing bacteria, the minimum inhibitory concentrations (MIC) are higher with bacteria which have reduced metabolic activity. Costerton et al. found an 800-fold increased MIC for Tobramycin in adhesive *Pseudomonas aeruginosa* compared to non-adhesive bacteria [11].

With antibiotics and the host immune system becoming ineffective against the adhering bacteria and no possibility to remove the bacteria from the implant surface, the replacement of a prosthesis is the only remedy in many cases.

For any treatment concept it is important that the microbiological cascade, including the biofilm production, is time-dependent. Hence, if the treatment starts early, before the planctonic bacteria become adhesive in large numbers and produce a protective glycocalix, the best results can be achieved.

Table 1. Infection rate in total hip arthroplasty

Technique	Follow up (years)	Infection rate %	Year / reference
Cemented	5	0.2 (AB*) – 0.8	1997 / [18]
Cemented	10	0.4 (AB*) – 0.7	2003 / [17]
Screwed cup	10	4	1998 / [1]
Screwed cup	5	1.2	1998 / [15]
Screwed cup	6.3	0	2003 / [53]
Press-fit	9.1	0.76	1998 / [3]
Press-fit	9	1.4	2001 / [2]
Press-fit	10.3	1.1	2001 / [27]

* antibiotic-loaded cement

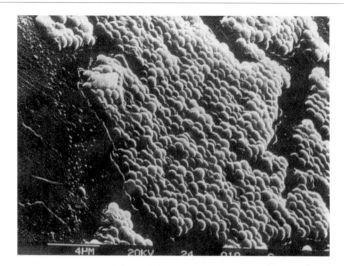

Fig. 1. *Staphylococcus epidermidis* adhesive on polyethylene (PE) (Photo: W. Mittelmeier, TU München)

Table 2. Revision concepts in infected arthroplasty

- Antibiotic treatment without surgery
- Debridement and irrigation with retention of the components
- One-stage revision
- Two-stage revision
- Multi-stage revision

The classification which correlates best with the microbiological process was published by Segawa et al [44] and Mont et al [39]. Early postoperative (acute) infection appears within the first four weeks after surgery, late chronic infection thereafter [39, 44]. Only in acute infection exists a realistic chance to eradicate the bacteria without removing or exchanging the implant. In chronic infection an exchange of the implant is mandatory.

However, the duration of infection is not the only parameter for the decision on a treatment concept. Age, comorbidity and immune response of the patient, sensitivity of the infecting bacteria and implant design [10] must be considered as well.

After taking all the details into account, the surgeon can decide which approach is the most promising. The different treatment options (Table 2) are described.

Revision Concepts

1. Antibiotic Treatment without Surgery

Conservative antibiotic therapy without an operative intervention should be restricted to patients which are not suitable for surgery because of their comorbidity or which disagree on a revision after informed consent. Cure from infection by conservative treatment cannot be expected, but a controlled *status quo* can be achieved.

Prerequisite for antibiotic therapy is that bacteria have been identified and oral antibiotics, according to the antibiogram, are available. To reduce the risk of inducing resistance, a double therapy should be used. The combination of rifampicin and ciprofloxacin was shown to be effective in septic TKA caused by *Staphylococcus epidermidis* [36].

2. Debridement and Irrigation with Retention of the Components

From a microbiological point of view, retention of the implant is only indicated if bacteria are still in a planctonic state and not yet adhesive to the components in large numbers.

As mentioned above, the time frame from the planctonic to the sessile status of bacteria with biofilm production is very small.

Good results with debridement, lavage and retention of components have been shown by Tsukayama et al [46]. In addition, Crockarell et al could clearly show that debridement and lavage were only successful within 4 weeks after primary hip arthroplasty and if debridement is performed early after the onset of symptoms (within 6 to 14 days) [12]. In all cases of late chronic infection the treatment was doomed to fail, while in acute infection 72 % were successfully treated after one year. However, after 6.7 years only 14 % were still free from infection [12]. In more recent trials success rates between 9 % [31], 32.6 % [45] and 35 % [14] in infected total knee arthroplasty were reported.

Radical debridement and lavage with retention of components should only be attempted in cases of early (acute) postoperative infection with a stable implant (Fig. 2). The surgical treatment is usually combined with IV antibiotics over 4 weeks followed by oral antibiotics for 6 weeks. Local antibiotics, like gentamicin-loaded collagen sheets can be used in addition [48]. If necessary, debridement can be repeated or a sequential therapy with Vacuum Assisted Closure (VAC) between two revisions performed [19].

Staphylococci have a high affinity to polyethylene (PE) components. In case of periprosthetic infection by these bacteria, exchange of PE components in combination with debridement and lavage is suggested [5].

In case of progression of infection, a second revision with exchange of the implants becomes necessary.

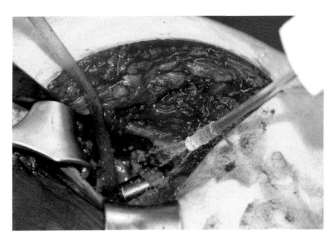

Fig. 2. Debridement and irrigation by jet-lavage with retention of cup and stem and exchange of head and inlay in infected total hip arthroplasty

3. One-stage Revision

Bacteria adhesive to the components and protected by a biofilm cannot be removed from the surface by any mechanical, antiseptic or antibiotic approach. In consequence, a revision arthroplasty becomes necessary in late chronic infection. Debridement alone and retention of components were shown to fail in all cases of chronic infection [12].

In the early eighties Buchholz and coworkers published their experience in one stage total hip revisions. Surgery included excision of soft tissue, removal of the implant and cement, replacement with an appropriate prosthesis using antibiotic-loaded cement and systemic antibiotics. Overall success rate after ten years was 77 % in 583 patients [5]. Hanssen and Rand could show that the use of antibiotic-loaded cement in one stage revisions is significantly more successful than usual cement (success rate 83 % vs. 60 %) [25]. More recent studies showed a higher success rate in small series of 90.9 % [6], 91.7 [7] and 100 % [47]. In a literature review including 12 reports overall success was 83 % [34].

Advantages of a one-stage revision are lower morbidity (single surgery), shorter hospital stay, lower costs and better functional outcome. The price for these advantages is the risk of recurrent infection, if not all infected tissue and necrotic bone have been meticulously removed and the "bacterial race for the surface of the components" can start again.

Careful selection of patients is important for a one-stage revision: good immune response, no comorbidity, no draining sinuses and bacteria sensible to oral antibiotics are in favor of this approach.

4. Two-stage Revision

Late chronic periprosthetic infections account for about 70 % of the cases, as compared to less than 30 % for acute postoperative infections [52]. Elderly patients with concomitant diseases and a low immune response are those more often affected. Moreover, infection generally starts long before the surgical treatment begins and draining sinuses exist over a long period.

With this difficult starting point, a one-stage revision is in our opinion too risky; the two-stage revision should be preferred. Two-stage salvage consists of removal of implants and cement, placement of local antibiotics (Gentamicin PMMA beads [48] or PMMA spacer), and appropriate intravenous antibiotic therapy followed by reimplantation usually with antibiotic-impregnated cement (Fig. 3) [13]. Time interval between implant removal and delayed revision surgery varies between one to two months. Antibiotic therapy should be stopped two weeks before surgery and revision arthroplasty only performed if blood test (WBC, CRP), clinical examination and / or cultures of a hip aspiration are negative for infection [40]. In literature success rates of two stage revisions are reported between 80 % [24] and 92 % [22] in septic THA.

After removal of the implant soft tissue contracture, arthrofibrosis, instability of the extremity and thus immobility of the patient are feared complications. To avoid these problems spacers have been introduced to the two-stage revision concept [9].

First, block spacers made of PMMA and gentamicin were used. In addition to serving as a drug delivery system, the antibiotic-impregnated spacer block gave mechani-

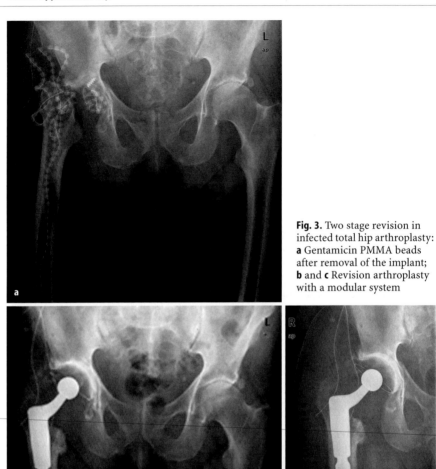

Fig. 3. Two stage revision in infected total hip arthroplasty: **a** Gentamicin PMMA beads after removal of the implant; **b** and **c** Revision arthroplasty with a modular system

cal stability to the joint [9]. Results were good with a recurrence rate of infection after revision TKA between 0 and 9 % [23, 26, 41, 49]. However, in some cases bone loss in the bone stock was observed [8]. This led to the frequent use of articulating spacers. In infected THA spacers are either hand molded of bone cement [50], fabricated in a Teflon mould (Fig. 4) [43] or preformed (Fig. 5) [38]. Dislocation of hip spacers has been reported, often in combination with a loosening of the shaft at the femur [37]. This can be avoided if a small amount of additional cement is used for the fixation of

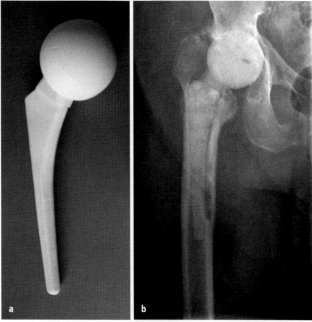

Fig. 4. Articulating, antibiotic loaded, cement hip spacers. Fabricated in a teflon mould (Biomet Deutschland, Berlin, Germany).

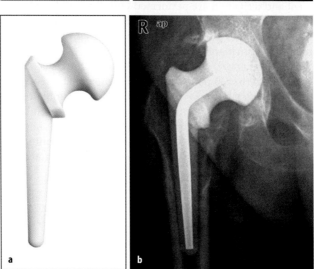

Fig. 5. Articulating, antibiotic loaded, cement hip spacers, preformed (Spacer-G – Tecres Spa, Italy)

the spacer [21]. Results for the use of articulating spacers in two-stage revisions are shown in Table 3.

In two-stage hip revision for infection a comparison of the interim use of antibiotic-loaded PMMA beads and spacer prostheses in 128 cases was performed. Interestingly, the recurrence of infection was not different in both groups (4.7 %). The use of a spacer was associated with a higher hip score, a shorter hospital stay, a decrease in

Number of patients	Recurrences of infection after THA revision	Follow-up (average in month)	Year / Reference
61	6 %	43	1997 [51]
10	20 %	35	2001 [38]
17	0 %	38	2003 [50]
42	2.5 %	55	2004 [28]
20	0 %	38	2004 [16]
24	0 %	50	2005 [30]

Table 3. Noncontrolled, non-randomized clinical studies on the efficacy of articulating, antibiotic-impregnated cement spacers in two stage revision after infected THA.

operative time, less blood loss and less postoperative dislocations [29]. This supports the safety and efficacy of articulating spacers.

5. Multi-stage Revision

A multi-stage revision concept may be used in "worst case situations", e.g. chronic infection caused by methicillin-resistant *Staphylococcus aureus* (MRSA) or *Staphylococcus epidermidis* (MRSE) [35] or an extensive system of draining sinus and abscesses. Surgical technique is equal to the two-stage revision concept, with the exception that between removal and reimplantation, surgical revisions with debridement and irrigation are performed [32]. During these "second" or "third" look surgeries, the surgical site can be explored, debridement and irrigation repeated, specimens for microbiological examinations taken and the time point and technique of reimplantation planned. To secure drainage of the surgical site, Vacuum Assisted Closure (VAC-therapy) should be used between the revisions [19].

In a trial (n = 30 patients) we could show that at every repetition of the debridement, less often bacteria were detected in the microbiological cultures (Fig. 6). In our opinion, the risk of a recurrent infection is minimized by the reduction of bacterial contamination of the surgical site before total hip re-implantation. Thus, not only in a "worst case situation", where the bacterial contamination is extremely high, but also in a young patient with no comorbidity sequential debridement combined with

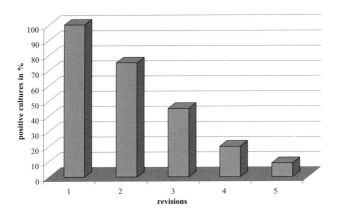

Fig. 6. Debridements and VAC-therapy after removal of the implants: positive bacterial cultures are reduced by every repetitive debridement (n = 30)

VAC-therapy may be appropriate to reduce the risk of recurrent infection. If a patient is suitable for repeated surgeries (no concomitant diseases, good general health, low risk profile), we suggest a multi-stage revision concept to keep the risk of recurrent infection as low as possible.

Conclusion

Decision on a treatment concept in infected THA must be based first on the clinical situation of the patient, especially his age, comorbidity and immune response, second on the chronicity of infection and third on the sensitivity of the infecting bacteria.

All these factors have to be carefully considered and an individual therapy planned.

Conservative antibiotic therapy should be restricted to patients not suitable for surgery. Debridement and retention of components might be successful in an early acute infection in combination with a good immune response of the patient and bacteria with low antibiotic resistance.

One-stage revision can be performed in early (acute) postoperative infection in a patient with no or little comorbidity.

Two-stage revision seems to become the standard procedure in chronic periprosthetic infection with the use of an antibiotic-loaded spacer during the interval between removal and reimplantation.

Multi-stage revisions can be performed in "worst case situations" like chronic periprosthetic infection caused by methicillin-resistant Staphylococci or to reduce the risk of recurrent infection in patients suitable for repeated surgeries.

References

1. Aigner C (1998) 10-Jahresergebnisse mit dem korundgestrahlten Reintitanring nach Zwymüller. Z Orthop (136):110–114
2. Aklin YP, Berli BJ, Frick W et al (2001) Nine-year results of Müller cemented titanum straight stems in total hip replacement. Arch Orthop Trauma Surg 121(7):391–398
3. Böhm P, Bösche R (1998) Survival analysis of the Harris-Galante I acetabular cup. J Bone Joint Surg (Br) 80(3):396–403
4. Brown MRW, Collier PJ, Gilbert P (1990) Influence of growth rate on susceptibility to antimicrobial agents: modification of the cell envelope and batch and continuous culture studies. Antimicrob Agents Chemother 34(9):1623–1628
5. Buchholz HW, Elson RA, Engelbrecht E et al (1981) Management of deep infection of total hip replacement. J Bone Joint Surg (Br) 63(3):342–353
6. Buechel FF, Femino FP, D'Alessio J (2004) Primary exchange revision arthroplasty for infected total knee replacement: a long-term study. Am J Orthop 33(4):190–8; disc. 198
7. Callaghan JJ, Kratz RP, Johnston RC (1999) One-stage revision surgery of the infected hip. A minimum 10 year followup study. Clin Orthop Rel Res (369):139–143
8. Calton TF, Fehring TK, Griffin WL (1997) Bone loss associated with the use of spacer blocks in infected total knee arthroplasty. Clin Orthop Relat Res (345):148–154
9. Cohen JC, Hozack WJ, Cuckler JM et al (1988) Two-stage reimplantation of septic total knee arthroplasty. Report of three cases using an antibiotic-PMMA spacer block. J Arthroplasty 3(4):369–377
10. Cordero J, Munuera L, Folgueira MD (1994) Influence of metal implants on infection. An experimental study in rabbits. J Bone Joint Surg (Br) 76(5):717–720

11. Costerton JW, Lewandowski Z, Caldwell DE et al (1995) Microbial biofilms. Annu Rev Microbiol (49):711–745. Review
12. Crockarell JR, Hanssen AD, Osmon DR, Morrey BF (1998) Treatment of infection with debridement and retention of the components following hip arthroplasty. J Bone Joint Surg (Am) 80(9):1306–1313
13. Cuckler JM (2005) The infected total knee: management options. J Arthroplasty 20(4 Suppl 2):33–36
14. Deirmengian C, Greenbaum J, Lotke PA et al (2003) Limited success with open debridement and retention of components of acute Staphyloccocus aureus infections after total knee arthroplasty. J Arthroplasty 18(7 Suppl 1):22–26
15. Delaunay CP, Kapandji AI (1998) Surviviorship of rough-surfaced threaded acetabular cups. 382 consecutive primary Zweymüller cups followed 0.2–12 years. Acta Orthop Scand 69(4): 379–383
16. Durbhakula SM, Czajka J, Fuchs MD et al (2004) Spacer endoprosthesis for the treatment of infected total hip arthroplasty. J Arthroplasty 19(6):760–767
17. Engesaeter LB, Lie SA, Espehaug B et al (2003) Antibiotic prophylaxis in total hip arthroplasty: effects of antibiotic prophylaxis systemically and in bone cement on the revision rate of 22,170 primary hip replacements followed 0–14 years in the Norwegian Arthroplasty Register. Acta Orthop Scand 74(6):644–651
18. Espehaug B, Engesaeter LB, Vollset SE et al (1997) Antibiotic prophylaxis in total hip arthroplasty. Review of 10,905 primary cemented total hip replacements reported to the Norwegian arthroplasty register, 1987 to 1995. J Bone Joint Surg (Br) 79(4):590–595
19. Fox MP, Fazal MA, Ware HE (2000) Vacuum assisted wound closure. A new method for control of wound problems in total knee arthroplasty. J Bone Joint Surg (Br) 82 (Suppl I):19
20. Gristina AG, Costerton JW (1985) Bacterial adherence to biomaterials and tissue. The significance of its role in clinical sepsis. J Bone Joint Surg (Am) 67(2):264–273
21. Haaker R, Senge A, Krämer J et al (2004) Osteomyelitis nach Endoprothesen. Orthopäde 33(4):431–438
22. Haddad FS, Murihead-Allwood SK, Manktelow AR et al (2000) Two-stage uncemented revision hip arthroplasty for infection. J Bone Joint Surg (Br) 82(5):689–694
23. Haleem AA, Berry DJ, Hanssen AD (2004) Mid-term to long-term followup of two-stage reimplantation for infected total knee arthroplasty. Clin Orthop Relat Res (428):35–39
24. Hanssen AD, Osmon DR (2002) Evaluation of a staging system for infected hip arthroplasty. Clin Orthop Relat Res (403):16–22
25. Hanssen AD, Rand JA (1999) Evaluation and treatment of infection at the site of a total hip or knee arthroplasty. Instr Course Lect (48):111–122. Review
26. Henderson MH, Booth RE (1991) The use of an antibiotic-impregnated spacer block for revision of the septic total knee arthroplasty. Semin Arthroplasty 2(1):34–39
27. Hinrichs F, Boudriot U, Griss P (2001) 10-Jahres-Ergebnisse einer Monobloc-Hüftendoprothesenpfanne mit mehrlagiger Reintitangitterschale zur zementfreien implantation. Z Orthop 139(3):212–216
28. Hsieh PH, Chen LH, Chen CH et al (2004) Two-stage revision hip arthroplasty for infection with a custom-made, antibiotic-loaded, cement prosthesis as an interim spacer. J Trauma 56(6):1247–1252
29. Hsieh PH, Shih CH, Chang YH et al (2004) Two-stage revision hip arthroplasty for infection: comparison between the interim use of antibiotic-loaded cement beads and a spacer prosthesis. J Bone Joint Surg (Am) 86(9):1989–1997
30. Hsieh PH, Shih CH, Chang YH et al (2005) Treatment of deep infection of the hip associated with massive bone loss: two-stage revision with an antibiotic-loaded interim cement prosthesis followed by reconstruction with allograft. J Bone Joint Surg (Br) 87(6):770–775
31. Husted H, Toftgaard Jensen T (2002) Clinical outcome after treatment of infected primary knee arthroplasty. Acta Orthop Belg 68(5):500–507
32. in Hofmann GO. Infektionen der Knochen und Gelenke in Traumatologie und Orthopädie. 2004. Urban und Fischer Verlag. München und Jena
33. Isaklar ZU, Darouiche RO, Landon GC, Beck (1996) Efficacy of antibiotic alone for orthopeadic device-related infections. Clin Orthop Relat Res (332):184–189

34. Jackson WO, Schmalzried TP (2000) Limited role of direct exchange arthroplasty in the treatment of infected total hip replacements. Clin Orthop Relat Res (381):101–105
35. Kilgus DJ, Howe DJ, Strang A (2002) Results of periprosthetic hip and knee infections caused by resistant bacteria. Clin Orthop Relat Res (404):116–124
36. Konig DP, Schierholz JM, Munnich U et al (2001) Treatment of staphylococcal implant infection with rifampicin-ciprofloxacin in stable implants. Arch Orthop Trauma Surg 121(5):297–299
37. Leunig M, Chosa E, Speck M et al (1998) A cement spacer for two stage revision of infected implants of the hip joint. Int Orthop 22(4):209–214
38. Magnan B, Regis D, Biscaglia R et al (2001) Preformed acrylic bone cement spacer loaded with antibiotics: use of two-stage procedure in 10 patients because of infected hips after total replacement. Acta Orthop Scand 72(6):591–594
39. Mont MA, Waldmann B, Banerjee C et al (1997) Multiple irrigation, debridment and retention of components in infected total knee arthroplasty. J Arthroplasty 12(4):426–433
40. Munjal S, Phillips MJ, Krackow KA (2001) Revision total knee arthroplasty: planning, controversies, and management – infection. Instr Course Lect (50):367–377
41. Nazarian DG, de Jesus D, McGuigan F et al (2003) A two-stage approach to primary knee arthroplasty in the infected arthritic knee. J Arthroplasty 18(7 Suppl 1):16–21
42. Nickel JC, Rureska I, Wright JB et al (1985) Tobramycin resistance of pseudomonas aeruginosa growing as a biofilm on urinary catheter material. Antimicrob Agents Chemother 27(4):619–624
43. Pearle AD, Sculco TP (2002) Technique for fabrication of an antibiotic-loaded cement hemi-arthroplasty (ANTILOCH) prosthesis for infected total hip arthroplasty. Am J Orthop 31(7):425–427
44. Segawa H, Tsukayama DT, Kyle RF et al (1999) Infection after total knee arthroplasty. A retrospective study of the treatment of eighty-one infections. J Bone Joint Surg (Am) 81(10):1434–1445
45. Silva M, Tharani R, Schmalzried TP (2002) Results of direct exchange or debridement of the infected total knee arthroplasty. Clin Orthop Relat Res (404):125–131
46. Tsukayama DT, Estrada R, Gustilo RB (1996) Infection after total hip arthroplasty. A study of the treatment of one hundred and six infections. J Bone Joint Surg (Am) 78(4):512–523
47. Ure KJ, Amstutz HC, Nasser S, Schmalzried TP (1998) An average ten-year follow up. J Bone Joint Surg (Am) 80(7):961–968
48. Walenkamp GH (2001) Gentamicin PMMA beads and other local antibiotic carriers in two stage revision of total knee infection: a review. J Chemother 13 Spec No 1(1):66–72
49. Wilde AH, Ruth JT (1988) Two-stage reimplantation in infected total knee arthroplasty. Clin Orthop Relat Res (236):23–35
50. Yamamoto K, Miyagawa N, Masaoka T et al (2003) Clinical effectiveness of antibiotic-impregnated cement spacers for the treatment of infected implants of the hip joint. J Orthop Sci 8(6):823–828
51. Younger AS, Duncan CP, Masri BA et al (1997) The outcome of two-stage arthroplasty using a custom-made interval spacer to treat the infected hip. J Arthroplasty 12(6):615–623
52. Zimmerli W, Ochsner PE (2000) Management of infection associated with prosthetic joints. Infection 31(2):99–108
53. Zweymüller K, Steindl M, Lhotka C. Die Bicon-Pfanne als Primärimplantat. In Effenberger H: Schraubpfannen, Effenberger, Grieskirchen:301–312.

29 Analysis of the Gait in Patients with Hip Spacers

C. Romanò[2], M. Ferrarin[1], M. Rabbuffetti[1], M. Recalcati[1], E. Meani[2]

[1] SAFLo Gait Laboratory – Don Gnocchi Foundation Research Center – Milan, Italy
[2] Department for Treatment of Osteoarticular Septic Complications (COS) –
Director: Prof. Enzo Meani
Operative Unit for Septic Prosthesis – Responsible: Prof. Carlo L. Romanò
"G. Pini" Orthopaedic Institute, Milan, Italy

Introduction

Two-stage revision is one of the most widely accepted procedures to eradicate infection and restore function in infected hip prosthesis [4–6, 7, 12]. However no objective data have yet been published regarding the function of the operated limb and the ability of the patients to walk during the period of permanence of the antibiotic-loaded spacer implant, that may range from few weeks to several months [8, 11]. The availability of a preformed hip spacers allows reproducibility of the intervention and known mechanical resistance of the implant [1–3] making possible, in the majority of cases, protected weight bearing and walking while the spacer is *in situ* [10, 11].

In this preliminary report we summarize some of the findings that we obtained with computerized gait analysis in patients with hip spacers implanted for hip prosthesis infection.

Materials and Methods

Gait analysis was performed in four patients (one male, 75 yrs, 180 cm, 85 kg; one female 53 yrs, 174 cm, 98 kg; one male, 25 yrs, 182 cm, 84 kg; one female, 65 yrs, 168 cm, 78 kg) in which an infected hip prosthesis had been previously removed and a preformed antibiotic-loaded spacer (Spacer-G – Tecres Spa, Italy) implanted.

Spacer-G is an off-the-shelf preformed antibiotic-loaded cement hip spacer. It is available in three different head sizes and two stem lengths, short (110 mm) and long (210 mm), that may be intra-operatively chosen. The inner part of the spacer features a stainless still rod that provides mechanical resistance. The cement is pre-loaded by the manufacturer with gentamicin at a concentration of 1.9 % (w/w).

All the hips in this series were operated through a lateral approach, with the patient laying in supine position. Two patients received a short-stem spacer, and two a long-stem spacer. In all the cases the spacer was fixed in the proximal part, to prevent implant rotation, with one pack of antibiotic-loaded cement (Cemex Genta – Tecres Spa, Italy) containing gentamicin 2.5 % and vancomycin 5 %. All patients were allowed touch-down weight bearing for one month and then partial weight bearing on the operated extremity with the assistance of two canadian crutches. Gait analysis was performed 6 to 10 weeks after spacer implantation.

Data Acquisition

Data acquisition was performed in the SAFLo gait laboratory of Don Gnocchi Foundation Research Center of Milano, Italy. The laboratory (Fig. 1) is equipped with an optoelectronic system for kinematic data acquisition (Elite system, BTS, Italy), a dynamometric platform (Kisler, Winterthur, Switzerland) for ground reaction force (GRF) measurement and a telemetric 8-channel system (TELEMG, BTS, Italy) for EMG signals acquisition.

Kinematic data were recorded by means of 8 TV cameras located around the calibrated volume of $2.5 \times 1 \times 2$ m^3, the three-dimensional position of subject's relevant body segments was determined by means of reflective markers (10 mm in diameter) glued on the following bony landmarks: sacrum, seventh thoracic vertebra, seventh cervical vertebra and, on both sides of the body, posterior superior iliac spines, lateral femoral condyles, lateral malleoli and fifth metatarsal heads (Fig. 2). After data acquisition (sampling frequency: 50 frames/sec), the marker coordinates were low-pass filtered (cut-off frequency 3–7 Hz) and individual anthropometric parameters were used to estimate the internal joint centers, according to a kinematic skeletal model (Fig. 2). These, in turn, enabled computation of trunk and lower limbs kinematics. Combining GRF data and kinematic data, lower limb joint moment and power were computed through inverse dynamic modelling. Surface EMGs were recorded using a telemetric 8-channel system (TELEMG, BTS, Milan, Italy) from Rectus Femoris (RF), Vastus Medialis (VM), SemiMembranosus (SM), Biceps Femoris Caput Longus (BFCL) e Tensor Fasciae Latae (TFL) muscles of the affected leg (implanted with hip spacer). Myoelectric signals were collected by pre-amplified Ag/AgCl electrodes (diameter: 25 mm, bipolar configuration, inter-electrode distance: 20 mm) and band-pass filtered (high$_{-pass}$ = 10 Hz, f$_{low-pass}$ = 200 Hz). Dynamic data and EMG signals were acquired at a sampling frequency of 1000 Hz and a resolution of 12 bit.

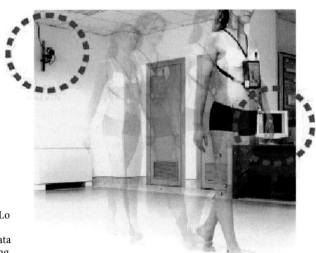

Fig. 1. Picture of the SAFLo lab. TV cameras and PC-based work station for data acquisition and processing are highlighted.

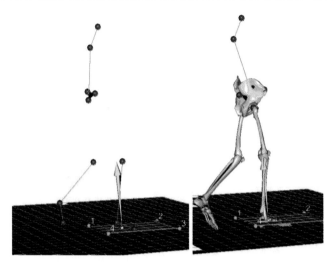

Fig. 2. Skeletal model of lower limb and pelvis and configuration of markers acquired with the motion capture system during the right limb stance phase of walking. The ground reaction forces (yellow arrow) measured by the force platform is superimposed.

The experimental protocol included: an upright quite standing posture, 10 walking trials where the platform was hit with one foot (5 trials for each foot) at natural walking speed, 4 walking trials where the platform was hit with one crutch (2 for each crutch). With the above protocol, the analysis of the load distribution between upper/lower limbs and between affected/unaffected side was allowed.

Specific data elaboration, performed with dedicated software developed by the Bioengineering Centre of the Don Gnocchi Foundation, provided gait parameters (mean gait velocity, cadence, stride and step length) and the time course of kinematic and dynamic variables (joint angles, moments and powers, absolute orientation of lower limb segments, pelvis and trunk.

Results

Kinematic Data

Kinematic data showed walking parameters that remained in the normal values, although in the slowest speed range. Mean velocity of the gait was in fact reduced from 20 % to 60 %, compared to normal subjects, in different patients. Reduction of mean velocity was due to an absolute reduction of the frequency and of the step and stride lengths. Compared to normal subjects, for the same velocity, we observed that the decrease of the cadence speed was mainly due to a decrease of the stride and step length, while the frequency was slightly increased.

Step lengths were asymmetrical, with an increase of the affected side and a decrease in the sound limb. Stance time and double support were also asymmetrical with an increase of the duration on the affected limb and a decrease on the contralateral side (Fig. 3).

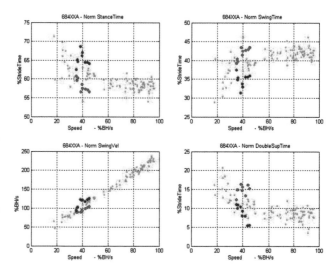

Fig. 3. Patient M1. In blue the limb with the spacer; in red the sound limb. The graphics show: Normalized Stance Time – Normalized Swing Time – Normalized Double Support Time. Stance phase is decreased in the affected side, while double support is prolonged.

Gait strategy may differ:

- Two-phase walking:
  - swing phase of the affected limb at the same time of the two crutches,
  - swing of the sound limb while the affected limb and the two crutches are supporting body weight.
- Three-phase walking:
  - Both two crutches are put forward
  - The affected limb is put forward, between the two crutches that are hold still
  - The sound limb is then put forward, slightly after the two crutches and the affected limb

Ground Reaction Forces

Ground reaction forces revealed that patients reduced vertical charge on the affected limb to 30 % – 50 % of body weight (Fig. 4), sharing the remaining weight equally to both crutches. The sound limb showed ground reaction forces in the normal range.

Kinetic Data and EMG

Postural adjustments and the use of crutches allowed the patients to reduce to nearly zero the frontal (Fig. 5) and sagittal moments around the affected hip, where only a very reduced extensor moments may be appreciated. Moments around the contralateral side are in the normal range. Calculated powers at the hip, knee and ankle joints in the affected limb are also near zero or zero. In this way stresses around the implant seems to be minimized and the requirements for abductor muscles activation are very low. According to this finding the electromyographic pattern of the recorded muscles of the thigh was normal as to concern timing and duration of activity, but recorded intensities were generally lower than in the contralateral side.

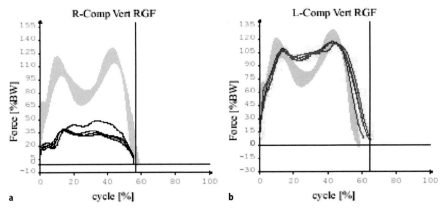

Fig. 4. Patient M1. Ground reaction forces in the affected side (**a**) is reduced to approximately 1/3 compared to normal side (**b**).

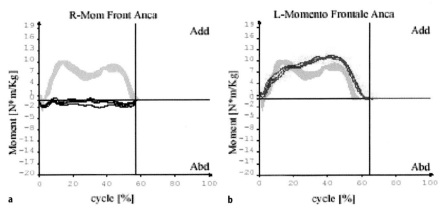

Fig. 5. Patient M1. Frontal moments around the affected hip (**a**) are reduced to nearly zero, while they remain in the normal range in the contralateral hip (**b**).

Joint Range of Motion

Joint range of motion was reduced at the hip, knee and ankle level from approximately 10 % to 50 %, compared with normal subjects and with the contralateral side. As to regard the timing, compared to normal subjects, the knee may anticipate flexion to start the swing phase. Hip extension is normal or slightly reduced and pelvis rotations are increased.

Discussion

This is the first report on gait analysis performed in patients that underwent hip spacer implant following the removal of a septic hip prosthesis.

Our data show that a well centered preformed hip spacer (no patients with spacer dislocation were included in the study), allows walking with two crutches with partial weight bearing on the operated limb. The non-operated limb usually shows kinematic and kinetic parameters in the normal range or only slightly reduced or altered. In the affected side the kinematic of the gait is substantially in the normal range, when compared to normal subjects walking at a low speed, but it clearly appears that different strategies are put in place by the patients to reduce the time of weight bearing on the operated limb, as it is observed in other conditions that affect the hip [9]. At the same time postural adjustments and weight balance between crutches and the sound limb reduce the ground reaction forces on the operated limb to 30–50 % of body weight, while moments and power around the hip spacers are decreased to nearly zero. In this way the patients are able to dramatically reduce the weight and muscular forces that act on the spacer implant, while the joint range of motion at the hip, knee and ankle is maintained, although reduced. This findings point out the ability of the body to provide useful postural modification, even in the absence of the proprioceptive input from a normal hip and even in the absence of a traditional total hip replacement. It is worth to note that the strategies put in place to reduce forces and moments around the operated hip (and ipsilateral knee and ankle) lead to a protection of the implant but they also may reduce muscular activation, leading, in the long run, to a progressive muscular atrophy. For this reason, even if a normal pattern of muscular activity was electromyographically recorded in our patients, the revision of the spacer should be performed as early as possible to prevent any unnecessary muscle wasting.

References

1. Affatato S, Mattarozzi A, Taddei P et al (2003) Investigations on the wear behaviour of the temporary PMMA-based hip Spacer-G. Proc Inst Mech Eng 217(1):1–8
2. Baleani M, Traina F, Toni A (2003) The mechanical behaviour of a pre-formed hip spacer. Hip International 13(3):159–162
3. Bertazzoni Minelli E, Benini A, Magnan B et al (2004) Release of gentamicin and vancomycin from temporary human hip spacers in two-stage revision of infected arthroplasty. J Antimicrob Chemother 53(2):329–334
4. Duncan CP, Masri BA (1995) The role of antibiotic-loaded cement in the treatment of an infection after a hip replacement. Instr Course Lect (44):305–313
5. Fehring TK, Calton TF, Griffin WL (1999) Cementless fixation in 2-stage reimplantation for periprosthetic sepsis. J Arthroplasty 14(2):175–181
6. Ivarsson I, Wahlstrom O, Djerf K et al (1994) Revision of infected hip replacement: Two-stage procedure with a temporary gentamicin spacer. Acta Orthop Scand 65(1):7–8
7. Kendall RW, Masri BA, Duncan CP et al (1994) Temporary antibiotic loaded acrylic hip replacement: a novel method for management of the infected THA. Semin Arthroplasty 5(4):171
8. Magnan B, Regis D, Biscaglia R et al (2001). Preformed acrylic bone cement spacer loaded with antibiotics. Use of two-stage procedure in 10 patients because of infected hips after total replacement. Acta Orthop Scand 72(6):591–594
9. Romano CL, Frigo C, Randelli G et al (1996) Analysis of the gait of adults who had residua of congenital dysplasia of the hip. J Bone Joint Surg (Am) 78(10):1468–1479
10. Romano CL, Meani E (2004) The use of pre-formed long stem antibiotic-loaded cement spacers for two-stage revisions of infected hip prosthesis. Multimedia Education Center American Academy of Orthopaedic Surgeons, San Francisco, CA – March 10–14, 2004
11. Romano CL, Meani E (2006) Long-stem pre-formed spacers followed by uncemented implants: a solution for wide femoral opening or bone loss in two-stage revision. (this book)
12. Younger AS, Duncan CP, Masri BA et al (1997) The outcome of two-stage arthroplasty using a custom-made interval spacer to treat the infected hip. J Arthroplasty 12(6):615–623.

Clinical Applications: Knee

Septic Knee Prosthesis Revision: A Challenging Surgery

E. Valenti

Orthopaedic and Traumatologic Unit, Buccheri La Ferla Fatebenefratelli Hospital, Palermo, Italy

Infections are a devastating complication in orthopaedic surgery and prosthetic surgery in particular. They can occur in the immediate post-operation period or after a prolonged period of time and have a higher incidence in patients with concomitant comorbidities such as diabetes and rheumatoid arthritis. Obesity also is an important risk factor [12], having an infection rate reported to be 6 times higher than normal patients, when the body mass index is > 35.

Progress has been made as far as prevention is concerned (antibiotic prophylaxis, asepsis of operating rooms, improvement of surgical techniques); however, the number of infections involving knee prostheses is increasing secondary to the increased number of primary implants being performed.

Treating a case of knee prosthesis infection is a difficult process, both for the patient and the surgeon. In the majority of cases the infection can be cleared (even if with functional results that are generally lower than the first implant) but there can be very serious outcomes, resulting in knee arthrodesis or amputation.

The economic aspect for both the hospital and society should also not be neglected. Often the costs, which can double those of an aseptical revision, are greater than the reimbursed.

In most acute cases, making the diagnosis is not difficult. Often in chronic cases, a differential diagnosis must take place, which is can be difficult and the clinical presentation can be confused with an aseptical loosening or with functional limitation due to other causes.

Lab data and imaging diagnostics are helpful but are not always definitive for the diagnosis. Even an examination of the synovial fluid, to find the eventual bacteria, can give false negative or false positive results. Calculating the number of white blood cells in the synovial fluid with the relative percentage of neutrophils is considered a good indication. A result of 70,000 leucocytes/mmc with a neutrophil percentage of over 80 % is considered diagnostic for infection [14]. Considerable progress has been made in molecular diagnostics, which enables the bacteria's identification quickly. False positives have been reported by this method but the rapid result and ability to start appropriate treatment quickly may be helpful. This method also is beneficial in identifying bacteria involved in chronic infections and currently reviewing antibiotic treatment [17]. According to recent studies [2], the genomic study of neutrophils in the synovial fluid can distinguish between a septical and aseptical inflammation.

Doubts on the eventual presence of an infection can remain even between operations. In this case, it is advisable to carry out an immediate histological test with a quantitative evaluation of polymorphonucleates for each field, which gives a result accuracy of 90 % [11, 19]. Involving an infectious disease consultant is advisable.

The treatment of acute infections generally consists of surgical irrigation and debridement, pulse lavage but keeping the pressure low to decrease damage to soft tissue and keep from driving the bacteria into the deeper tissue [7] and prolonged antibiotic therapy, with good results in most cases.

In chronic infections this treatment is certainly less efficient. The surgical irrigation and debridement and prolonged antibiotic therapy is not able, in most cases, to eradicate the infection [16]. Studies on biofilm, on the various bacteria and on their capability to increase their resistance after an antibiotic treatment have been the subject of recent studies [1, 3, 4, 13] and may, in the near future, change our current therapeutic approach. The complete mechanical removal of the biofilm is today an essential requirement for successful treatment and for the antibiotic's efficacy in the preoperation period. Since this is almost impossible, while retaining the prosthesis, it is necessary to remove it. This procedure can be carried out in one stage or in two stages.

The one-stage treatment is easier on the patient and less expensive. For a good result, with a one-stage procedure, it is necessary to know the bacteria accurately and this, is not always possible before the operation. But its result on the germ's identification cannot be immediate. It should also be noted that in over 10 % of cases, according to some authors, the infection can be caused by multiple germs. Furthermore, international literature normally reports better results for two-stage rather than one-stage procedures, except in very few highly specialized centres where the one-stage procedure showed excellent results [5, 6, 15, 18].

In the two-stage procedure the antibiotic continues to be given for at least six weeks, on the basis of the bacteria that was identified and the antibiotic essay. However, some centres refer similar results with a normal, brief perioperational antibiotic prophylaxis [8].

In the two-stage procedure, in order to improve the patient's comfort during the period in between the two operations, an articulated antibiotic-loaded spacer has been introduced. This allows a reasonable ambulation, with the aid of a crutch or walker, while keeping the knee's movement. This simplifies the second operation and potentially improves the final functional result. There are various systems that enable mobility with the antibiotic-loaded spacer, both with preformed spacers and with various methods of extemporaneous preparation. Among the various possibilities, the Hofmann method is worth special mention due to its simplicity, affordability and efficacy [9, 10].

Another advantage of the two-stage technique is to proceed with the definitive revision when clinical and lab data indicate the absence of infection, or to proceed with a second irrigation and debridement and placement of a second antibiotic spacer. A late infection treated with the one-stage technique needs to have the implant removed and may lead to excessive bone loss.

The loss of bone-stock is a major problem in the treatment of knee prosthesis infections. This is generally more severe than with aseptical revisions. Bone loss can be filled in with metallic spacers, bone grafting or cement. In the most serious cases using a tumoral type of prosthesis may be necessary or arthrodesis.

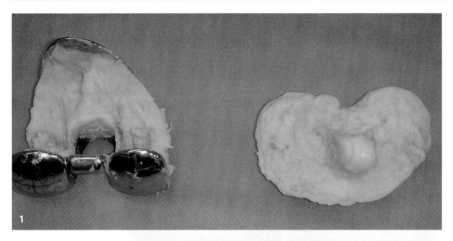

Fig. 1–2. Articulated spacer according to Hofmann before and after positioning

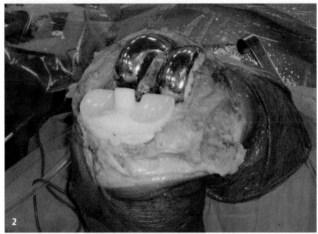

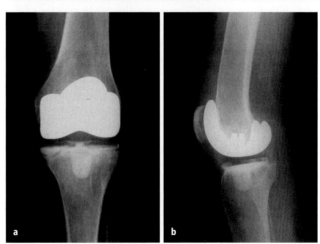

Fig. 3a, b. X-ray control of a spacer according to Hofmann

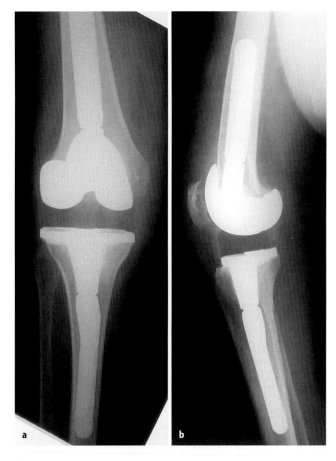

Fig. 4a, b. Definitive implant

Obtaining ligament stability can be difficult in revisions for infection. In cases where a satisfactory balance is not achieved, constrained prosthesis may be needed. In some cases, it may be difficult to re-establish an acceptable range of motion.

The treatment of knee prosthesis infections can be challenging for both the surgeon and patient. Successful treatment requires experience and a multi-disciplined approach.

References

1. Costerton JW (2005) Biofilm theory can guide the treatment of device-related orthopaedic infections. Clin Orthop Relat Res (437):7–11
2. Deirmengian C, Lonner JH, Booth RE (2005) White blood cell gene expression. Clin Orthop Relat Res (440):38–44
3. Donlan RM (2005) New approaches for the charaterization of prosthetic joint biofilms. Clin Orthop Relat Res (437):12–19
4. Ehrlich GD, Hu FZ, Shen K et al (2005) Bacterial plurality as a general mechanism driving persistence in joint infection. Clin Orthop Relat Res (437):20–24

5. Goodman TR, Scuderi GR, Insall JN (1996) Two-stage reimplantation for infected total knee replacement. Clin Orthop Relat Res (331):118–124

6. Haleem AA, Berry DJ, Hanssen AD (2004) Mid-term to long term follow up of two stage reimplantation for infected total knee arthroplasty. Clin Orthop Relat Res (428):35–39

7. Hassinger SM, Harding G, Wongworawat MD (2005) High-pressure pulsatile lavage propagates bacteria into soft tissue. Clin Orthop Relat Res (439):27–31

8. Hoad-Reddick DA, Evans CR, Norman P et al (2005) Is there a role for extended antibiotic therapy in a two-stage revision of the infected knee arthroplasty? J Bone Joint Surg (Br) 87(2):171–174

9. Hofmann AA, Kane KR, Tkach TK et al (1995) Treatment of infected total knee arthroplasty using an articulating spacer. Clin Orthop Relat Res (321):45–54

10. Hofmann AA, Goldberg T, Tanner AM et al (2005) Treatment of infected total knee arthroplasty using an articulating spacer (2- to 12-year experience). Clin Orthop Relat Res (430): 125–131

11. Ko PS, Ip D, Chow KP et al (2005) The role of intraoperative frozen section in decision making in revision hip and knee arthroplasties in a local community hospital. J Arthroplasty 20(2):189–195

12. Namba RS, Paxton L, Fithian DC et al (2005) Obesity and perioperative morbidity in total hip and total knee arthroplasty patients. J Arthroplasty 20(7 Suppl 3):46–50

13. Patel R (2005) Biofilms and antimicrobical resistance. Clin Orthop Relat Res (437):41–47

14. Patel R, Osmon DR, Hanssen AD (2005) The diagnosis of prosthetic joint infection. Clin Orthop Relat Res (437):55–58

15. Raut VV, Siney PD, Wroblewski BM (1995) One-stage revision of total hip arthroplasty for deep infection. Clin Orthop Relat Res (321):202–207

16. Schoifet SD, Morrey BF (1990) Treatment of infection after total knee arthroplasty by debridement with retention of the components. J Bone Joint Surg (Am) 72(9):1383–1390

17. Tarkin IS, Dunman PM, Garvin KL (2005) Improving the treatment of musculoskeletal infections with molecular diagnosis. Clin Orthop Relat Res (247):83–88

18. Whiteside LA (1994) Treatment of infected total knee arthroplasty. Clin Orthop Relat Res (299):169–172

19. Wong YC, Lee QJ, Wai YL et al (2005) Intraoperative frozen section for detecting active infection in failed hip and knee arthroplasties. J Arthroplasty 20(8):1015–1020.

Management of TKA Infection – One-stage Exchange

T. Gehrke[1], S.J. Breusch[2]

[1] Depatment of Orthopaedics, ENDO-Clinic, Hamburg, Germany
[2] Depatment of Orthopaedics, University of Edinburgh, United Kingdom

Introduction

The management of periprosthetic infection remains a challenge to any arthroplasty surgeon. Several treatment options are available depending on the clinical situation, the local set-up, the surgeon's preference and expertise. In the most frequent scenario, where revision surgery with prosthesis exchange is necessary, controversy still exists between single and two-stage approach to the problem. With the introduction of articulating spacers, the functional outcome of two-stage exchange has significantly improved [8, 19, 26, 36]. However, one-stage exchange offers certain advantages including the need for only one operation (if no recurrence), shorter hospitalisation, lower overall cost and high patient satisfaction [3, 10, 11]. In this review the authors will describe their management strategy and experience with direct exchange. Particular emphasis is given to the requirements that provide the basis for success. Furthermore, 8 year outcome data of 100 consecutive patients following one-stage revision TKA for infection with no lost to follow-up are provided and discussed.

Pathophysiology and Etiology

Periprosthetic infection is a foreign body associated infection. It must be clearly differentiated from other bone infections, like osteomyelitis. Not only bacteria are recognized by the host defense as "enemies", but also foreign bodies. Both, micro-organisms and foreign materials induce inflammation as a reaction to tissue injury and are handled in the same manner by the human body. More than 90 % of infections during the first year after implantation are due to bacterial contamination during surgery [30]. Hematogenous infections and infections which reach the site of infection from other sources are less frequent. In the presence of foreign bodies, a contamination as low as 100 colony-forming units (CFU) is sufficient to induce an infection in contrast to 10,000 cfu without foreign material [6, 31]. This effect is due to the diminished clearing capacity of phagocytosis by leukocytes in the presence of foreign material [44]. Macrophages as the first line of defence try to degrade these materials by enzymatic digestion. But if the foreign body is too large for our little macrophage, fibroblasts are stimulated to form granulation tissue around the foreign body. Just like fibroblasts, a number of bacteria, in particular staphylococci are able to colonize the surface of the foreign body. The competition between the fibroblasts, activated by the macrophages, and the bacteria to colonize the foreign body has been given a very descriptive term by Gristina: "The race for the surface". The bacteria are anchored to the surface by forming a biofilm. This biofilm protects from the host's defence mechanisms and these sessile bacteria are also highly resistant to antimicrobial agents [5, 18, 44]. But colonization and formation of slime alone do not cause an infection or an infectious disease. Periprosthetic infection begins when some of the sessile bacteria switch back to planktonic forms and induce infection in the adjacent tissue – periprosthetic osteomyelitis [11]. The period between colonization and clinically detectable infection may last for months, even up to about three years. Signs of infection may occur very late when the bacteria leave the interface, invade surrounding tissue and induce a secondary osteomyelitis. It is important to realise that periprosthetic infection is not only an infection of the prosthetic interface, but also an infection of bone and surrounding soft tissues. This understanding is of utmost importance for the surgical management.

Diagnosis

The diagnosis of periprosthetic infection can be simple, but occasionally most difficult to establish. In the case of immediate postoperative infection the first symptoms can be seen around day 4 to 8 after TKA. If purulent secretion is present the diagnosis is obvious. However, prolonged wound discharge (> 7 – 10 days), continued soft tissue swelling and induration, or wound dehiscence should be taken seriously, considered as infection until proven otherwise and managed with a pro-active and aggressive attitude. If an early infection (within 3 weeks) occurs after patient discharge from hospital, often superficial wound healing problems, hematomas and seromas are evident. However, this is not always obvious and the clinical signs can be more subtle. Monitoring of C-reactive protein (CRP) is probably the most useful parameter in this scenario. CRP values are highest with a peak on day 2 – 3 postop, and should return to normal, preoperative values within 3 weeks. In some patients CRP normalisation can take up to 6 weeks and there is no reason for concern or panic, as long as CRP values show a continuing decline. Failure to do so should result in prompt action. In our experience patients with good (non-indurated) soft tissues, dry wounds and CRP levels below 60 to 90 mg/dl on day 5 – 6 can be considered "safe", but all others (or if in doubt) warrant early follow-up in order not to miss the window of opportunity for early aggressive debridement and suction/irrigation [38].

Whereas clinical symptoms are the main parameters for diagnosing periprosthetic infection in its early stages, laboratory and radiological investigations become more important in late infection. Erythrocyte sedimentation rate has a longer lag time than CRP and is probably only a useful additional tool in the management of patients with rheumatoid arthritis with chronically raised CRP (and ESR) levels. ESR and CRP have a specificity and sensitivity of about 90 %. In contrast, leukocytosis is unspecific and rarely present. Other more sophisticated parameters like Interleukin 6, Procalcitonin or the Interleukin 2 receptor are expensive and generally give us no additional clinically relevant information.

The most important clinical parameter in late infection is the presence (or recurrence !) of pain. Although rarely described in the literature local skin and deep soft tissue induration are poor prognostic indicators in our experience. A "woody" leg should raise the level of suspicion ! Serial radiographic comparison can be of value and bone scans are non-specific although highly sensitive. Bone scans can stay hot for several years following arthroplasty, can represent bone remodeling and may be misleading. Recently, antigranulocyte scintigraphy was reported with a sensitivity of 1.0, a specificity of 0.83, a positive prediction value of 0.83 and a negative prediction value of 1.0. In contrast, preoperative joint aspiration and culture, was less sensitive, but showed a specificity and positive prediction value of 1.0 [28].

In our own practice joint aspiration with prolonged culture time of at least 10 – 14 days is considered mandatory and gold standard. This must be done under strictly sterile conditions without the use of local anaesthetic and saline, which both can exhibit bactericidal effects. The accuracy of aspiration in the Endoclinic in Hamburg has been higher than 95 % [40] in more than 7500 periprosthetic infections treated. However, some special aspects in the investigation of the aspirated fluid have to be considered. The number of bacteria is very small so culture must last for a minimum of 10 – 14 days and not only 3 days as is usual for blood cultures. Fast transport of the aspirated fluid in a sterile container – swabs are inadequate – to the laboratory, rapid processing and an experienced microbiologist with an interest in this demanding problem are important pre-requisites and of utmost importance for success. In some cases repeated aspiration can increase the capture rate, particularly if the patients have been treated with antibiotics previously. A minimum period of 14 days off any antibiotics is required before aspiration in this instance.

Management Strategy – One Stage Exchange

Only in the presence of a positive culture and with the respective antibiogram at hand should a one-stage procedure be considered and offered to the patient. A cemented fixation using antibiotic loaded acrylic cement (ALAC) is considered treatment of choice to achieve high local therapeutic levels of antibiotic elution from ALAC [12]. The secret of success not only depends on complete removal of all foreign material (including intramedullary cement and restrictors) and the use of ALAC, but in particular on the aggressive and complete debridement of the soft tissues and bone. A full synovectomy also in the posterior aspects of the knee is considered of importance and performed routinely. To gain access this invariably means sacrificing the posterior cruciate ligament, if still existing, and not infrequently the collateral ligaments, which will result in the need for hinged implants (see below).

The ALAC should be regarded as a means to prevent re-colonization of the new implants and not seen as the "killer" and cure for infection. It is the surgeon's knife above all, which will determine success. Surgery in periprosthetic infection should be carried out as a tumor procedure and no comprise should be made during debridement: if in doubt cut it out !

General Pre-Operative Planning

Anaesthesia:

- Clinical and anaesthesiological assessment of operative risk
- Adequate quantity of additional donor blood
- In case of long exchange operations preoperative administration of fibrinolysis inhibitors (e.g. Trasilol®) is recommended. Cave: risk of anaphylactic shock!

Radiological Preparation

- Conventional x-rays in two or three planes (patella skyline) in a standardized position are usually adequate. Imaging of hips and entire femur if ipsilateral hip replacement. Long leg alignment films are recommended.
- In some cases calibrated x-rays may have to be taken with a radiopaque scale, especially when special, extra small, custom-made implants or megaprostheses (e.g. total femoral replacement) are required.

Patient Information – Specific Risks

- Risk of recurrent or new infection – about 10–15 %
- Re-operation for haematoma, wound debridement or persistent infection
- Damage to peroneal nerve or main vessels
- Postoperative stiffness and loss of function (extensor mechanism)
- Risk of intra- and postoperative fracture
- Increased risk of aseptic loosening

Surgeon's Planning and Preparation

Choice of Implants and Cement:

- The surgeon should have knowledge of the implant in situ and be familiar with its removal and disassembly (e.g. hinge mechanism). Occasionally it is useful to order and use the implant-specific instrumentation, if available for the particular implant
- A variety of implants must be at hand, ranging from primary total condylar to stemmed hinges, depending on the requirements for reconstruction.
- Ligament deficient knees will require constraint implants, but ligament deficiency may also result during intraoperative debridement – hence the need for rotating of fixed hinge implants. **Due to the aggressive soft tissue debridement strategy of both authors this is the case in almost all cases of one stage exchange.**
- Loss of bone stock, the possibility of intraoperative complications such as shaft fractures, perforations of the cortex, windows and tibial/femoral disintegration must be taken into consideration when choosing the implant. Always have a second line of defence available!
- Distal femoral or proximal tibial replacement implants may have to be chosen in patients with significant bone deficiency. Bone loss is always significantly more extensive than radiographically evident. Custom made implants with extra long

Bacteria	Antibiotics	Dosage per 40 g PMMA cement
Gram positive		
Staphylococci	Lincomycin	3.0 g
Streptococci	Gentamicin	1.0 g
Propionibacteria		
Staphylococci	Cefuroxim	3.0 g
Streptococci	Gentamicin	1.0 g
Propionibacteria		
Staphylococci	Vancomycin	2.0 g
(highly resistant)	Ofloxacin	1.0 g
Enterococci	Vancomycin	2.0 g
	Ampicillin	1.5 g
Gram negative		
Enterobacteriaceae	Cefotaxim	3.0 g
	Gentamicin	1.0 g
Pseudomonas aeruginosa	Cefoperazon	2.0 g
	Amikacin	2.0 g
Acid-fast rods		
Mycobacteria	Streptomycin	2.0 g

Table 1. Combinations of antibiotics recommended for addition to PMMA cement. (Selected according to the susceptibility of the pathogen)

or narrow stems may have to be ordered prior to surgery. The potential need for total femoral replacement implants should also be considered.

- In patients where significant damage to the extensor mechanism is pre-existing or can be anticipated an arthrodesis nail should be available as a last resort (patient consent!)
- ALAC with additional antibiotics (AB) in powderform to be added intraoperatively should be available (Table 1). Invariably at least 2 – 3 mixes of cement (80 – 120 g) per femur and also per tibia are required. Large mixing systems and appropriate cement guns are required. In patients with a narrow diaphysis extra narrow nozzles allow for appropriate retrograde cementing technique.
- The surgeon should know which type of ALAC was been used at the index operation, as resistance of the organism to the previously used AB must be expected [34, 42] and a different ALAC should be chosen. In individual cases an industrially pre-manufactured ALAC cement may be appropriate. The antibiogram and ideally a recommendation from the microbiologist should be available (Table 1) including the AB for cement impregnation and for postoperative i.v. administration.

Operative steps

Skin Incision and Debridement:

- Old scars in the line of the skin incision should be excised (Fig. 1).
- If a prior incision does not lie in this line, keep sufficient distance between it and the new incision. Use the incision from the last approach if technically feasible. Avoid raising a subcutaneous flap.
- Crossing the old scar at an acute angle or deviating from it should be avoided.

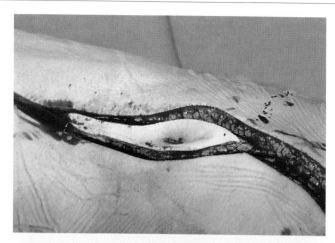

Fig. 1. Skin incision and fistulectomy

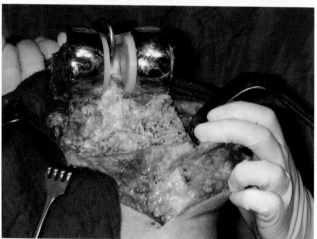

Fig. 2. Complete synovectomy and debridement

- Fistulae should be integrated into the skin incision if possible and radically excised all the way to the joint (Fig. 1). If the fistulae lie too far laterally or posteriorly they are handled by means of a separate excision, following down the fistula tract. Methylene blue staining can be helpful in this case.
- If the need for muscular-cutaneous flaps can be anticipated, a plastic surgeon should be available. However, if the surgeon is familiar with a medial gastrocnemius transfer, most situations can be handled.
- As the operative time commonly exceeds 2 hours an above knee tourniquet is applied but not inflated. The procedure is started without tourniquet so that all bleeders can be coagulated on the way in. Furthermore, without tourniquet the boundary between infected tissue, scar and healthy bleeding soft tissue (and bone) can be distinguished better during debridement. All non bleeding tissue and bone should be excised. Particular emphasis should be given to perform a complete synovectomy and debridement in the posterior compartment (Figs 2 and 3).

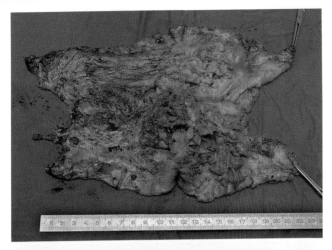

Fig. 3. Removed sinovia and debrided tissue

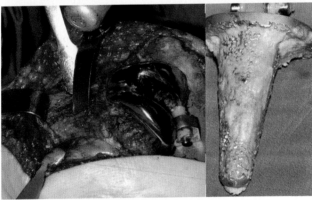

Fig. 4. Prosthesis removal may require a dedicated instrumentarium

- Biopsy material, preferably 5–6 samples, should be taken as a routine measure from all relevant areas of the operation site for microbiological and histological evaluation [1, 39]. Then the chosen i.v. AB are administered. This commonly comprises a broad spectrum cephalosporin and additionally one or two others according to the antibiogram.

Implant Removal and Completion of Debridement

- Removing cemented implants stems is generally much easier and less invasive than removing cementless components, in particular when these are stemmed and ingrown.
- In cases of well fixed uncemented components with stem, often cortical windows are required to gain access to the interface. High speed burrs and curved saw blades aid removal (Fig. 4). Unfortunately even in experienced hands occasionally significant destruction and loss of bone stock will occur.
- Using narrow straight osteotomes with asymmetrically honed blade remove all

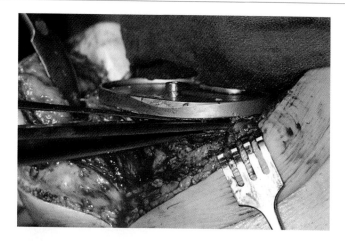

Fig. 5. Implant and cement removal with osteotomes

accessible bone cement (if cemented implant), that can be removed without causing further loss of bone stock

- A Gigli say can be useful to cut around the femoral shield and the tibial base plate of the implant. A full range of narrow and wide osteotomes of various thicknesses (Lambotte osteomes) should be available. By using multiple osteotomes, which are carefully driven between tibial base plate and cement from medial and lateral the tibial component, even if stemmed, can be gradually wedged/forced out from its cement mantle (Fig. 5). This is less destructive than aggressive extraction with hammer blows.
- Extract the implant using special or universal extraction instruments, if available. Otherwise punches are required.
- Cement removal is completed using special cement chisels, long rongeurs, curretting instruments, long drills and cement taps, as well as ball headed reamers. The particular technique of cement removal has been described elsewhere [13, 14].
- Final debridement of bone and posterior soft tissues must be as radical as possible. It should include areas of osteolysis and non-viable bone (Fig. 6).
- Copious pulsatile lavage should be used throughout the procedure.
- After another thorough lavage the intramedullary canals are packed with Chlorhexidine soaked swabs (Lavasept®) and large Chlorhexidine soaked packs are placed, before the wound is covered with a clean incisional film or closed temporarily.
- The entire surgical team should now re-scrub and new instruments are used for re-implantation after re-draping.
- A second dose of i.v. AB is given after 1.5 hrs operating time or if blood loss at this point exceeds 1 l.

Reimplantation

- After completion of debridement and implant removal, it can be helpful to then inflate the tourniquet to aid final intramedullary cement removal and in particular for re-cementation and closure. In short legs or if proximal soft tissue expo-

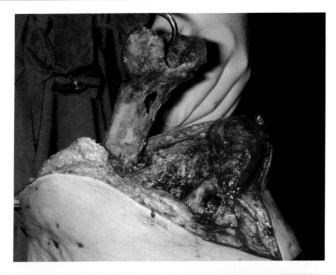

Fig. 6. Radical soft tissues and bone debridement

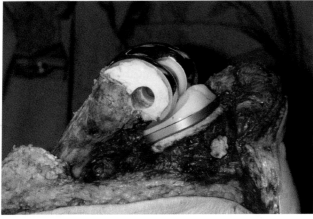

Fig. 7. Bone defect reconstruction and prosthesis fixation with antibiotic-loaded acrylic cement

sure is extensive no tourniquet can be used, unless a sterile one can be made available.

- Reconstruction of bone stock may require the use of allograft, although ideally this should be avoided. We prefer to fill large defects with ALAC if biomechanically acceptable (Fig. 7).
- If morcellized allograft is used, it should be thoroughly lavaged (pulsatile lavage with hot saline !) and impregnated with antibiotics [22] prior to impaction grafting
- Antibiotic loaded cement is prepared. It is mandatory to only use suitable antibiotics which need to fulfill the following criteria:
  - Appropriate AB, antibiogram, good elution characteristics from cement [43].
  - Bactericidal (exception Clindamyin)
  - Powder form (never use liquid AB !)

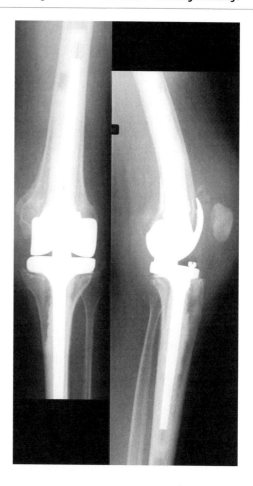

Fig. 8. Post-operative X-rays. One-stage revision with antibiotic-loaded hinged prosthesis

- Pharmaceutical admixing of AB powder to PMMA powder using a fine sieve before mixing
- Maximum addition of 10 %/PMMA powder (e.g. 4 g AB/ 40g PMMA powder
- in MRSA: Vancomycin plus Ofloxacin [29].
 Cave: Some antibiotics (e.g. vancomycin) will change the polymerization behavior of the cement causing acceleration of cement curing !
- The principle of modern cementing techniques should be applied. As mentioned above a better cement bone interface can be achieved if the tourniquet is inflated prior to cementing (Fig 8).
- Postoperatively, i.v. AB are administered according to the treatment recommendations given by the microbiologist. Commonly not more than 14 days are required. The value of prolonged AB given orally thereafter is not proven.
- Serial CRP levels are the most important tool for postoperative monitoring.

Discussion

One stage exchange for infected TKA is less popular than two stage procedures [22]. Higher success rates for two stage have been postulated and with articulating spacers the functional outcome and patient satisfaction [17, 32] have improved significantly [8, 19, 26, 36]. Furthermore, the operative approach is less demanding due to minimal contractures [7, 9, 17, 25] and the rate of extensor mechanism complications has been reduced [19, 27]. Far more studies have been published about two stage revision and fewer series, usually with small patient numbers treated with one stage exchange are available.

In the non-English literature, the early Endoclinic experience from 1976 to 1985, including 118 one stage revision TKAs for infection – followed for 5–15 years – showed a 73 % chance of cure of infection [10]. An English literature review in 2002 of direct exchange [38] revealed that there were only 8 studies on this topic reporting a total of 37 knees – 32 treated with ALAC -, of which 18 were part of one series [15]. All other quoted studies reported patient numbers below 6 and therefore should be considered case reports [38]. The overall success rate, i.e. control of infection was calculated as 89.2 %, but no information was provided regarding the respective length of follow-up. The largest cohort of 69 patients was excluded from the metaanalysis as no distinction from two stage outcomes was possible [38].

A more recent study [4] of 22 consecutive patients treated with direct exchange, radical debridement, ALAC, i.v. AB for 4–6 weeks followed by 6–12 months oral AB showed a 90.9 % rate free of infection after 1.4 to 19.6 years (mean 10.2 years). The authors concluded that their results compare favorably with delayed exchange revision TKA.

Apart from use of ALAC [21, 38] aggressive debridement of all infected tissue [3, 15, 38] the absence of sinus formation [38] and Gram-positive organisms [38] are considered factors associated with success. Our results and experience would support that Gram-positive organisms are more benign, but fistulae have not been associated with poorer outcome. On the contrary, if sinus formation is present (i.e. draining infection) the extent of soft tissue infection is usually less pronounced. Multiple previous surgeries have been reported to adversely affect the chance of success [23]. This, however, was not the case in our series.

The duration of postoperative intravenous antibiotics ranged from 2–4 weeks (mean 2.4) in the metaanalysis of direct exchange [38]. A prolonged administration of intravenous AB for 6 weeks is particular common in the interval between first and second stage [16]. However, the rationale for this has been questioned most recently [24] and the authors concluded from their experience in 38 patients, that a prolonged course of AB does not seem to alter the incidence of recurrent or persistent infection after two stage revision. Interestingly, if patients are re-aspirated prior to re-implantation positive cultures can be found in almost 10 %, thus providing the rationale and justification for pre-revision cultures [33]. In the Endoclinic protocol of direct exchange a duration of 10 days is rarely exceeded now.

In our series of 100 consecutive patients with infected TKA, which were treated with one stage exchange, all required hinge prostheses. This fact both reflects the degree of aggressive debridement and the patient material. Furthermore, at the time the use of fixed hinges was policy, but since then the majority of patients are treated with rotating hinges (ratio 70:30). In a recent report using the same implant for sal-vage revision TKA, 23 cases were done for infection, which showed encouraging out-come at midterm, however inferior compared to aseptic patients [37]. A similar expe-rience with this implant used for salvage of limb threatening cases has also been reported [41]. The functional outcome with this design has been encouraging, although in general stiffer knees have to be expected in septic two stage exchange compared to aseptic revision TKA [2]. In our series there was a 3 % amputation rate, this has dropped , however since to 0.5 % in the last 7 years.

The overall rate of patients free of infection at 8.5 years was 90 % in this consecu-tive Endoclinic series and can be regarded as more than acceptable. If one includes the 3 patients who required a "second-stage" (further direct exchange) then the suc-cess rate is 93 %. Long-term observation is important, as the implant survival rates can deteriorate significantly over time, for both mechanical failure, but also recurrent infection requiring re-operation. In a series of 96 knees, followed for a mean of 7.2 years after two stage revision TKA, the survivorship free of implant removal for re-infection was 93.5 % at 5 years, but dropped to 85 % at 10 years [20].

In conclusion, the Endoclinic results presented here further support the philoso-phy of direct exchange for infected TKA. Patient satisfaction is high as hospitalisation is rarely over 2 weeks and only one operative procedure is required in 90 % of cases. Decreased morbidity for the patient by eliminating the need for a second major pro-cedure with high risk of repeated blood transfusion [35] and associated prolonged inpatient stay are further arguments in favor of a one stage strategy [3]. It remains the more cost-effective approach [4] and can offer similar if not better cure and survival rates even in the longer term.

References

1. Atkins BL, Bowler IC (1998) The diagnosis of large joint sepsis. J Hosp Infect 40(4):263 – 274
2. Barrack RL, Lyons TR, Ingraham RQ et al (2000) The use of a modular rotating hinge compo-nent in salvage revision total knee arthroplasty. J Arthroplasty 15(7):858 – 866
3. Buechel FF (2004) The infected total knee arthroplasty: just when you thought it was over. J Arthroplasty 19(4 Suppl 1):51 – 55
4. Buechel FF, Femino FP, D'Álessio J (2004) Primary exchange revision arthroplasty for infected total knee replacement: a long term study. Am J Orthop 33(4):190 – 198
5. Costerton JW, Stewart PS, Greenberg EP (1999) Bacterial biofilm: a common cause of persis-tent infections. Science 284(5418):1918 – 1322. Review
6. Elek SD, Conen PE (1957) The Virulence of Staphylococcus pyogenes for man: a study of the problems of wound Infection. Br J Exp Pathol 38(6):573 – 586
7. Durbhakula SM, Czajka J, Fuchs MD et al (2004) Antibiotic loaded articulating cement spacer in the 2-stage exchange of infected total knee arthroplasty. J Arthroplasty 19(6): 768 – 774
8. Evans RP (2004) Successful treatment of total hip and knee infection with articulating antibi-otic components: a modified treatment method. Clin Orthop Relat Res (427):37 – 46
9. Fehring TK, Odum S, Calton TF et al (2000) Articulating versus static spacers in revision total knee arthroplasty for sepsis. The Ranawat Award. Clin Orthop Relat Res (380):9 – 16
10. Foerster v. G, Klueber GD, Kaebler U (1995) Mittel – bis langfristige Ergebnisse nach Behand-lung von 118 periprothetischen Infektionen nach Kniegelenkersatz durch einzeitige Aus-tauschoperationen. Der Unfallchirurg, 225:146 – 157
11. Frommelt L (2000) Periprosthetic infection – Bacteria and the interface between prosthesis and bone. In: Learmonth ID (ed). Interfaces in total hip arthroplasties. Springer, London. pp. 153 – 161

12. Gehrke T, Frommelt L, v. Foerster G (1998) Pharmacokinetic study of a gentamycin/clinda-mycin bone cement used in one stage revision arthroplasty
13. In Walenkamp GH, Murray DW (eds): Bone cement and cementing technique. Springer, 1998
14. Gehrke T (2004) Behandlung infizierter Hüft- und Kniegelenksendoprothesen. *In* Schnettler R, Steinau, HU (eds): Septische Knochenchirurgie, Georg Thieme Verlag, Stuttgart New York: 224 – 57:2004
15. Gehrke T (2005) Revision is not difficult. *In* Breusch SJ, Malchau H (Eds). The well cemented total hip arthroplasty. Chapter 18, Springer Verlag, Heidelberg, New York, Tokyo, 2005
16. Goksan SB, Freeman MA (1992) One-stage reimplantation for infected total knee arthro-plasty. J Bone Joint Surg Br 74(1):78 – 82
17. Goldman RT, Scuderi GR, Insall JN (1996) 2-stage reimplantation for infected total knee replacement. Clin Orthop Relat Res (331):118 – 124
18. Goldstein WM, Kopplin M, Wall R et al (2001) Temporary articulating methymethacrylate antibiotic spacer (TAMMAS). A new method of intraoperative manufacturing of a custom articulating spacer. J Bone Joint Surg (Am) 83(Suppl 2 Pt 2):92 – 97
19. Gristina AD (1987) Biomaterial-centred infection: microbial adhesion versus tissue integra-tion. Science 237:1588 – 1595
20. Haddad FS, Masri BA, Campbell D et al (2000) The PROSTALAC functional spacer in two-stage revision for infected knee replacements. Prosthesis of antibiotic acrylic cement. J Bone Joint Surg (Br) 82(6):807 – 812
21. Haleem AA, Berry DJ, Hanssen AD (2004) Mid-term to long term follow up of two-stage reimplantation for infected total knee arthroplasty. Clin Orthop Relat Res (428):35 – 39
22. Hanssen AD, Rand JA, Osmon DR (1994) Treatment of the infected total knee arthroplasty with insertion of another prosthesis. The effect of antibiotic-impregnated bone cement. Clin Orthop Relat Res (309):44 – 55
23. Hanssen AD (2002) Managing the infected knee: as good as it gets. J Arthroplasty 17(4 Suppl 1):98 – 101
24. Hirakawa K, Stulberg BN, Wilde AH et al (1998) Results of 2-stage reimplantation for infected total knee arthroplasty. J Arthroplasty 13(1):22 – 28
25. Hoad-Reddick DA, Evans CR, Norman P et al (2005) Is there a role for extended antibiotic therapy in a two-stage revision of the infected knee arthroplasty? J Bone Joint Surg (Br) 87(2):171 – 174
26. Hofmann AA, Kane KR, Tkach TK et al (1995) Treatment of infected total knee arthroplasty using an articulating spacer. Clin Orthop Relat Res (321):45 – 54
27. Hofmann AA, Goldberg T, Tanner AM et al (2005) Treatment of infected total knee arthro-plasty using an articulating spacer: 2- to 12-year experience. Clin Orthop Relat Res (430):125 – 131
28. Insall JN, Thompson FM, Brause BD (1983) Two-stage reimplantation for the salvage of infected total knee arthroplasty. J Bone Joint Surg (Am) 65():1087 – 1098
29. Kordelle J, Klett R, Stahl U et al (2004) Infection diagnosis after knee-TEP-implantation. Z Orthop 142(3):337 – 343
30. Kordelle J, Frommelt L, Kluber D et al (2000) Results of one stage endoprosthesis revision in periprosthetic infection caused by methicillin-resistant Staphylococcus aureus. Z Orthop 138(3):240 – 244
31. Lidwell OM, Lowbury EJL, Whyte W et al (1982) Effect of ultraclean air in operating rooms on deep sepsis in the joint after total hip or knee replacement: a randomised study. Br Med J (Clin Res Ed) 285(6334):10 – 14
32. Mangram AJ, Horan TC, Pearson ML et al (1999) The Hospital Infection Control Practices Advisory Committee. Guidelines for prevention of surgical site infection. Infect Control Hosp Epidemiol 20:247 – 280
33. Meek RM, Dunlop D, Garbuz DS et al (2004) Patient satisfaction and functional status after aseptic versus septic revision total knee arthroplasty using the PROSTALAC articulating spacer. J. Arthroplasty 19(7):874 – 879
34. Mont MA, Waldman BJ, Hungerford DS (2000) Evaluation of preoperative cultures before second stage reimplantation of a total knee prosthesis complicated by infection. A compari-son-group study. J Bone Joint Surg (Am) 82(11):1552 – 1557
35. Neut D, van de Belt H, Stokroos I et al (2001) Biomaterial-associated infection of gentamicin-

loaded PMMA beads in orthopaedic revision surgery. J Antimicrob Chemother 47(6): 885–891

36. Pagnano M, Cushner FD, Hansen A et al (2004) Blood management in two-stage revision knee arthroplasty for deep prosthetic infection. Clin Orthop Relat Res (367):238–242
37. Pietsch M, Wenisch C, Traussnig S et al (2003) Temporary articulating spacer with antibiotic-impregnated cement for an infected knee endoprosthesis. Orthopade 32(6):490–497
38. Pradhan NR, Bale L, Kay P et al (2004) Salvage revision total knee replacement using the Endo-model rotating hinge prosthesis. Knee 11(6):469–473
39. Silva M, Tharani R, Schmalzried TP (2002) Results of direct exchange or debridement of the infected total knee arthroplasty. Clin Orthop. Relat Res (404):125–131
40. Spanghel MJ, Masri BA, O'Connell JX et al (1999) Prospective analysis of preoperative and intraoperative investigations for the diagnosis of infection at the sites of two hundred and two revision total hip arthroplasties. J Bone Joint Surg (Am) 81(5):672–683
41. Steinbrink K, Frommelt L (2005) Treatment of periprosthetic infection of the hip using one stage exchange surgery. Orthopade 24(4):335–343
42. Utting MR, Newman JH (2004) Customised hinged knee replacements as a salvage procedure for failed total knee arthroplasty. Knee 11(6):475–479
43. van de Belt H, Neut D, Schenk W et al (2001) Staphylococcus aureus biofilm formation on different gentamicin-loaded polymethylmethacrylate bone cements. Biomaterials 22(12): 1607–1611
44. Walenkamp G (2001) Gentamicin PMMA beads and other local antibiotic carriers in two-stage revision of total knee infection: a review. J Chemother 13 Spec No 1(1):66–72
45. Zimmerli W, Lew PD, Waldvogel FA (1984) Pathogenesis of foreign body infection – evidence for a local granulocyte defect. J Clin Invest 73(4):1191–1200

Antibiotic-loaded Bone Cement Spacers for the Two-stage Revision in Total Knee Replacement

R.P. Pitto

Department of Orthopaedic Surgery; University of Auckland, New Zealand

Introduction

The most feared complication for any total knee replacement (TKR) surgeon and for their patient is deep infection. The treatment often results in prolonged hospitalisation, a period of marked limitation of mobility for the patient and the prospect of a major reconstructive procedure with a compromised outcome. The infection rate after primary TKR is usually reported to range from 0.5 to 2 percent [1, 34]. This is a serious problem despite modern technology and rigorous prophylaxis. Peersman et al. [28] reported recently a 0.43 % rate of deep infection in a consecutive series of 6439 total knee replacements performed with vertical laminar airflow and body-exhaust suits. This is encouraging, however, considering the increasing number of patients with TKR, infection is still a complication of major concern [2, 3, 29, 30, 38, 41].

A variety of techniques and devices have been developed to improve the management of the infected TKR. Antibiotic-loaded bone cement spacers in two-stage reimplantation technique allow early joint and patient mobilisation, a shorter hospital stay and potentially a reduced rate of re-infection. In this article we have reviewed the use of joint spacers and outlined their potential benefits and drawbacks.

The Infected Total Knee Replacement

The choice of management for patients with infected TKR depends on many factors; nevertheless the clinical presentation of infection can be used as a guide to the treatment. Segawa et al [36] proposed a classification based on the clinical presentation of prosthesis-related infections, focusing on the severity of symptoms and the temporal relationship between the index operation and the infection.

The classification recognizes 4 types of infections: 1) early postoperative infection; 2) late chronic infections; 3) acute haematogenous infections and; 4) sub-clinical infections with positive cultures. The early postoperative infection (type 1) is defined as a wound infection (superficial or deep) developing less than four weeks after the index operation. The treatment for superficial infection is extra-articular soft-tissue debridement and a course of antibiotics [26]. Deep infection extend into the joint and require aggressive treatment including debridement, exchange of the polyethylene insert of the tibial component and intravenous administration of antibiotics. Intra-articular placement of antibiotic-loaded cement beads has been also advocated [27].

Retention of prosthesis is possible in early postoperative deep infection if the implant appears well fixed. Late chronic infections (type 2) develop four weeks or more after the index operation and has an insidious clinical presentation. These infections are most commonly treated with debridement, implant removal and placement of antibiotic-impregnated cement spacer or antibiotic-impregnated cement beads. This is followed by a course of systemic antibiotics for six weeks and a delayed-exchange arthroplasty (two-stage reimplantation technique). The acute haematogenous infection (type 3) is associated with a documented or suspected antecedent bacteraemia and is characterised by an acute onset of severe pain and swelling. These infections are treated with debridement, exchange of the polyethylene insert of the tibia component, retention of prosthesis if it is well fixed and intravenous antibiotics for six weeks. The non-specific symptoms and signs of subclinical infection (type 4) generally lead to the patient proceeding to revision surgery for presumed aseptic loosening of the implant. The patient is then treated with intravenous antibiotics for six weeks often without requiring repeated revision surgery, essentially because of the wide antibiotic susceptibility of the infecting organisms.

Two-stage Revision

It is been widely accepted that the most reliable outcome for the treatment of late chronic infection is obtained by a two-stage technique, involving implant removal followed by a 6-week course of systemic antibiotics and delayed exchange arthroplasty. The success rate has been reported at around 90 % [14, 22, 35, 39, 41]. The two-stage reimplantation has become a procedure of choice to eradicate the infection and maintain a functional extremity. The major disadvantage of this method is the period between stages which is often associated with pain, difficult mobility and knee instability [13, 17]. Furthermore, reimplantation is often difficult because of scar formation, shortening of the extensor mechanism, and retraction of the joint capsule and ligaments. To overcome these difficulties, temporary joint spacers has been introduced [15, 25].

Spacers

The spacers have been reported successful in preserving the length of the limb and minimising soft-tissue contracture, therefore facilitating re-implantation [7, 16, 41]. Furthermore, the insertion of an antibiotic-loaded cement spacer, in addition to the elution of high levels of antibiotic into the joint, allow ambulation, rehabilitation and earlier discharge from the hospital between stages [12]. Essentially, there are two types of temporary spacers: 1) block spacers (also known as non-articulating or static); 2) articulating spacers (also known as mobile spacers).

Block Spacers

The use of block spacers was first reported in 1988 by Cohen et al [7] and Wilde and Ruth [39]. Antibiotic-impregnated polymethylmethacrylate cement blocks are hand-made in the operating room and are fashioned to fit the bone stock defect left after removal of the infected prosthesis. A small cement stem can be added to the spacer block to achieve adequate fixation. The impregnated cement allows higher local concentrations of antibiotics and the block itself maintains the articulating space and prevents retraction of the collateral ligaments. These factors facilitate easier re-implantation. Static knee spacers are better option for knees with severe bone loss as the mobile spacers cannot maintain stability in these settings [4, 5, 10, 11, 18]. Block spacers presents several disadvantages: patients are not allowed to move the knee and require cast immobilisation between stages. The spacer can dislodge and cause bone erosion. Moreover, second-stage surgery is still difficult due to scar formation, tissue adherence and quadriceps shortening.

Articulating Knee Spacers

To overcome disadvantages of the block spacers and to ease reimplantation surgery several authors have independently introduced articulated spacers in two-stage revision for infected knee replacements [20, 21]. Emerson et al.[10] compared static block spacers (26 knees) with articulating spacers (22 knees) and found an improved postoperative range of motion in the articulating spacer group (108° compared with 94°) with no significant difference in the reinfection rate at 36 months (9% compared with 7.6%).

Essentially, there are three types of articulating spacers: 1) Temporary prosthesis from re-sterilised components or new components (also called spacer prosthesis); 2) Cement spacers moulded during operation; 3) Preformed cement spacers.

Temporary Prosthesis

Scott et al [35] reported cementing the original prosthesis between stages after resterilisation in autoclave. The cement was loaded with antibiotics. After 6 weeks, the final stage was performed fixing the definitive prosthesis using antibiotic-loaded bone cement according to the sensitivity profile of the infecting organism.

In 1995 Hoffmann et al [20] used the removed and sterilised femoral and tibial components, a new polyethylene tibial insert, and a new all-polyethylene patellar component for the 2-stage revision of TKR. Partial weight-bearing and range of motion exercises were allowed after surgery. There was no recurrence of infection in a series of 25 patients at an average follow-up of 30 months. The drawback of the temporary prosthesis is the presence of metallic and plastic components which can, in theory, favour bacterial adhesion [14]. Also, current infection disease control policies prohibit in many countries the use of removed and resterilised prosthetic implants. Moreover, the use of a new prosthesis as a spacer is an additional factor increasing the high costs of management of patients with infected TKR [19].

Cement Spacers Moulded During Operation

McPherson et al [25] presented the technique of using a handmade mould of a TKR made of antibiotic-loaded cement as a temporary spacer in two-stage revision. Although this allowed some function of the knee, stability was difficult to maintain.

Duncan et al [8, 9] also introduced an intra-operatively moulded cement spacer. This spacer had smooth articular surfaces obtained with the utilization of plastic moulds. The spacer is a facsimile of a TKA prosthesis made entirely of antibiotic-loaded bone cement (Prostalac – Prosthesis of Antibiotic-Loaded Acrylic Cement – Smith & Nephew, USA). Haddad et al [16] reported the use of Prostalac spacer in two-stage revision for infected TKR in 45 consecutive patients. The mean follow-up was for 48 months. At the final review, there was no evidence of infection in 41 patients (91 %); only one had a recurrent infection with the same organism. There was improvement in the Hospital for Special Surgery knee score at final review. The range of movement was maintained between stages. According to the authors, complications were primarily related to the extensor mechanism, wear and stability of the knee between stages. These problems have been addressed with refinement of the design of the implant. The new generation of Prostalac has femoral and tibial components made of antibiotic-loaded bone cement with a small metal-on-polyethylene articular surface, with a posterior stabilised design. Emerson et al [10] suggested the use of 3.6g of tobramycin and 2g of vancomycin per 40g of cement. Haddad et al [15] confirmed that the normal limit of antibiotic comprising 5 % of the whole cement mass does not necessarily apply in temporary spacers. This doesn't seem to affect the mechanical properties of such constructs. Generally, patients with these spacers *in situ* are allowed to walk with partial weight-bearing and free knee motion is encouraged with or without a brace. One of the advantages of the Prostalac system is the ability to add relatively large amount of antibiotic powder to the bone cement [23]. Again, the presence of metal and plastic, although in small amounts, could in theory favour bacterial adhesion between the stages of the revision. Also, an objection can be made that this "custom made" cement spacer cannot warrant reproducible mechanical properties. Molds for articulating knee spacers are not always readily available.

MacAvoy and Ries [24] treated 13 infected total knee arthroplasties with large bone defects or collateral ligament loss using the rubber bulb portion of an irrigation syringe and a bipolar trial to create a ball and socket articulating spacer. This technique was successful in controlling infection in 9 of 13 knees. All patients were able to ambulate independently with the spacer in place using a walker or crutches, including one patient with bilateral spacers. At an average follow-up of 28 months after reimplantation, average knee flexion was 98 degrees.

Preformed Cement Spacers

Castelli et al [6] recently introduced a preformed articulating spacer. The spacers are manufactured in the factory with ultra-congruent condylar knee prosthesis design made exclusively of acrylic cement impregnated with gentamicin antibiotic (Spacer-K – Tecres Spa, Italy) no additional reinforcement device is used (Fig. 1). Both components, femoral and tibial, are produced in three sizes. Experimental studies on

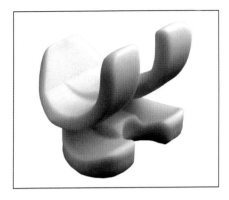

Fig. 1. The Spacer-K preformed articulating spacer

mechanical and pharmacological behaviour of this spacer have demonstrated good mechanical properties and standardised antibiotic release. In theory, good mechanical properties without the presence of metal or plastic are an advantage in the treatment of infected TKR. Like other articulating spacers, Spacer-K is fixed to the bone with cement, loaded with antibiotics of the surgeon's choice. It allows partial weight-bearing and knee motion exercises between stages (Fig. 2).

A multicentre prospective study on Spacer-K [34] showed no recurrence of infection at a minimum follow-up of 6 months. A recent 2-year minimum follow-up [30] of articulating spacers showed that the preoperative range of motion remained unchanged between stages and improved after reimplantation of the final prosthesis. No patient had recurrence of infection at latest follow-up. Neither breakage, nor clinically relevant wear of the spacer were detected, and no complications related to the spacer were observed.

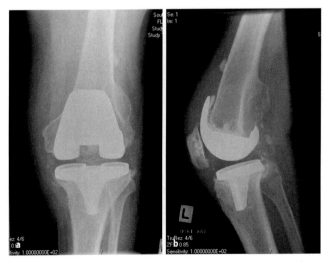

Fig. 2. a Preoperative antero-posterior and **b** lateral radiographs of a 60-year-old male with late infection and loosening of the total knee replacement.

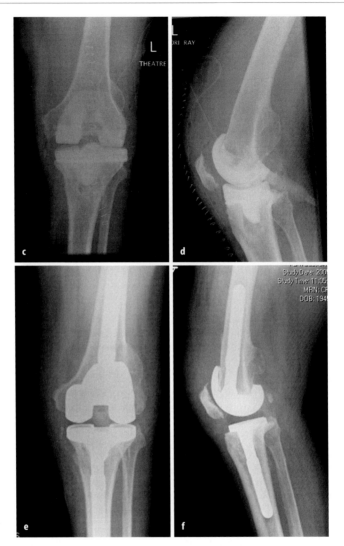

Fig. 2. c Postoperative antero-posterior and **d** lateral radiographs after first stage revision show a cemented antibiotic-loaded articulating Spacer-K. **e** Postoperative antero-posterior and **f** lateral radiographs one year after second stage revision show revision total knee replacement with acceptable bone stock and satisfactory alignment of the implant.

Conclusion

Infected TKR is a devastating complication, both for the patient and the surgeon. It causes major morbidity, and presents a difficult surgical management issue with possible unsatisfactory outcome, prolonged hospitalisation, and a period of marked limitation of mobility for the patient. Hebert et al [19] reported that the surgical treatment of an infected TKR is three to four times as expensive as a primary procedure. Most of the cost was related to the hospitalisation and antibiotic treatment. Knee spacers used in the two-stage surgical management of infected TKR, at present the gold standard of treatment [12, 15, 21], can improve mobilisation and hasten recovery of patients, with shorter hospital stay between stages. Furthermore, in addition to the local delivery of high levels of antibiotics, spacers facilitate the second stage procedure by maintaining the joint space and, in case of articulating devices, maintaining knee range of motion. It has been shown that the patients with the articulating spacers, when compared with the block spacers, have better mobility after reimplantation with a similar complication rate and infection rate in the long term [12, 21, 23]. Last but not the least, the cost of spacers represents a relatively small fraction of the total expenses for the management of the infected TKR.

References

1. Abudu A, Sivardeen KAZ, Grimer RJ et al (2002) The outcome of perioperative wound infection after total hip and knee arthroplasty. Int Orthop 26(1):40–43
2. Bengtson S, Knutson K, Lidgren L (1986) Revision of infected knee arthroplasty. Acta Orthop Scand 57(6):489–494
3. Bengtson S, Knutson K (1991) The infected knee arthroplasty. A 6-year follow-up of 357 cases. Acta Orthop Scand 62(4):301–311
4. Booth RE, Jr, Lotke PA (1989) The results of spacer block technique in revision of infected total knee arthroplasty. Clin Orthop Relat Res (248):57–60
5. Calton TF, Fehring TK, Griffin WL (1997) Bone loss associated with the use of spacer blocks in infected total knee arthroplasty. Clin Orthop Relat Res (345):148–154
6. Castelli C, Martinelli R, Ferrari R (2002) Preformed all-cement knee spacer in two-stage revision for infected knee replacement. Proceedings of the SICOT XXII World Congress, 327c
7. Cohen JC, Hozack W, Cuckler JM et al (1988) Two-stage reimplantation of septic total knee arthroplasty. Report of three cases using an antibiotic-PMMA spacer block. J Arthroplasty 3(4):369–377
8. Duncan CP, Beauchamp C, Masri BA (1992) The antibiotic loaded joint replacement system: a novel approach to the management of the infected knee replacement. J Bone Joint Surg (Br) Suppl III 74:296
9. Duncan CP, Beauchamp C (1993) A temporary antibiotic-loaded joint replacement system for management of complex infections involving the hip. Orthop Clin North Am 24(4): 751–759
10. Emerson RH, Jr, Muncie M, Tarbox TR et al (2002) Comparison of a static with a mobile spacer in total knee infection. Clin Orthop Relat Res (404):132–138
11. Fehring TK, Odum S, Calton TF et al (2000) Articulating versus static spacers in revision total knee arthroplasty for sepsis. Clin Orthop Relat Res (380):9–16
12. Fehring TK (2003) Techniques for the infected knee: Molded Acrylic Spacer. Proceedings of the Knee Society meeting, New Orleans, LA, 19
13. Goksan SB, Freeman MA (1992) One-stage reimplantation for infected total knee arthroplasty. J Bone Joint Surg (Br) 74(1):78–82
14. Goldman RT, Scuderi GR, Insall JN (1996) 2-stage reimplantation for infected total knee replacement. Clin Orthop Relat Res (331):118–124
15. Haddad FS, Masri BA, Duncan CP (2001) Cement spacers in knee surgery. In: Insall JN, Scott WN (Eds) Surgery of the knee, Churchill-Livingstone, Philadelphia 2:1891–1913
16. Haddad FS, Masri BA, Campbell D et al CP (2000) The Prostalac functional spacer in two-stage revision for infected knee replacements. J Bone Joint Surg (Br) 82(6):807–812
17. Hanssen AD, Rand JA, Osmon DR (1994) Treatment of the infected total knee arthroplasty with insertion of another prosthesis. The effect of antibiotic-impregnated bone cement. Clin Orthop Relat Res (309):44–55
18. Hanssen AD (2003) Techniques for the infected knee: Static Spacers for the infected knee replacement. Proceedings of the Knee Society meeting, New Orleans, LA, February, 18
19. Hebert CK, Williams RE, Levy RS et al (1996) Cost of treating an infected total knee replacement. Clin Orthop Relat Res (331):140–145

20. Hofmann AA, Kane KR, Tkach TK et al (1995) Treatment of infected total knee arthroplasty using an articulating spacer. Clin Orthop Relat Res (321):45–54
21. Hofmann AA (2003) Techniques for the infected knee: 10-year experience in the treatement of infected total knee arthroplasty using an articulating spacer. Proceedings of the Knee Society meeting, New Orleans, LA, 17
22. Insall JN, Thompson FM, Brause BD (1983) Two-stage reimplantation for the salvage of infected total knee arthroplasty. J Bone Joint Surg (Am) 65(8):1087–1098
23. Masri BA, Duncan CP, Campbell D et al (2000) Prostalac two-stage exchange for infected knee replacements: a prospective analysis. Proceedings of the 10th combined meeting of the Orthopedic Associations of the English-speaking World, Auckland, NZ, J Bone Joint Surg (Br) Suppl II, 82:153
24. MacAvoy MC, Ries MD (2005) Articulated antibiotic impregnated cement spacers. J Arthroplasty. 20(6):757–762
25. McPherson EJ, Lewonowski K, Dorr LD (1995) Techniques in arthroplasty. Use of an articulated PMMA spacer in the infected total knee arthroplasty. J Arthroplasty 10(1):87–89
26. Mont MA, Waldman B, Banerjee C et al (1997) Multiple irrigation, debridement, and retention of components in infected total knee arthroplasty. J Arthroplasty 12(4):426–433
27. Nelson CL, Evans RP, Blaha JD et al (1993) A comparison of gentamicin-impregnated polymethylmethacrylate bead implantation to conventional parenteral antibiotic therapy in infected total hip and knee arthroplasty. Clin Orthop Relat Res (295):96–101
28. Peersman G, Laskin R, Davis J et al (2002) Infection in total knee replacement: a retrospective review of 6489 total knee replacements. Clin Orthop Relat Res (392):15–23
29. Pitto RP, Spika I (2004) Antibiotic-loaded bone cement spacers in two-stage management of infected total knee arthroplasty. Int Orthop 28(3):129–133
30. Pitto RP, Castelli CC, Ferrari R et al (2005) Pre-formed articulating knee spacer in two-stage revision for the infected total knee arthroplasty. Int Orthop 29(5):305–308
31. Rand JA, Bryan RS, Morrey BF et al (1986) Management of infected total knee arthroplasty. Clin Orthop Relat Res (205):75–85
32. Rand JA, Fitzgerald RH, Jr (1989) Diagnosis and management of the infected total knee arthroplasty. Orthop Clin North Am 20(2):201–210. Review
33. Resig S, Saleh KJ, Bershadsky B (2002) The outcome of perioperative wound infection after total hip and knee arthroplasty. Int Orthop 26(4):257
34. Salvati EA, Robinson RP, Zeno SM et al (1982) Infection rates after 3175 total hip and total knee replacements performed with and without a horizontal unidirectional filtered air-flow system. J Bone Joint Surg (Am) 64(4):525–535
35. Scott IR, Stockley I, Getty CJ (1993) Exchange arthroplasty for infected knee replacements. A new two-stage method. J Bone Joint Surg (Br) 75(1):28–31
36. Segawa H, Tsukayama DT, Kyle RF et al (1999) Infection after total knee arthroplasty. A retrospective study of the treatment of eighty-one infections. J Bone Joint Surg (Am) 8110: 1434–1445
37. Spika IA, Castelli C, Ferrari R et al (2004) Articulating spacers in two-stage revision of the infected total knee replacement. J Bone Joint Surg [Suppl IV], 86-B:471–472
38. Whiteside LA (1994) Treatment of infected total knee arthroplasty. Clin Orthop Relat Res (321):169–172
39. Wilde AH, Ruth JT (1988) Two-stage reimplantation in infected total knee arthroplasty. Clin Orthop Relat Res (236):23–35
40. Windsor RE, Insall JN, Urs WK et al (1990) Two-stage reimplantation for the salvage of total knee arthroplasty complicated by infection. Further follow-up and refinement of indications. J Bone Joint Surg (Am) 72(2):272–278
41. Windsor RE, Bono JV (1994) Infected total knee replacements. J Am Acad Orthop Surg 2(1):44–53

33 Key Points in Two-stage Revision for Infected Knee Arthroplasty: Bone Loss, Quality of Life Between Stages and Surgical Approach at Second Stage

C.C. Castelli, R. Ferrari

Departments of Orthopaedics and Traumatology, Ospedali Riuniti of Bergamo, Italy

Introduction

Total knee replacement is one of the most common and successful procedures in orthopaedic surgery. Excellent long-term results are reported both in young adult patients and elderly people [23, 25, 26]. However, infection remains, notwithstanding rigorous prophylactic protocols, an important cause of failure. The incidence rate ranges from 0.5 to 5 % in different case reports, with an increased risk in revision surgery or in patients with certain risk factors, such as rheumatoid arthritis diabetes mellitus or compromised immune status [24, 27, 29]. The treatment of this devastating complication is still controversial today, and in the literature many therapeutic options are reported, ranging from simple parenteral antibiotic therapy, repeated joint lavage without joint removal, and resection arthroplasty, to one-stage or two-stage re-implantation and finally to arthrodesis or amputation [8, 19, 24]. The choice of the treatment depends upon many variables: the type of infection and the type of the organism responsible, the general conditions of the patients and his life expectancy. Prosthetic infections are classified, using chronological criteria, into four types as early post-operative infection, late chronic infections, acute Hematogenous infections and sub clinical infections with positive cultures [29]. In the treatment of late chronic infections the best results, both for the eradication of the disease and for function recovery, have been obtained with either one-stage or two-stage exchange arthroplasty. The two-stage technique, has been shown to be more effective, with a success rate ranging from 90 to 96 % [4, 31, 32]. This procedure requires primary implant removal, followed by a six-week course of systemic antibiotics and delayed exchange arthroplasty. The use of an impregnated antibiotic cement spacer block was introduced to maintain the joint space, prevent retraction of the collateral ligaments and to provide local antibiotic release [4, 7, 31, 32]. Despite encouraging results in infection eradication the block spacer presents several disadvantages: knee movement is restricted by cast immobilization between stages and the spacer may dislodge resulting in bone erosion. Second stage surgery is still difficult secondary to a scar formation, tissue adherence and quadriceps shortening. To overcome the disadvantages of block spacers, and to facilitate reimplantation surgery, articulating spacers were introduced. Emerson et al [12] compared static block spacers with articulating spacers and reported an improvement in post operative ROM with no significant difference in the reinfection rate.

Essentially there are three types of articulating spacers: temporary [12, 18, 28], utilizing re-sterilized components or new components (also called spacer prostheses);

cement spacer molded during operation [10, 14, 16, 21], and preformed cement spacers [6] . The first two techniques showed advantages and disadvantages both with mechanical and biological points of view: the presence of hardware could theoretically favour bacterial adhesion, and the cement spacer moulded in the operative room do not have reproducible mechanical characteristics, and therefore a potential risk of component fracture [22]. We have reported our experience with the preformed articulating knee spacer. In the years 2000, we established a protocol for the two stage treatment for patients who have a late chronic deep infection of the knee. Between March 2000 and December 2005 a preformed articulating spacer (Spacer-K – Tecres Spa – Italy) was implanted in the management of infected total knee arthroplasty. The rehabilitation program between stages is the same as for a primary implant, with resulting shorter hospitalization and costs. The second stage surgical procedure is easier without an increase in bone loss.

Materials and Methods

Study Group

From March 2000 to December 2005 twenty-eight consecutive patients underwent two-stage exchange arthroplasty for infection at the site of a total knee arthroplasty, using a preformed articulating knee spacer. Two of these required arthrodesis (for medical problems). Another was unable to complete his functional questionnaires adequately because of language difficulties. Thus, twenty-five patients were available for inclusion in the present study.

Mean patient age was sixty-seven (range 54 – 77). The patients included seventeen women and eight men, with an average duration of follow-up of thirty-eight months (range twelve to sixty-nine months). Coagulase-negative staphylococci were detected in 75 % and in two cases the bacteria was not detected (Table 1).

Basing upon Mc Pherson's classification [20], fifteen were type A and ten type B. The diagnosis of infection was confirmed on the basis of positive culture of a pre operative aspiration and intra operative tissue specimen and increase c-reactive protein levels and an elevated erythrocyte sedimentation rate. According to Segawa infection classification [29], all cases were late chronic infections. All these knees had a functioning of extensor mechanism and collateral ligaments (medial): according to Engh's classification the bone loss was type I & II [13].

Treatment Protocols

Spacer-K (Tecres Spa, Italy) was used in all the knees. The device is manufactured in three sizes, with the characteristics of an ultra-congruent condylar knee-prosthesis.

Table 1. Average pre-operative, interim & last follow-up of ROM, IKSS clinical & function, Womac pain & function

	Pre-op average	Interim average	Last FU average
ROM	83° (40° – 120°)	77° (45° – 100°)	90° (75° – 125°)
IKSS c	35.38	72.92	75.38
IKSS f	37.96	76.04	80.58
Womac p	17.38	8.92	8.67
Womac f	60.67	34.25	31.04

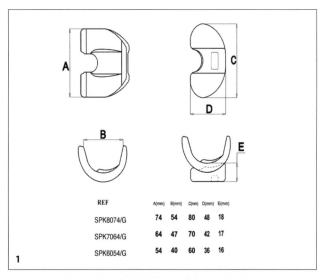

REF	A(mm)	B(mm)	C(mm)	D(mm)	E(mm)
SPK8074/G	74	54	80	48	18
SPK7064/G	64	47	70	42	17
SPK6054/G	54	40	60	36	16

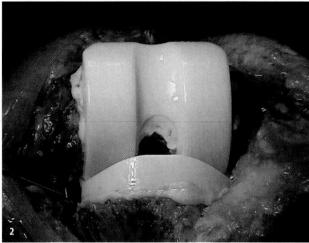

Fig. 1, 2. Device dimensions and intra-operative photograph obtained after the application of the Spacer-K

It is made of antibiotic-loaded acrylic bone cement (gentamicin 2.5 % w/w), and ready to use (Figs. 1, 2).

The mechanical properties have been tested [30] and validated. The antibiotic content and release mechanism is known and standardized [2]. The first stage is an aggressive debridement of all the infected or devitalized tissues and after an extensive pulsating lavage , the preformed articulating spacer, is inserted, always secured with proper antibiotic-loaded cement (Figs. 3, 4), based upon the culture exam. To each patient a systemic antibiotic therapy (minimum two types of antibiotic) was administered, for six weeks under the guidance of an infectious diseases consultant. Patients were encouraged to actively mobilize the knee immediately after surgery with partial weight bearing. The spacer was left in place until clinical healing of the soft tissue and

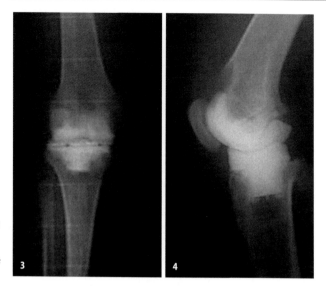

Fig. 3, 4. Antero-posterior and lateral radiograph showing the preformed articulating spager before the second stage

normal laboratory parameters. Joint aspiration for microbiological investigation was carried out one week after completion of the antibiotic therapy. The mean time in which the spacer has been left in situ is 12 weeks; in two patients it had been left longer: the first was the patient's choice and the second was a minor skin necrosis in a knee that had undergone several previous operations with multiple scars.

Evaluation

With the ethical committee board's approval, the study outcomes were assessed on the basis of the patients' responses to the Western Ontario and McMaster Universities Arthritis Center (WOMAC) questionnaire, the IKSS and satisfaction questionnaire. The satisfaction score has been based upon the answers regarding post operative pain, activities of daily living, ability to walk and use of crutches. Daily activities were scored on four different levels: excellent, good, fair, and poor.

The ability to walk is scored on unlimited (> one km), good (up to 800 meters), fair (less than 400 meters), poor (only at home). The postoperative range of motion has been recorded before the arthroplasty removal, while the device was working and at the last follow-up of the definitive implant. Bone loss was assessed radiographically and defined intraoperatively, according to the classification system of Engh [13] at both, the first and the second stage of the revision. Reinfection was defined as a recurrence of inflammation with a positive culture or clear serological evidence of infection.

Results

Standard surgical approach is performed at the second stage. Tibial tubercle or quadriceps snip osteotomy is never utilized.

Germ	Percentage
CNS MS	50
CNS MR	15
CNS MR + MS	15
MSSA	5
Others	5
Not detected	10

Table 2. Infecting organisms.

CNS MS = Coagulase-negative *Staphylococcus* methicillin-susceptible; CNS MR = Coagulase-negative *Staphylococcus* methicillin-resistant; MSSA = Methicillin-susceptible *Staphylococcus aureus*

The first stage bone loss was classified, according to the Engh system, as type 1 for seven femora (14 %); nine tibiae (18 %); as type 2A for thirteen femora (26 %); eleven tibiae (22 %); as type 2B for five femora and tibiae (10 % each). The spacer removal has always been easy without any change in previous Engh's classification and in the shape of the bone itself. No spacer wear or breakage has been shown.

During the interim period the use of crutches is mandatory and the patients' begin to walk after two days post surgery.

Two weeks later seventy seven per cent of patients went on one crutch, but one third of this percentage of patients had stated that they were capable of walking without crutches. Seventy-one per cent of patients reported no pain; twenty-nine percent reported mild discomfort. Brace was used for the first post-operative week just in three patients. The ability to walk was unlimited in six patients (24 %), good in thirteen (52 %), fair in four (16 %), poor in two (8 %). The range of motion remained unchanged between the first and second stage or improved after definitive reimplantation.

Patients judged the result as excellent or good in 76 % of cases, fair in 16 %, and poor in 8 %. Mean IKSS clinical was 35.38 (clinical) and 37.6 (function) on presentation; it improved to a mean of 72.92 (clinical) and 76.04 (function) after the first stage and to a mean of 75.38 (clinical) and 80.58 (function) at final review. Mean WOMAC (function and pain scores) were 17.38 and 60.67 on presentation respectively; it improved to a mean of 8.92 and 34.25 after the first stage and to a mean of 8.67 and 31.04 at final review (Table 2) . We have at the first stage the following prosthesis : 24 % of PS, 38 % CR. 19 % M. bearing, 14 % M. bearing UCOR, 5 % hinge. At the second stage a PS type revision implant was used in 30 % of patients. In 55 % was CCK and in 15 % a hinge implant was required. One case (4 %) had a recurrence of infection.

Discussion

Two stage reimplantation is the preferred option treatment in late chronic infection following total knee replacement. The use of spacers between stages has become the accepted practice. The purpose of the current study was to determine whether a preformed articulating spacer could reduce or avoid bone loss, improve quality of life between stages, ease surgical exposure at second stage and increase functional results, without a concomitant increase in infection rate. The removal of the spacer proved uncomplicated, and in no case was a progression in osseous defect, either on the femoral or tibial side noted. Other authors [12, 16] do not evaluate specifically the bone loss, but Fehring et al [14] performed comparison of static spacer blocks with an articulating spacer and reported that 60 % of the patient with static spacers had either tibial or femoral bone loss . At the same time the authors were unable to measure any bone loss between stages in the 30 patients who underwent reconstruction with an articulating spacer.

The quality of life using a preformed spacer between stages, has been satisfactory and the ability to bend the knee between stages improves patient lifestyle without compromising the overall results. With the exception of the first three cases where we had used a brace for the first seven days post operatively, we never immobilized the knee. The knee motion was pain free in most of the cases with a range of motion that remained unchanged between first and second stage or improved after definitive reimplantation in the stiff knee at the first stage. Of the 77 % of the patients who went on only one crutch, at least one third admitted that they could walk without crutches. Few authors report details of finding regarding ROM and quality of life between first and second stage. Duncan et al [16] report that the average HSS (Hospital for Special Surgery) score during the interim period was 55.9 with a mean flexion of 76.1°. Unfortunately the cement spacers molded in the operating room do not have reproducible mechanical characteristics, and there is a potential risk of fracture of the components [22]. The Spacer-K works in a similar fashion to the intermediate prosthesis, but the major drawback of the intermediate prosthesis, is the presence of hardware that could theoretically favor glycocalyx formation and bacterial adhesion [15] . In many countries, current infectious disease control policies prohibit the use of removed and re-sterilized prosthetic implants. It is difficult to make comparisons with the non-articulating spacer block where the patient is not allowed to move the knee or apply any significant weight during the interim period always using two crutches and brace. Because of quadriceps shortening caused by 6 to 8 weeks of immobilization, surgeons still are faced with a knee with significant scarring and capsular contracture at the time of re-implantation. Surgical exposure at second stage is difficult and often requires quadriceps snip, V-Y turn-down, or tibial tubercle osteotomy. Regarding the surgical technique, all the knees were surgically exposed at second stage through the previous incision using a medial parapatellar arthrotomy. A quadriceps snips or tibial tubercle osteotomy at the second stage has never been necessary, but we used it at the first stage in two knees with a flexion under 50°. The quadriceps snips have always been used at the second stage by other surgeons [17, 18]. For the revision implant, we used a PS type in 30 % of patients. In 55 % we used CCK and in 15 % a hinge implant was required. These results demonstrate that a good ligament balance is possible also at the second stage. The hinge implant was used in knees which have been stiff from the first stage . Still today our reinfection rate is 4 % . These results are similar to that achieved by other surgeon with a follow-up like ours. Duncan and colleagues [10] based on 45 patients with knee infection the recurrence of infection occurred in 9 % at mean follow-up of 48 months. Hofmann et al [17, 18] reported on fifty patients a 12 % recurrence of infection at mean follow-up 73 months, Emerson [12] looking only at the patients with the static block spacers, with a follow up to 12.7 years reported a re-infection rate of 30 %. We agree that the ability to bend the knee between stages improves patient satisfaction without compromising the eradication of infection, but the definition of complete healing of the infectious process would, however require a longer period of observation. It is remarkable that the re-infection rate depends more on time elapsed rather than on surgical technique.

References

1. Bengtson S, Knutson K, Lidgren L (1986) Revision of infected knee arthroplasty. Acta Orthop Scand 57(6):489–494
2. Bertazzoni Minelli E, Benini A, Biscaglia R et al (1999) Release of gentamicin and vancoycin alone and in combination from polymethylmethacrylate (PMMA) cement. J Antimicrob. Chemoter 44(suppl A):55–56
3. Booth RE Jr, Lotke PA (1989) The results of spacer block technique in revision of infected total knee arthroplasty. Clin Orthop Relat Res (248):57–60
4. Borden LS, Gearen PF (1987) Infected total knee arthroplasty: A protocol for management. J Arthroplasty 2(1):27–36
5. Calton TF, Fehring TK, Griffin WL (1997) Bone loss associated with the use of spacer blocks in infected total knee arthroplasty. Clin Orthop Relat Res (345):148–154
6. Castelli C, Martinelli R, Ferrari R (2002) Preformed all-cement knee spacer in two-stage revision for infected knee replacement. Proceedings of the SICOT XXII World Congress, 327c
7. Cohen JC, Hozack W, Cuckler JM, Booth RE Jr (1988) Two-stage reimplantation of septic total knee replacement. Report of three cases using an antibiotic-PMMA spacer block. J Arthroplasty 3(4):369–377
8. Cuckler JM, Star AM, Alavi A, Noto RB(1991) Diagnosis and management of the infected joint arthroplasty. Clin. Orthop North Am (229):523–530
9. Diduch DR, Insall JN, Scott WN et al (1997) Total knee replacement in young active patients. Long Term of follow-up and functional outcomes. J Bone Joint Surg (Am) 79(4):575–582
10. Duncan CP, Beauchamp C (1993) A temporary antibiotic-loaded joint replacement system for management of complex infections involving the hip. Orthop Clin North Am 24(4):751–759
11. Duncan CP, Beauchamp C, Masri BA (1992) The antibiotic loaded joint replacement system: a novel approach to the management of the infected knee replacement. J Bone Joint Surg (Br) (Suppl III) 74:296
12. Emerson RH, Jr, Muncie M, Tarbox TR et al (2002) Comparison of a static with a mobile spacer in total knee infection. Clin Orthop Relat Res (404):132–138
13. Engh GA (1997) Bone defect classification: Eng GA, Rorabeck CH, Editors. "Revision total knee arthroplasty. Baltimore: Williams and Wilkins; 1997. p 63–120
14. Fehring TK, Odum S, Calton TF, Mason JB (2000) Articulating versus static spacers in revision total knee arthroplasty for sepsis. Clin Orthop Relat Res (380):9–16
15. Goldman RT, Scuderi GR, Insall JN (1995) Two stage reimplantation for infected total knee replacement. Clin Orthop Relat Res (331):118–124
16. Haddad FS, Masri BA, Campbell D et al (2000) The Prostalac functional spacer in two-stage revision for infected knee replacements. J Bone Joint Surg (Br) 82(6):807–812
17. Hofmann AA, Goldberg T, Tanner AT et al (2005) Treatment of infected total knee arthroplasty using an articulating spacer. 2 to 12 year experience. Clin Orthop Relat Res (430):125–131
18. Hofmann AA, Kane KR, Tkach TK et al (1995): Treatment of infected total knee arthroplasty using an articulating spacer. Clin Orthop Relat Res (321):45–54
19. Insall JN (1986) Infection of total knee arthroplasty. Instr Course Lect. (35):319–324
20. McPherson EJ, Patzakis MJ, Gross JE et al (1997) Infected total knee arthroplasty: Two stage reimplantation with a gastrocnemius rotational flap. Clin Orthop Relat Res (341):73–81
21. McPherson EJ, Lewonoswski K, Dorr LD (1995) Use of an articulated PMMA spacer in the infected total knee arthroplasty. Clin Arthroplasty 10(1):87–89
22. Pitto RP, Spika IA (2004) Antibiotic-loaded bone cement spacers for two-stage management of the infected total knee arthroplasty. Int Orthop (28)3:129–133
23. Ranawat CS, Flynn WF Jr, Saddler S et al (1993) Long-term results of the total condylar knee arthroplasty. Clin Orthop Relat Res (286):94–102
24. Rand JA, Fitzgerald RH (1989) Diagnosis and management of the infected total knee arthroplasty. Clin Orthop North Am 20(2):201–210. Review
25. Rand JA (1993) Alternatives to reimplantation for salvage of the total knee arthroplasty complicated by infection. J Bone Joint Surg (Am) 75(2):282–289
26. Robertsson O, Knutson K, Lewold S et al (1997) Knee arthroplasty in rheumatoid arthritis. A report from the Swedish Knee Arthroplasty Register on 4381 primary operations 1985–1995. Acta Orthop Scand 68(6):545–553

27. Salvati EA, Robinson RP, Zeno SM et al.(1982) Infection rates after 3175 total hip and total knee replacements performed with and without a horizontal unidirectional filtered air-flow System. J Bone Joint Surg (Am) 64(4):525–535

28. Scott IR, Stockley L, Getty CJM (1993) Exchange arthroplasty for infected knee replacements. J Bone Joint Surg (Br) 74(1):28–31

29. Segawa H, Tsukayama DT et al (1999) Infection after total knee arthroplasty. A retrospective study of the treatment of eighty-one infections. J Bone Joint Surg (Am) 81(10):1434–1445

30. Villa T, Pietrabissa R (2003) Evaluation of the mechanical reliability of a knee spacer. 2003 Summer Bioengineering conference June, Key Biscaine (FL)

31. WalkerRH, Schurman DJ (1984) Management of infected total knee arthroplasties. Clin.Orthop Relat Res (186):81–89

32. Wilde AH, Ruth JT (1988) Two-stage reimplantation in infected total knee arthroplasty. Clin Orthop Relat Res (236):23–35

33. Windsor RE, Insall JN, Urs WK et al (1990) Two-stage reimplantation for the salvage of total knee arthroplasty complicated by infection. Further follow-up and refinement of indications. J Bone Joint Surg (Am) 72(2):272–278

Two-stage Revision with Preformed Knee Spacers and Modular Knee Prosthesis

E. Meani, C.L. Romanò

Department for Treatment of Osteoarticular Septic Complications (COS) –
Director: Prof. Enzo Meani
Operative Unit for Septic Prosthesis – Responsible: Prof. Carlo L. Romanò
"G. Pini" Orthopaedic Institute, Milan, Italy

Introduction

Infection after total knee arthroplasty may require different therapeutical solutions: one- or two-stage revision, surgical debridement and suppressive antibiotic therapy, knee arthrodesis, amputation. Two-stage reimplantation using an interval spacer of antibiotic-impregnated bone-cement has been investigated previously as a method to eradicate infection, prevent limb shortening and stiffness [1, 2, 7, 8, 10, 12, 13, 18, 19, 21].

Our indication for this surgical treatment is based on the following conditions:

1. Chronic infection
2. Delayed (onset after 8 – 12 weeks from surgery) or late (onset after one year from prosthesis implant) acute infection
3. Diagnosis confirmed by clinical history and examination, germ isolation.
4. Presence of extensor apparatus and local conditions allowing the surgical approach.
5. General conditions of the patient allowing a double surgery.
6. Informed consent of the patient and agreement on following the therapeutical indications.

Preformed antibiotic-loaded spacers (Spacer-K – Tecres Spa, Italy) (Fig. 1) offer predictable antibiotic release [3, 4] and tribological qualities that allow partial weight-bearing and joint mobility.

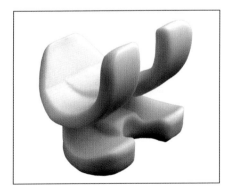

Fig. 1. Preformed antibiotic-loaded spacer (Spacer-K – Tecres Spa, Italy)

Medium term results of a consecutive series of patients with chronically infected total knee prosthesis, treated according to a same protocol are reported. The protocol included a two-stage revision using a preformed antibiotic-loaded cement spacer, cemented modular revision prosthesis and prolonged systemic antibiotic therapy after first and second stage.

Materials and Methods

From year 2001 to 2006 40 patients, affected by septic knee prosthesis, underwent two-stage revision in our Department according to the same protocol. For the purpose of this study we have considered the first 21 consecutive patients, at a follow-up ranging from 2 to 4 years from revision. Two patients were lost to follow-up. In all the cases the infected prosthesis was removed and a preformed antibiotic-loaded spacer was implanted. Spacer-K is an off-the-shelf preformed antibiotic-loaded cement knee spacer, available in three different femoral and tibial sizes, not interchangeable, that may be intra-operatively chosen. The cement is pre-loaded by the manufacturer with gentamicin at a concentration of 1.9 % (w/w). Two to three months after implant, the spacer was removed and the patients underwent reconstruction using cemented modular prosthesis (PFC TC3, Johnson & Johnson-DePuy Inc.).

There were 6 men and 12 women. Mean age at the time of the operation was 63.5 years (range, 58 – 76). The interval between the previous index operation and the revision ranged from 1 to 4 years. Five patients underwent a previous revision operation.

Specimens for culture were obtained from wound drainage in 4 patients, from knee aspirate in 10 patients, only intra-operatively in 3 patients. In two patients the cultural examinations were always negative.

After prosthesis removal and accurate bone and soft tissues debridement, the Spacer-K was inserted. In all the cases the spacer was fixed with one or two packs of antibiotic-loaded cement (Cemex Genta – Tecres Spa, Italy – gentamicin 2.5 %) to which vancomycin (5 %) was also intra-operatively added. To this aim the vancomycin powder was thoroughly mixed with the cement powder before the addition of liquid monomer. Postoperatively, patients were allowed partial weight-bearing on the operated extremity with two crutches until re-implantation.

All the patients received a minimum of 6 weeks of organism-specific antibiotics postoperatively and returned for clinical follow-up at the completion of their antibiotic course. Patients were scheduled for removal of the spacer and revision arthroplasty 2 to 4 weeks after completion of intravenous antibiotics or 8 to 12 weeks after spacer implant.

Patients with successful eradication of their infection, as evidenced by complete blood count with differential and C-reactive protein within the normal ranges underwent the second stage of their reconstruction. If clinical suspicion of persistent infection remained despite negative laboratory studies, joint aspiration before reimplantation was performed for cultural examination and white blood cells count. In all cases, intraoperative cultures were obtained at the time of the second stage procedure.

At revision the knee was exposed through the same surgical approach and the spacer was removed without difficulty. When necessary (in 5 patients) an osteotomy of the anterior tibial apophysis was performed, to allow knee flexion and placement of the patella. All the knees were treated with modular cemented (Cemex Genta – Tecres Spa, Italy) revision prosthesis (PFC-TC3, Johnson&Johnson DePuy). Cement was not applied in the femoral or tibial canal or around the prosthesis' stems. Touch-down weight-bearing was allowed for 6 weeks followed by 50 % weight-bearing for 6 weeks. Full weight-bearing was usually permitted at 12 – 16 weeks after surgery, depending on muscular strength. After operation, parenteral antibiotics were administered for 6 weeks. After each procedure closed suction drainage was inserted and removed after 48 hours.

Our primary outcomes included eradication of infection, spacer stability and integrity and implant stability. Failure of treatment was a recurrence of infection, defined as the occurrence of clinical signs of infection (redness, swelling, pain, fistulae) whenever at follow-up.

Preoperative and post-operative hematologic studies included the determination of erythrocyte sedimentation rate, white blood cell count, and C-reactive protein level. Plain radiographs included anteroposterior and lateral views of the knee joint. Radiographic examination was performed at 2, 6 and 12 months postoperatively, followed by yearly intervals thereafter. Knee range of motion pre- and post-operatively was recorded.

Results

The 21 patients included in this study were followed for an average of 32 months (range, 24 – 48 months). Two patients were lost to follow-up at, respectively, 36 and 40 months post-operatively, without any sign of infection.

Identified organisms were the following: *S. aureus* in 9 patients and *S. epidermidis* in 6 patients (methicillin-resistant staphylococci strains: 10), *Pseudomonas aeruginosa* in 2 patients, *Escherichia coli* in 1 patient, no isolates in 2 patients.

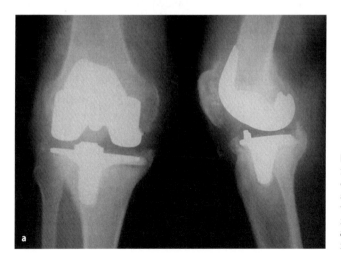

Fig. 2. 63-year-old female who had chronic infection with a draining sinus in total knee replacement
a pre-operative plain radiograph

The interval between the first-stage and second-stage operations ranged from 8 to 12 weeks (mean 83 ± 16 days). During the interval 18 patients had no pain and 3 patients reported mild pain. All the patients were able to walk with partial weight-bearing, with two crutches.

At the time of the latest follow-up no patient showed clinical evidence of infection recurrence and no patient required revision for any reason (Fig. 2). The range of motion was improved from 60.8 and –5.1 to 81.1 to –3.1 flexion and extension range, respectively.

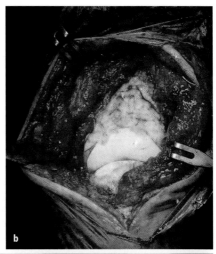

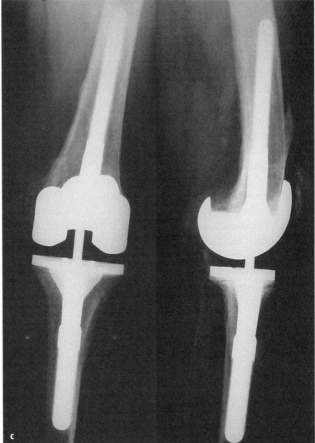

Fig. 2b. Intra-operative view of the spacer. Note the large amount of cement used to fix the implant
c control 4 years from revision

Postoperative complications included: one spacer dislocation; one femoral and tibial fracture, treated with osteosynthesis; two knee lateral instability > 5 degrees.

Two patients had side effects during antibiotic treatment (gastrointestinal tract dysfunction), that required temporary withdrawal of antibiotics.

Discussion

Two-stage revision of septic knee prosthesis has been reported to provide a success rate ranging from 80 % to 100 % and a mean success rate of 92 % in 246 patients at a mean follow-up of 3.4 years, according to a meta-analysis of different studies (cf. Table 1). Our results, when compared to the literature data, are encouraging, even if the number of our series is still relatively low.

The use of antibiotic-loaded cement, as it has been shown in many studies, allows to obtain bactericidal local antibiotic levels [3–5, 9, 11, 14–17, 20], even if some authors pointed out possible inconvenience connected with the toxic effect of poly-methylmethacrylate on polymorphonuclear cells [22, 23], the risk of developing resistant strains and of cement fragilization. In this regard, the possibility of using in cement spacers antibiotic combinations with concentrations higher than those permitted in one-stage revision surgery, may reduce the risk of occurrence of resistant bacteria and of small colony variants.

Many Gram-positive and Gram-negative organisms are resistant to gentamicin, that currently is the antibiotic added by the manufacturer to the preformed spacers that we have used. In our series vancomycin was added in the cement used to fix the spacer implant. Therapeutic levels of vancomycin and gentamicin, have been found *in vitro* and in drainage fluid after they were used with cement [4, 5, 9, 11, 14, 17]. Systemic antibiotic administration has also been performed for approximately six weeks after the first and second stage operation. The antibiotic choice has been made on the basis of cultural examination and antibiogram and two antibiotics have been administered parentally and orally during the first 3 or 4 weeks and then only orally for the remaining 2 or 3 weeks in all the patients. In the lack of comparative studies it is not possible to drive any conclusion either if this prolonged systemic antibiotic treatment was an over-treatment or, on the contrary and as we suggest, if it may have played a role in the overall good success rate in this series of patients. Two of our patients (11 %) had side effects due to antibiotics. These side effects might be related to post-operative intravenous antibiotics or antibiotics used in the cement spacer (or both). However, the safety of the antibiotic delivery from the cement spacer has been previ-

Table 1

Author	FU	# Cases	% Success
Masri BA et al. (1994)	2.2	24	91.7
Wilde AH et al. (1988)	1.5	15	80.0
Haddad FS et al. (2000)	4.0	45	91.0
Barrack RL et al. (2000)	3.0	28	94.0
Fehring (2000)	2.5	15	100.0
Emerson RH (2002)	4.0	22	90.9
Meek RM (2003)	4.0	47	96.0
Hofmann AA et al. (2005)	6.0	50	92.0

ously established [6] and the side effects resolved after temporary withdrawal of intravenous antibiotics in all the patients.

Our surgical technique included in rigid knees the osteotomy of the tibial apophysis. This technique, that allows optimal surgical exposure and placement of the patella, did not lead to non-unions in our series, although this remains a possible complication.

In conclusion, our results show, in a limited but homogeneous series of patients, that a preformed articulated spacer and a cemented modular revision prosthesis allow to achieve infection eradication and a significant increase in the joint range of motion.

References

1. Wilde AH, Ruth JT (1988) Two-stage reimplantation in infected total knee arthroplasty. Clin Orthop Relat Res (236):23–35
2. Barrack RL, Engh G, Rorabeck C et al (2000) Patient satisfaction and outcome after septic versus aseptic revision total knee arthroplasty. J Arthroplasty 15(8):990–993
3. Bertazzoni Minelli E, Benini A (2000) "Modalità di rilascio di antibiotici da cemento" Da Atti del Congresso "Cementi Ossei nell'anno 2000. Attualità e prospettive"Varese 7 Aprile 2000
4. Bertazzoni Minelli E, Benini A, Magnan B et al (2004) Release of gentamicin and vancomycin from temporary human hip spacers in two-stage revision of infected arthroplasty. J Antimicrob Chemother 53(2):329–334
5. Chapman MW, Hadley KW (1976) The effect of poymethylmethacrylaye and antibiotic combinations on bacterial viability. J Bone Joint Surg (Am) 58(1):76–81
6. Duncan CP, Masri BA (1995) The role of antibiotic-loaded cement in the treatment of an infection after a hip replacement. Instr Course Lect (44):305–313. Review
7. Emerson RH Jr, Muncie M, Tarbox TR et al (2002) Comparison of a static with a mobile spacer in total knee infection. Clin Orthop Relat Res (404):132–138
8. Fehring TK, Odum S, Calton TF et al (2000) Articulating versus static spacers in revision total knee arthroplasty for sepsis. The Ranawat Award. Clin Orthop Relat Res (380):9–16
9. Grassi FA (2000) Razionale d'impiego del cemento con antibiotico. Da Atti del Congresso "Cementi Ossei nell'anno 2000. Attualità e prospettive", Varese 7 Aprile 2000
10. Haddad FS, Masri BA, Campbell D et al (2000) The PROSTALAC functional spacer in two-stage revision for infected knee replacements. Prosthesis of antibiotic-loaded acrylic cement. J Bone Joint Surg (Br) 82(6):807–812
11. Hill L, Kienerman L, Trustey S et al (1977) Diffusion of antibiotics from acrylic bone-cement in vitro. J Bone Joint Surg (Br) 59(2):197–199
12. Hofmann AA, Goldberg T, Tanner AM et al (2005) Treatment of infected total knee arthroplasty using an articulating spacer: 2- to 12-year experience. Clin Orthop Relat Res (430):125–131
13. Hofmann AA, Kane KR, Tkach TK et al (1995) Treatment of infected total knee arthroplasty using an articulating spacer. Clin Orthop Relat Res (321):45–54
14. Kuechle DK, Landon GC, Musher DM et al (1991) Elution of vancomycin, daptomycin, and amikacin from acrylic bone cement. Clin Orthop Relat Res (264):302–308
15. Levin PD (1975) The effectiveness of various antibiotics in methyl methacrylate. J Bone Joint Surg (Br) 57(2):234–237
16. Marks KH, Nelson CL, Lautenschlager EP (1976) Antibiotic-impregnated acrylic bone cement. J Bone Joint Surg (Am) 58(3):358–364
17. Masri BA, Duncan CP, Beauchamp CP (1998) Long-term eliution of antibiotics from bone-cement. J Arthroplasty (13):331–338
18. Masri BA, Kendall RW, Duncan CP et al (1994) Two-stage exchange arthroplasty using a functional antibiotic-loaded spacer in the treatment of the infected knee replacement: the Vancouver experience. Semin Arthroplasty 5(3):122–136

19. Meek RM, Masri BA, Dunlop D et al (2003) Patient satisfaction and functional status after treatment of infection at the site of a total knee arthroplasty with use of the PROSTALAC articulating spacer. J Bone Joint Surg (Am) 85(10):1888–1892

20. Murray WR (1984) Use of antibiotic-containing bone cement Clin Orthop Relat Res (190):89–95

21. Nijhof MW, Oyen W JG, Van Kampen A et al (1997) Hip and knee arthroplasty infection. Acta Orthop Scand 68(4):332–336

22. Panush RS, Petty W (1978) Inhibition of human lymphocyte responses by methylmethacrylate. Clin Orthop Relat Res (134):356–363

23. Petty W (1978) The effect of methylmetacrylate on bacterial phagocytosis and killing by human polymorphonuclear leukocytes. J Bone Joint Surg (Am) 60(6):752–757.

Arthrodesis for the Treatment of Severe Knee Disease

C. Sandrone, G. Moraca, G. Casalino Finocchio

Department of Orthoaedics, Section of Osteo-articular Inflammatory Disease, Santa Corona Hospital, Pietra Ligure (SV), Italy

Introduction

Knee arthrodesis is a surgical procedure performed in order to salvage a limb in which the knee joint is compromised in a way to preclude any possibility to re-create a new articulation through a prosthetic replacement. This is especially true in severe periprosthetic septic cases.

The etymology comes from Greek language: arthron (= articulation) + desis (= block, constraint).

Known as well as "joint fusion", arthrodesis is an artificially-induced ankylosis with a surgical procedure, normally irreversible (dis-arthrodesis has been exceptionally performed – Figure 1).

Aims of arthrodesis are: 1) pain elimination; 2) search for a joint stability which is compromised; 3) re-alignement of the articular ends displaced by severe osteoarthritis.

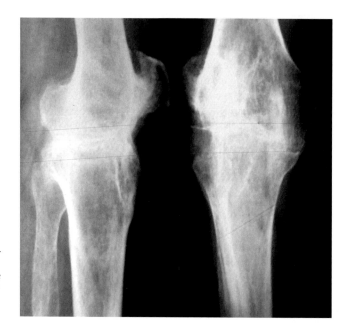

Fig. 1. If dis-arthrodesis is performed, it is necessary to re-create an adequate articular midline (thin lines) and have the patella

Henry Park (1745–1831) was the first surgeon to perform a knee arthrodesis in a 33-year-old sailor affected by tubercular gonilitis [1].

Park resected the distal end of the femur and the proximal end of the tibia and then joined together the two ends. The wound healed and the extremities fused. The patient was left with a 3-inch shorter limb, a limb which was anyway functional.

On September 18, 1782 he wrote to his mentor and friend Sir Percivall Pott, explaining the rationale of the intervention: "The cure is the complete removal of the articulation, and of the whole or the largest part possible of the capsule; in this way healing is achieved through the formation of a callus which joins the femur to the tibia, when this intervention is performed at knee level" [2].

Park and the French surgeon Moreau collaborated strictly to develop the technique of articular resection for tuberculosis [3].

Excision or arthrodesis of the knee was a simple technique, which corrected the deformities and produced wide flat surfaces of cancellous bone which just needed to be kept firm, while fusion occurred.

Initially surgeons used only external braces for the immobilization. Morrant Baker in 1887 introduced the use of crossed nails for the internal fixation [4]. In 1915 Melvin Henderson published the experience at the Mayo Clinic [5]. In 1932 Albert Key introduced the concept of compression (= positive pressure) [6]: indeed, after the resection of the articular ends of the tibia and the femur, fixed them using long nails passing through the proximal tibia and the distal femur. The screws were fixed with tighteners, which allowed to achieve a positive pressure between the resected surfaces, immobilizing them rigidly.

Sir John Charnley made public the usefulness and the technique of arthrodesis [7, 8, 9, 10]. Nelson and Evarts (1971) first described arthrodesis as election treatment for failed total knee arthroplasty [11]. Since then knee prosthesis failure have become the main indication for knee arthrodesis. [12, 13]

Stulberg and Rand clearly described the indications for knee arthrodesis following a failed total knee replacement:

- high functional demand
- disease involving a single joint
- relatively young age
- deficient extensor mechanism
- inadequate soft tissue coverage
- immunocompromised condition
- the presence of a highly virulent microorganism causing infection that requires highly toxic antimicrobial therapy [14, 15].

The surgical technique foresees:

a. accurate removal of the residues of cartilage and of the fibrous and membranous adherences from both articular surfaces
b. compression and fixation of the bone ends, as in fracture
c. bone graft (possible with local auto-graft), useful for bone fusion stimulation

The main complication of knee arthrodesis is pseudo-arthrosis ("non-union").

The causes of pseudoarthrosis are:

- bone deficit (bone-loss)
- infection persistence
- insufficient apposition of bone grafts
- mal-alignement of the bone segments
- inadequate immobilization

The optimal positioning of the knee requires:

- negligible valgism
- extra-rotation of 10°
- a flexion ranging from 0 to 20°

Contraindications to arthodesis are considered:

- a severe septic bilateral arthopathy of the knee
- a severe septic ipsilateral arthropathy of the hip and of the ankle
- a severe bone segmental deficit
- the amputation of the controllable limb

The methods of achieving fixation for a knee arthrodesis following a failed knee replacement include including external and internal fixation [25].

External fixation can be performed taking advantage of a number of medical devices, ranging from orthopaedic braces and casts, Kirschner wires and Steinmann pins (percutaneously inserted), and external fixators (monoaxial, quadrilateral, circular, hybrid) [16].

Internal fixation can be achieved using an intramedullary nail or a plate [17, 18, 19].

The use of an endomedullary nail (Fig. 4) provides a reliable union rate even in the setting of major bone defects and septic failure [25]. The use of bone graft is useful and helpful to restore lost bone stock or to augment fusion [26].

Staged debridement prior to intramedullary nail arthrodesis, with removal of all the prosthetic components and infection control, is mandatory to avoid re-infection before proceeding with the fusion [16, 18, 22, 23, 25]. Intramedullary nailing is also the preferable technique to repair considerable limb shortenings (over 6 cm) and the best choice when arthrodesis is necessary and sepsis is not present (as in the irreparable lesions of the knee extensor apparatus).

Nonetheless there are some contraindications to the use of the endomedullary nail:

a. active infection for the risk of diffusion into the diaphyseal canal of femur and tibia;
b. presence of angular deformities of the femoral or tibial diaphysis.

The complications described in literature are quite high (from 40 % to 55 %) and go from breakage to migration of the nail till bone fracture. Therefore external fixation is to be preferred in those cases in which infection resolution is not sure, whereas internal fixation finds its indication when infection has healed and a limited limb shortening is required [20, 21, 22, 23].

A further problem is to decide whether arthrodesis should be performed at the time of prosthesis removal (one stage) or be delayed (two stages).

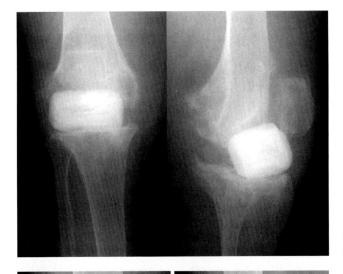

Fig. 2. Intra-operative moulded spacer

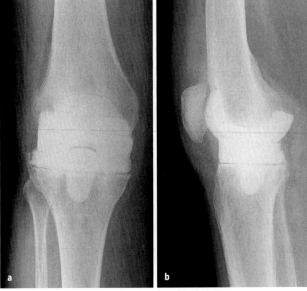

Fig. 3a, b. Preformed knee spacer (Spacer-K – Tecres Spa, Italy)

In our experience, fixation with endomedullary nail (4 cases) was always performed in two stages, external fixation instead was performed in one stage or two stages. One stage was performed 1) due to age or patient conditions; 2) due to local conditions or lack of clinical signs; 3) due to a direct request of the patient. When a two-stage approach was performed, a temporary PMMA spacer supplemented with antibiotic (spacer block) was used.

Until 2001 spacers were hand made in the operating theatre (Fig. 2) adding 1 or 2 g of vancomycin to a 40 g cement dose, which could also be already supplemented with antibiotic (gentamicin, tobramycin, erithromycin).

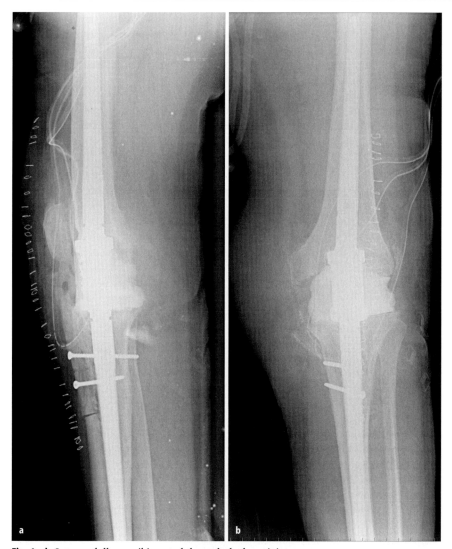

Fig. 4a, b. Intramedullary nail inserted through the knee joint

From 2002 a preformed cement spacer (Tecres Spa) has been used (Fig. 3). The spacer is fixed with cement supplemented with tobramycin, and sometimes a second antibiotic (vancomycin, imipenem, others) if suggested by the antibiogram.

Surgical Technique

The success of arthrodesis depends mainly on the width of the two surfaces of cancellous bone well aligned and from the stability of the fixation. Special attention is given to the removal of prosthesis components and cement, using proper saws and chisels. Bone cement and all devitalized and granulation tissues must be removed, without injuring the bone in good condition, essential to achieve a good contact with the bone surfaces and the right alignement. The "good" bone wrongly removed should be reused; often the bone of the patella is used, preserving the integrity of the extensor apparatus.

To increase the contact between the bone surfaces, the fragments of cancellous bone (chips) are inserted among them. Generally neither grafts taken far from the arthrodesis site (iliac crest, contralateral pre-tibial apophysis), nor bone from bank, nor synthetic bone substitutes is used.

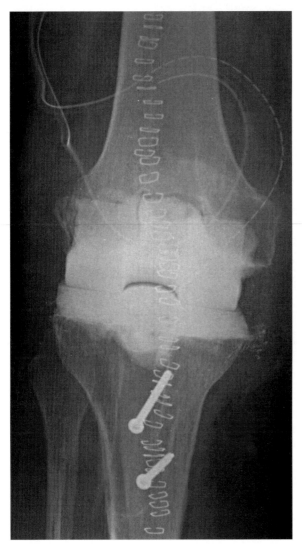

Fig. 5a. first stage with knee spacer application

The preparation of the surfaces is quite demanding, especially after the removal of highly invasive prosthesis, such as constrained or revision ones, or when large geodic cysts or sclerotic areas are present [24, 25]: in this last case several revitalizing bone perforation are performed (Beck's style).

After the preparation of the bone surfaces, fixation must be performed with much attention, especially with severe osteoporosis or bone loss. For increasing the stability, the external fixator is reinforced with further pins.

Before performing the fixation with external axial fixator, another fixation with Kirschner wires or crossed Steinman pins is done (Fig. 5), entering percutaneously into the proximal tibia and proceeding through the diaphyseal canal till to transpass the cortical bone of the distal femur from inside to outside.

The fixation with crossed wires is left generally for one month – one month and a half, and then it is easily removed. Weight-bearing is given quite early, except when the pre-tibial apophysis is detached and the osteosynthesis is performed, in these cases weight bearing is delayed of 15 days.

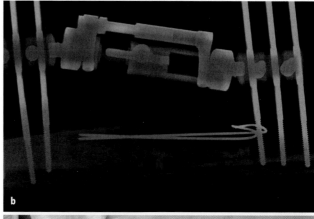

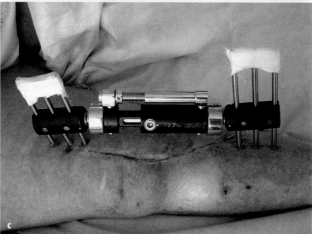

Fig. 5b. second stage with external fixator and Kirschner wires; **c** clinical aspect of the second stage

Case Series

Materials and Methods

From January 2002 and April 2006, 25 patients (6 M, 19 F) underwent knee arthrodesis. The average age was 67 (range 35–84). 4 patients were treated with endomedullary nail and 21 with external fixation (3 with Ilizarov with trochanteric pins, 18 with monoaxial external fixator).

Reason for arthrodesis were: peri-prosthetic sepsis (20 cases), tubercular gonilitis (2 cases); severe septic arthritis following osteosynthesis (2 cases); severe polimicrobic osteoarthritis with long-term fistula following homoplastic transplant of ACL.

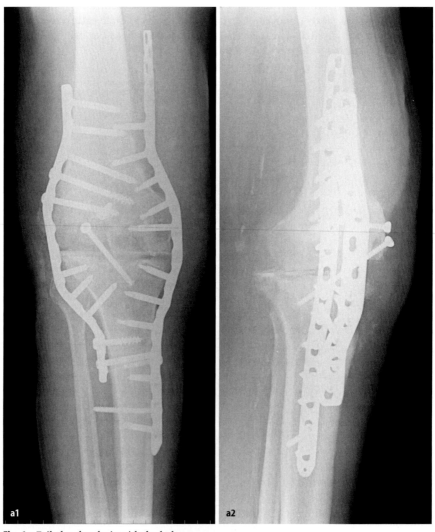

Fig. 6a. Failed arthrodesis with dual plate

The 4 cases treated with endomedullary nails (2 cemented and 2 uncemented), introduced in retrograde fashion, were performed in two stages.

One-stage procedure (direct arthrodesis) was performed in 11 patients (2 tubercular gonilitis; 2 post-traumatic osteoarthritis, 4 failed arthrodesis (Fig. 6), 1 secondary osteoarthritis following ACL transplant, 2 peri-prosthetic infections following TKR); two-stage procedure was performed in the remaining 14 patients, all showing a peri-prosthetic infection.

In 7 cases a preformed spacer (Spacer-K – Tecres Spa, Italy) was implanted: 4 were then treated with an endomedullary nail.

In the other 7 cases an hand-made spacer was implanted (in one case only the tibial component of the prosthesis was removed and therefore the spacer had a reduced thickness).

In the patients treated with a two-stage procedure, arthrodesis ha been performed at least 6 months after spacer implantation.

3 patients, which underwent the first stage of the procedure (prosthesis removal and Spacer-K implantation) have not yet completed the second stage of the procedure after 2 years and are in a stand-by situation (possible definitive spacer?) and therefore are not considered in the present series.

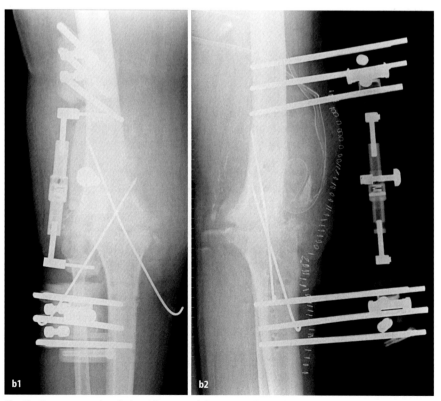

Fig. 6b. One-stage arthrodesis with external fixation and Kirschner wires

One patient is affected by a severe dilatative miocardiopathy, another is affected by severe renal insufficiency, the third is affected by sclerodermy, with extended femoral bone alterations of infarct-type following a prolonged cortisone therapy. All of them can walk with a crutch and are satisfied of their functionality.

Results

Bone fusion occurred on average in 7–8 months (range 6–9 months) in 17 patients; 3 patients (all females) died during the treatment for different causes and 5 still need to complete the treatment. Limb shortening was on average of 3.8 cm (1.5–6.2 cm) and this was compensated satisfactorily with a proper support.

No recurrence of infection was observed in the 17 patients which completed the treatment at a mean follow-up of 14 months (2–39).

All the patients had some reduction in limb functionality: 2 patients walk without any need of crutches and do not have any pain, 10 generally use a crutch when they leave their home, but without pain; 5 often need to be helped when they walk or need two crutches or use the walking frame, but without much pain. Both groups are satisfied in respect to the situation prior to arthrodesis.

Complications

The observed complication were:

1. spacer dislocation, with rotation of the device due to wide osteolysis due to debris formation. The case was successfully solved with the arthrodesis;
2. oblique fracture of the femoral diaphysis where the fiches were applied: the femur was extremely osteoporotic due to the prolonged inactivity of the patient. The case was surgically solved with additional osteosynthesis with a plate. The patient subsequently died for cardiac problems.
3. anaemia following the intervention for the lesion of three perforating arterioles of the femur due to transfixion of the fiches: the case was solved with selective embolization of the arterioles;
4. mal-positioning of the femoral component of the nail with proximal protrusion from the diaphyseal canal: nonetheless the patient is fine even during walking as the cemented endodiaphyseal part of the stem does guarantee stability.

Conclusions

In the present experience external monoaxial fixators pin tract infections resulted negligible, the management did not resulted problematic and the patients showed a good tolerance and compliance.

Two-stage arthrodesis with the use of an antibiotic-loaded spacer, the possibility to perform proper surgical debridement and adequate specimens retrieval for microbiological evaluation in both surgical acts and consequently the proper tailored systemic antibiotic therapy allowed to optimize the treatment with arthrodesis of the irretrievably septic failures of the knee prosthesis, reducing extremely the main causes for insuccess of this treatment, i.e. recurrence and pseudo-arthrosis.

References

1. D'Arcy Power (1936) Henry Park, who excised joints in 1781. Brit J Surg 24:2057
2. Park H, Moreau PF (1806) Cases of the excision of carious joints. Glasgow University Press, 3 sc
3. Moreau PF (1803) Observation pratiques relatives à la résection des articulations affectés de carie. Farge, Paris
4. Morrant Baker (1887) Remarks on method of fixing the bones in the operation of excision of the knee joint. Brit Med J 321–324
5. Henderson MS (1915) Resection of the knee for tuberculosis. JAMA (64):140–145
6. Key JA (1932) Positive pressure in arthrodesis for tuberculosis of the knee joint. South Med J (25):909–915
7. Charnley J (1948) Arthrodesis of the knee joint. J Bone Joint Surg (Br) 30:478–486
8. Charnley J, Lowe HG (1958) A study of the end results of compression arthrodesis of the knee. J Bone Joint Surg (Br) 40(4):633–635
9. Charnley J, Houston JK (1964) Compression arthrodesis of the shoulder. J Bone Joint Surg (Br) (46):614–620
10. Charnley J (1951) Compression arthrodesis of the ankle and shoulder. J Bone Joint Surg (Br) 33(2):614–620
11. Nelson CL, Evarts CM (1971) Arthroplasty and arthrodesis at the knee-joint. Orthop Clin North Am 2(1):245–264
12. Brodersen MP, Fitzgerald RH Jr, Peterson LFA et al (1979) Arthrodesis of the knee following failed total knee arthroplasty. J Bone Joint Surg (Am) 61(2):181–185
13. Hagemann WF, Woods GW, Tullos HS (1978) Arthrodesis in failed total knee replacement. J Bone Joint Surg (Am) 60(6):790–794
14. Stulberg SD (1982) Arthrodesis in failed total knee replacements. Orthop Clin North Am 13(1):213–234
15. Rand JA (1993) Alternatives to reimplantation for salvage of the total knee arthroplasty complicated by infection. J Bone Joint Surg (Am) 75(2):282–289. Review
16. Knutson K, Bodelind B, Lidgren L (1984) Stability of external fixators used for knee arthrodesis after failed knee arthroplasty. Clin Orthop Relat Res (186):90–95
17. Nichols SJ, Landon GC, Tullos HS (1991) Arthrodesis with dual plates after failed total knee arthroplasty. J Bone Joint Surg (Am) 73(7):1020–1024
18. Donley BG, Matthews LS, Kaufer H (1991) Arthrodesis of the knee with intramedullary nail. J Bone Joint Surg (Am) 73(6):907–913
19. Stiehl JB, Hanel DP (1993) Knee arthrodesis using combined intramedullary rod and plate fixation. Clin Orthop Relat Res (294):238–241
20. Vander Griend R (1983) Intramedullary arthrodesis of the knee after failed total knee arthroplasty. Clin Orthop Relat Res (181):146–150
21. Harris CM, Froehlich J (1985) Knee fusion with intramedullary rods for failed total knee arthroplasty. Clin Orthop Relat Res (197):209–216
22. Wilde AH, Stearns KL (1989) Intramedullary fixation for arthrodesis of the knee after infected total knee arthroplasty. Clin Orthop Relat Res (248):87–92
23. Ellingsen DE, Rand JA (1994) Intramedullary arthrodesis of the knee after total knee arthroplasty. J Bone Joint Surg (Am) 76(6):870–877
24. Wiedel JD (2002) Salvage of infected total knee fusion: the last option. Clin Orthop Relat Res (404):139–142
25. Petty W (1999) Knee arthrodesis in the treatment of failed total knee replacement. Med Gen Med 1(1) [formerly published in Medscape Orthopedics and Sports Medicine Journal 1998 2(3)]
26. MacDonald JH, Agarwal S, Lorei MP et al (2006) Knee arthrodesis. J Am Acad Orthop Surg 14(3):154–163

36 Arthrodesis and Amputation in Knee Joint Infections

R.A. LAUN

Department of Trauma and Reconstructive Surgery, General Hospital Centre Neukölln of Capital Berlin, Germany

Introduction

Infection is certainly one of the most menacing complications of total knee arthroplasty. Infection causes pain, limited function and prolonged hospitalization with additional series of surgery [1, 8, 10].

Similar problems and treatment algorithms exist in cases of severe bone or soft tissue defects of the knee area with or without joint affection. Soft tissue defects of the knee that require reconstructive surgery may occur after trauma or following a surgical procedure, for example a failure due to severe infection [2, 3, 5, 7, 9]. Wound breakdown and infection control is a challenge for both patient and orthopaedic surgeon.

More aggressive treatment is necessary for severe infection with resistant organisms and/or an immuno-suppressed host and/or in cases of general sepsis [6,7, 8].

As a final option knee amputation is indicated in the presence of a life-threatening sepsis, especially with multi-resistant or gas-forming microorganisms. To the surgeon infection is still a diagnostic and therapeutic dilemma, especially in cases of acute or chronic knee joint infection [4, 5, 6, 10].

Main

Between October 2003 and March 2006 ten patients underwent a knee arthrodesis after an infect-defect situation. One patient required an above knee amputation soon after the surgical procedure.

Common indications for knee arthrodesis include failed total knee arthroplasty, peri-articular tumor (mostly osteosarcoma), post-traumatic arthritis, and chronic joint infection [1, 9, 10]. The primary contraindications to knee arthrodesis are bilateral involvement or an ipsilateral hip arthrodesis. In case of a damaged knee and exclusion of other reconstructive measures the contraindications are relative [9, 10].

A wide variety of arthrodesis techniques have been described, including external fixators, internal fixation by compression plates, intramedullary fixation through the knee with a modular nail, and antegrade nailing through the pertrochanteric area. Allograft or autograft are described to restore lost bone stock or to augment fusion [2, 3, 9, 10].

In this series a knee arthrodesis with an intramedullary modular nail passing through the knee joint with a coupling module for the femoral and tibial nail components was used.

This procedure allows a direct approach to the joint, simple intra-operative length and rotational control, immediate bony compression and stable fixation of the long bones femur and tibia – and lead in a trained team to short operative procedures. Bone grafting was not used.

The indication to knee arthrodesis were found in patients with severe septic osteoarthritis (5), after failed knee arthroplasty (3) and with severe soft tissue defects around the knee in combination with deep infection (2). The indication was based on the microbiological evidence of the joint infection, mostly caused by *Staphylococcus aureus* or mixed flora with Gram-positive and/ or Gram-negative cocci. In all ten cases (including the above knee amputation) an outpatient antibiotic therapy was done without success.

The surgical management was in all cases two-staged.

In the first stage local and systemic infection was treated with surgery, antibiotic therapy [6, 7, 8] and simultaneous knee joint stabilization with an external fixator. In a failed prosthesis or osteosynthesis the simultaneous removal of all implants and bone cement was performed. In the cases of osteoarthritis total removal of articular cartilage in combination with pulsed irrigation was performed. Intermittent revision debridements with pulsed lavage followed every two days. A vacuum wound occlusion was performed when possible. Accompanying systemic antibiotic treatment started from day one and was modified according to the antibiogram.

In a second stage the definitive knee arthrodesis followed if microbiological and histological examination were negative for three consecutive times.

All arthrodeses were performed with a trans-articular knee joint approach, reamed retrograde nailing of the femur and reamed antegrade nailing of the tibia. Limb length adjustment, rotational adjustment and bone compression of the femoral and tibial parts were achieved with a modular coupling module.

In all cases we used the modular knee arthrodesis system of the Peter Brehm Company (Erlangen, Germany).

Figures 1–7 show a case of 32-year-old man with severe osteoarthritis and osteomyelitis with subchondral abscesses left knee treated successful with two staged management of knee joint arthrodesis.

For carefully selected patients with realistic expectations, knee revision prosthesis may represent a therapeutic option in a controlled infection. In our patient group it did not exist indication for a knee revision prosthesis replacement. Reasons for these decisions were: old aged patients, long serial revision surgery, soft tissue defects, functional arthrodesis caused by long period of knee joint transfixation and lack of patient compliance.

Reports of knee arthrodesis indicate approximately 90 % success in eradication of infection [2, 3, 9, 10]. The encouraging results, better functional outcome and better patient convenience using the operative method of an intramedullary device with a coupling module have expanded the role of this operative treatment option to refractory cases and to severe infections with major soft-tissue loss. No reinfection after arthrodesis was seen, and wound and bone healing was normal in all nine patients.

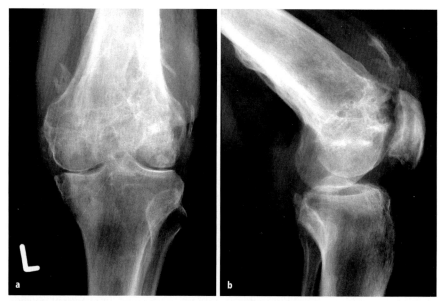

Fig. 1a, b. X-rays of a 32 year old man with severe post-traumatic arthritis and osteomyelitis by accompanying infection. Infect-defect situation of the left knee joint

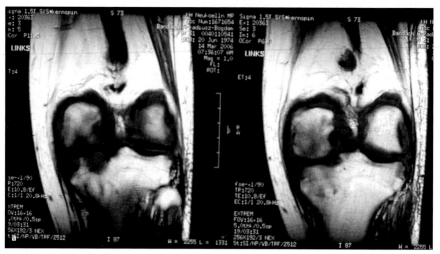

Fig. 2a, b. MRI of left knee joint shows severe post-traumatic arthritis with deep sub-chondral abscesses in the medial part of the tibia

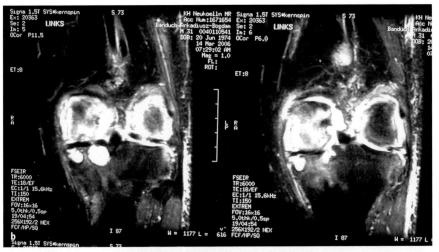

Fig. 2b

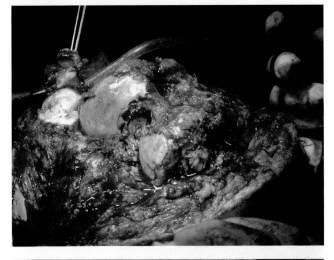

Fig. 3. Intra-operative site with deep defects, chronic chondritis and synovialitis, typical signs of chronic osteomyelitis with accompanying joint infection. Pre-operative and operative antibiogram show mass of *S. aureus*

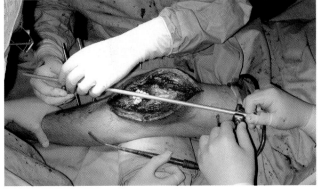

Fig. 4. Intra-operative site: resection debridement, pulsed irrigation and spacer with antibiotic bead chain, temporary stabilization of the knee joint with external fixator

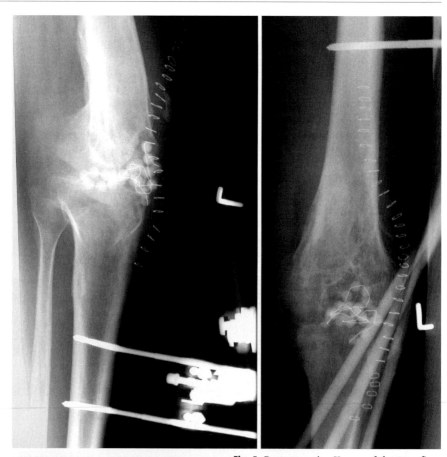

Fig. 5. Post-operative X-rays of the transfixation of the knee joint with external fixator

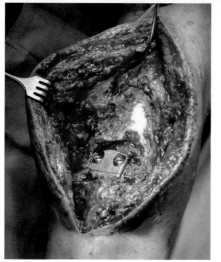

Fig. 6. Two staged management: intra-operative sight of the finished knee arthrodesis with a modular nail system with coupling module

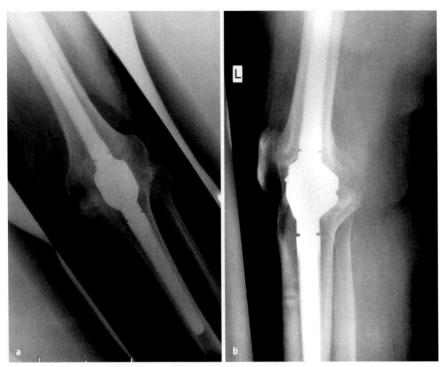

Fig. 7a, b. Post-operative X-rays of the knee arthrodesis with the modular nail system with coupling module showing correct axis and a closed gap by bone compression

Post-operative care was similar for all patients. External splints or casts were not used. All patients started mobilization using two crutches and half weight-bearing on day two. Average length of complete hospital stay was 48 days (range, 17–118 days). Hospital stay after arthrodesis averaged 12 days. No patient developed pseudo-arthrosis, normal bone healing and fixed bony fusion was seen within eight weeks postoperatively. At this time all patients were allowed full weight-bearing without crutches.

An 84 years old female patient with a severe infection of knee prosthesis with a multi-resistant *S. aureus* despite immediate prosthesis removal, temporary stabilization with an external fixator developed a necrotizing fasciitis around the knee. Renal and hepatic insufficiency along with bad general conditions forced us within two days to the above knee amputation. The patient died after 4 months.

Clinical results are shown in Table 1.

Table 1. Clinical results of nine knee arthrodeses and one case of a knee amputation after infect-defect-situations due to different causes in a 30-month period.

Pt.	Sex	Age	Diagnosis	Pathogen/s	N° of previous operations	N° of red blood cell concentrates (300 ml)	Complications	Hospital stay (days)	Walking with crutches at dismissal
1	F	78	Infected knee prosthesis	S.aureus	5	9	none	41	yes
2	M	81	Infected patellar osteosynthesis with severe soft tissue defect	Mainly S. aureus and mixed flora with Gram-positive and Gram-negative cocci	7	4	none	46	no
3	M	32	Osteoarthritis and osteomyelitis	S. aureus	7	4	none	37	yes
4	M	39	Post-traumatic osteoarthritis	S. aureus	4	---	none	19	yes
5	F	79	Infected knee prothesis after peri-prosthetic femoral fracture	Mainly S. aureus and mixed flora with Gram-positive and Gram-negative cocci	9	16	Delayed infection with multi-resistant S. aureus	72	yes
6	M	51	Severe soft tissue defect above knee area	Mainly mixed flora with Gram-positive and Gram-negative cocci	16	25	Schizophrenia leading to delayed mobilization and remittance to psychiatric rehab	67	yes
7	M	45	Post-traumatic osteoarthritis	S.aureus	3	---	none	17	yes
8	M	29	Osteoarthritis and osteomyelitis	S. aureus	8	---	none	34	yes
9	M	62	Osteoarthritis after arthroscopy	S. aureus and Gram-negative cocci	5	4	none	29	yes
10	F	84	Infected knee prothesis	Multi-resistant S. aureus and mixed flora with Gram-positive cocci	2	8	Above knee amputation on day 2, long period on ICU	118	no
Mean		58			6.6	7		48	

Conclusion

In the described small series knee arthrodesis was the therapeutic option in severe different infect-defect situations of the knee joint. Respecting the patient request for a safe and convenient method in all the cases the trans-articular intramedullary fixation with a modular nail system and a coupling module was used. This method of knee arthrodesis allows to obtain a stable and painless knee in a short healing time in case of a damaged knee joint that is not amenable to other reconstructive measures.

Arthrodesis resection arthroplasty is in all other cases of a severe infection the method of choice to end serial surgery. Above knee amputation is limited to absolute refractory cases or a life-threatening situation [2, 3, 9, 10].

References

1. Berbari EF, Hanssen AD, Duffy MC et al (1992) Risk factors for prosthetic joint infections: case control study. Clin Infect Dis 27(5):1247–1254
2. Damron TA, McBeath AA (1995) Arthrodesis following failed total knee: comprehensive review and metaanalysis of recent literature. Orthopedics 18(4):361–368
3. Ellingsen DE, Rand JA (1994) Intramedullary arthrodesis of the knee after failed total knee arthroplasty. J Bone Joint Surg (Am) 76(6):870–877
4. Garvin KL, Hanssen AD (1995) Infection after total hip replacement Past, present and future. J Bone J Surg (Am) 77(10):1576–1588
5. Hansis M, Meeder PJ, Weller S (1984) Die Behandlung des Kniegelenkempyems Zentralbl Chir 109(22):1431–1436
6. König DP, Randerath O, Hackenbroch MH (1999) Nosokomiale Infektionen mit Methicilin-resistenten Staphylococcus aureus (MRSA) und -epidermidis (MRSE) Stämmen Unfallchirurg 102(4):324–328
7. Nelson CL, Evans RP, Blaha JD et al (1993) A comparison of gentamicin-impregnated polymethylmethacrylate bead implantation to conventional parenteral antibiotic therapy in infected total hip and knee arthroplasty. Clin Orthop Relat Res (295):96–101
8. Ryan MJ, Kavanagh R, Wall PG, Hazleman BL (1997) Bacterial joint infections in England and Wales: analysis of bacterial isolates over a four year period. Br J Rheumatol 36(3): 370–373
9. Vlasak R, Gearen PF, Petty W (1995) Knee arthrodesis in the treatment of failed total knee replacement. Clin Orthop Relat Res (321):138–144
10. Wilson MG, Kelley K, Thornhill TS (1990) Infection as a complication of total knee-replacement arthroplasty: Risk factors and treatment in sixty-seven cases. J Bone Joint Surg (Am) 72(6):878–883

37 Salvage Procedures in Exposed Septic Knee Prothesis

L. Vaienti, A.O. Menozzi, J. Lonigro, A. Di Matteo, D. Zilio

Unit of Plastic & Reconstructive Surgery, Policlinico S. Donato, University of Milan, Italy

Introduction

Many factors are responsible and predispose to infection and failed wound healing in knee arthroplasty. During the preoperative phase presence of scars around the knee for previous menisectomy or synovectomy [20], diabetes, tabagism, autoimmune diseases, steroid therapy may lead to complicated wound healing. Moreover patients with rheumatoid disorders are more prone to deep sepsis [2]. During the operative phase wrong operation planning and surgical technique (including the prosthesis type selection; e.g. constrained prosthesis is a predisposing factor in comparison with unconstrained prosthesis) [17, 19] or wrong skin incisions may cause infection and failed wound healing [20]. Because of many conditions, the incidence of complications reported in knee arthroplasty is very high, if compared with hip arthroplasty [20]. The main complications of knee arthroplasty are deep venous thrombosis [20, 22, 24], pulmonary embolism [24], tibial loosening [31], supracondylar fractures of the femur [6], peroneal nerve injury [28], wound failure [16] and deep infection [2, 12]. From a reconstructive point of view, the worse consequence is wound breakdown with exposed prosthesis.

Deep infection and failed wound healing are the main causes of exposed prosthesis, making sometimes critical the patient management. The laminar flow systems in the operative theater should not be underestimated too: laminar flow systems was thought to reduce intraoperative concentration of airborne bacteria and wound contamination. Unfortunately some authors noticed an increased rate of sepsis in total knee arthroplasty, while in total hip arthroplasty a sensible improvement was observed. Their conclusion was that personnel positioning around the operating table was a determinant factor of the rate of sepsis [21]. During the post-operative phase late mobilization and continuous passive motion, no antibiotic prophylaxis and haematoma are risk factors. Several reconstructive procedures, depending on the the wound coverage size and shape, are described to manage complex wounds around the knee with preservation of the joint and extremity: local skin flaps, local traditional fasciocutaneous flaps, muscle flaps (pedicled or free) and neurocutaneous flaps 10]. For superficial damage local skin flaps should be considered, but if deep structures are exposed and a bacterial agent is identified the result could be partial or total flap loss. Traditional local fasciocutaneous flaps, as described by Ponten [26], have been described for coverage of even large, but superficial skin loss around the knee These flaps can be raised in different orientations as the parafascials vessels are supplied by a collateral vascular network around the knee, but they can be effective only if the underneath joint capsule is intact. In addition, local fasciocutaneous flaps do not have enough freedom for transfer because the pedicle is short and wide, hence their indication is limited. The development of deep wound infection is also very dangerous. This is the most devastating complication resulting in pain, discharge and loss of function. The diagnosis, without wound breakdown can be difficult, because pain, swelling, knee effusion and wound inflammation often occur after arthroplasty. The main pathogens are *Staphylococcus aureus* and *Staphylococcus epidermidis*. Sometimes fungal infections or *Pseudomonas aeruginosa* (infection or superinfection) are present.

Three main portals of entry for infection have been suggested [2]:

- **intra-operative contamination** due to skin commensals (*S. epidermidis*) or pathogens present in the atmosphere of the operating site (principally *Micrococcus* spp. and *Diphteroids*). In both cases, they can survive, in the wound, hidden in the prosthetic material despite a correct antibiotic prophylaxis [1, 2, 18, 20];
- **post-operative inoculation** of the joint by puncture wound or dehiscence of the operative wound [2];
- **hematogenous seeding** related to distant foci of infection [2, 3]. Urinary tract and gastrointestinal infections, but also dental procedures, are involved [2, 18];

Some Authors even recognized an association between the pathogens and the prosthetic material: *S. aureus* and metallic prosthesis, *S. epidermidis* and polyethylene [11].

A reliable method for soft-tissue coverage around the knee is represented by muscle flaps. These flaps offer several advantages providing obliteration of the dead space around the prosthesis and enhancing humoral defense by improving vascularity, draining collections and effusions [33].

Muscle flaps can take the form of local flaps or free vascularized flaps. Local muscle flaps (e.g. gastrocnemius muscle, soleus muscle) have the important advantage over free flaps of requiring shorter operative, assuring minimal donor site morbidity, furthermore microsurgery is not necessary and post-operative care is simple. However free flaps are more amenable to coverage of massive defects than pedicled muscle flaps [33]. The gastrocnemius muscle has been a mainstay for soft tissue coverage of the knee and the upper tibia: it is safe, versatile and easy to conform to different size and shape defect, moreover sometimes it may be unable to provide coverage for large defects around the knee, particularly the supra-patellar region [29].

Perforator flaps represent an alternative useful method for reconstruction of the knee, resulting in excellent aesthetic and functional results, but their dissection is tedious and tiring for surgeons, especially if untrained, as they require extremely long and proper (atraumatic) pedicle dissection technique. In addition a reliable perforator vessel could not be found during dissection in patient with considerable anatomical variations. But a non-underestimable drawback is the presence of scars in the lower third of the leg and knee.

As reported in literature, and tested in our clinical experience, neurocutaneous pedicled flaps, as described by Masquelet [23], could be a valuable alternative for soft tissue coverage around the knee providing different advantages over gastrocnemius muscle flap: greater flexibility of size and shape, longer arc of rotation, provision of skin with protective sensation, less swelling at recipient site and avoidance of a flap twitch [29].

Our surgical experience in salvaging exposed knee prosthesis using island sural neurocutaneous flaps is described.

Materials and Methods

The series refers to 15 patients (6 M, 9 F). Among these, 4 patients had diabetes, 2 immunologic diseases and 2 were under corticosteroid treatment.

In all cases cultures were positive. The detected pathogens were *S. aureus* and *P. aeruginosa*. Teicoplanin, amikacin and cephalosporins were administered.

All patients had post-surgical antithrombotic prophylaxis (LMWH). Subsequently they underwent passive motion (Kinetec 0° – 30°) for two weeks, followed by active rehabilitation.

In all cases, after surgical debridement, an island fasciocutaneous flap based on the vascular network accompanying the sural nerve was used for soft tissue coverage. The flap is raised with a midline axis, the distal margin is incised through the deep fascia and the midline neurovascular pedicle identified. The sural nerve and accompanying vessels are tied up and cut, and the deep fascia is included elevating the flap from distal to proximal, the flap is then transposed and inserted in the recipient site.

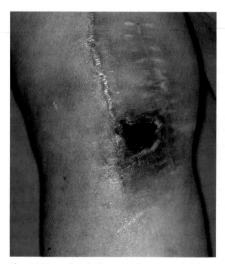 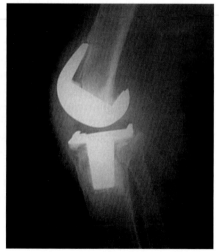

Fig. 1. View of right knee with a necrotic tissue of 3.5 × 3 cm localized in the inferior part of normal tissue between two vertical scars

Fig. 2. X-ray immmage of the knee prosthesis

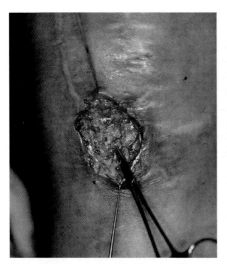

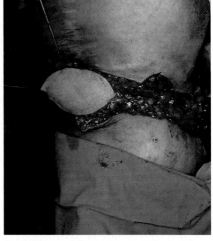

Fig. 3. Right knee after debridement. The knee prosthesis is showed by the surgical instrument

Fig. 4. The sural fasciocutaneous is turned from the back to the anterior side of the knee to reconstructing the skin wound

Fig. 5. The post-operative result after 11 months

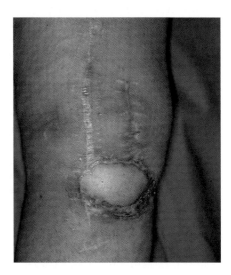

Results

At a mean follow-up of 18 months all flaps survived.

Neither venous congestion, nor suffering of the edges of the incision intended for raising the flap were observed.

In two cases an hematoma occurred two weeks after surgical procedure due to heparin. Both cases healed with primary closure, after surgical evacuation.

One case of recurrence, with formation of a small fistula, occurred in a patient with RA treated with steroids.

Discussion

Knee prosthesis exposure is due to wound dehiscence, skin necrosis, marginal wound necrosis, skin steeping, sinus tract formation and hematoma [16], but early tissue breakdown with exposure of the prosthesis is a severe, but rare, complication following knee arthroplasty [7]. Moreover total knee arthroplasty requires major handling and extensive undermining of the soft tissues, followed by early post-operative mobilization: this may result in a damage to the skin. Skin breakdown generally occurs in the region of the patella and the tibia, also because the soft tissues are poorly vascularized [8]. In this area, the position of the prosthesis just under the skin may result in exposure [5].

Other risk factors are diabetes, previous local radiotherapy, inflammatory rheumatic diseases, prior scars [5]. Infection increases if the damage to the skin is not closed. Different studies suggest that revision surgery, rheumatoid arthritis, surgery with conflicting skin incision and post-operative superficial wound infection are all predisposing factors [15]. Insall and Johnson's studies confirm the association of deep infection with the use of constrained prosthesis [15, 19]. Design modifications have greatly reduced the incidence of problems associated with early constrained and semi-constrained total knee prosthesis. Nonetheless, post-operative infections continue to be a serious problem [4]. The management of the infected knee prostheses is often obscure. Attention should therefore be focused on prophylactic measures directed towards gentle handling of the periarticular soft tissues. The most effective and practical way to reduce the risk of deep infection is by achieving first wound healing. For this reason the parapatellar incision is ideal for the knee prosthesis insertion as it is parallel to the skin cleavage lines of the knee and subjected to considerably minor wound tension during knee flexion. Long-term antibiotic treatment suppresses symptoms and reduce discharge, but usually does not eradicate deep infection in a cemented prosthesis, with persisting wasting of bone stock, pain and functional disability. Long-term antibiotic suppression is generally limited to patients which cannot undergo surgical intervention and in patients with a limited life expectancy [19]. On the contrary, antibiotic prophylaxis is crucial for infection prevention, and establishes the finest pre-operative and post-operative conditions for first wound healing. Incorporation of antibiotics, usually gentamicin, into the methyl-methacrylate cement is used as a prophylactic means against infection [5]. In this way antibiotics can be effective against organisms resistant to the levels reached by parenteral administration because of their extremely elevated local concentration [5]. Studies reported in literature suggest that in most cases careful, an early and adequate surgical management can be an effective choice for salvaging an exposed knee prosthesis [4].

Surgical management must be planned to achieve a painless knee. Many different surgical techniques can be performed for the management of an exposed prosthesis: arthrodesis, surgical debridement without prosthetic removal [4], spacer positioning, reimplantation of a new prosthesis [4, 5] and, as last option, amputation. Following arthrodesis, fusion is reachable in a small proportion of cases as suggested by Hagemann et al [13]. More recent studies [31] confirm that the technique of immobilization with Charnley compression clamps is inadequate for arthrodesis following infection. A two-stage intramedullary nail, combined with additional bone grafting, appears to be the most effective technique in order to obtain fusion [25, 32, 34]. Eventually Bigliani suggested the use of pulsing electromagnetic fields to increase fusion rate [2].

Immediate exchange prosthesis following radical debridement has proven to give unpredictable results. A radical debridement, including prosthetic components and cement removal as the first stage of a two-stage reimplantation arthroplasty, appears to be more promising [2, 3, 11, 27]. Several authors' opinion is that a two-week interval between removal of the prosthesis and replacement is inadequate [2, 4, 19, 27]. In most cases when the prosthesis is replaced after six weeks, painless walking is achievable [2, 19]. Usually antibiotic-impregnated methyl-methacrylate beads are positioned in the knee cavity after debridement and prosthetic components removal till the time of reimplantation [4]. Antibiotic selection is based on organisms sensitivity and phlogosis indexes. During the period following removal of the prosthesis, length is maintained with an external fixation-device or a long-leg cast [4] or a spacer. Generally antibiotic impregnated cement is used for the reimplantation; in well fixed uncemented knee replacement good results were also reported in a small series just with drainage and antibiotics [7]. In spite of positive results of revision surgery, the prospect of amputation or even death remain a possibility as suggested by Hood and Insall [14], and Grogan [12]. It seems that in most cases early coverage of the soft tissue defect with a flap can avoid and neutralize exposure and infection [5]. According to our surgical experience the fascioneurocutaneous sural flap is a good and useful flap for the salvage of knee prosthetic exposure, offering several distinct advantages: it is capable of covering large defects; it can be tailored to the defect size and shape, providing less swelling at the recipient site and outlined anywhere on the suprafascial course of the nerve; it provides skin with protective sensation as reported by Masquelet [23]. Other advantages of this flap include ease of re-elevation from the recipient site for subsequent orthopedic procedures and the absence of a flap twitch at the recipient site; it is possible to raise either a proximally or distally based pedicle flap [5]. The most significant drawback of this flap is the cosmetic deformity at the donor site, moreover the sural nerve is divided and an area of sensory loss in the lateral aspect of the foot is produced, eventually a risk of neuroma formation is reported [2, 29]. In our patients we have not observed any the above described complications. In our opinion, the island neurofasciocutaneous sural flap represents a reasonable reconstructive alternative for providing fine and useful soft tissue for covering skin defects around the knee.

References

1. Alexakis PG, Feldon PG, Wellisch M et al (976) Airborne bacterial contamination of operative wounds West J Med 124(5):361–369
2. Bigliani LU, Rosenwasser MP, Caulo N et al (1983) The use of pulsing electromagnetic fields to achieve arthrodesis of the knee following failed total knee arthroplasty. A preliminary report. J Bone Joint Surg (Am) 65(4):480–485
3. Blomgren G, Lindgren U (1981) Late hematogenous infection in total joint replacement: Studies of gentamicin and bone cement in the rabbit. Clin Orthop Relat Res (155):244–248
4. Borden LS, Gearen PF (1987) Infected total knee arthroplasty. A protocol for management. J Arthroplasty 2(1):27–36
5. Casanova D, Hulard O, Zalta R et al (2001) Management of wounds of exposed or infected knee prostheses. Scand J Plast Reconstr Surg Hand Surg 35(1):71–77

6. Delport PH, Van Audekercke R, Martens M et al (1984) Conservative treatment of ipsilateral supracondylar femoral fracture after total knee arthroplasty. J Trauma 24(9):846–849
7. Freeman MA, Sudlow RA, Casewell MW et al (1985) The management of infected total knee replacements. J Bone Joint Surg (Br) 67(5):764–768
8. Gerwin M, Rothaus KO, Windsor RE et al (1993) Gastrocnemius muscle flap coverage of exposed or infected knee prostheses. Clin Orthop Relat Res (286):64–70
9. Goodfellow JW, O'Connor J (1986) Clinical results of the Oxford knee. Clin Orthop Relat Res (205):21–42
10. Gravvanis AI, Tsoutsos DA, Karakitsos D (2006) Application of the pedicled anterolateral thigh flap to defects from the pelvis to the knee. Microsurgery 26(6):432–438
11. Gristina AG (1987) Biomaterial-Centered infection: microbial adhesion versus tissue integration. Science 237(4822):1588–1595
12. Grogan TJ, Dorey F, Rollins J et al (1986) Deep sepsis following total knee arthroplasty. Ten-year experience at the University of California at Los Angeles Medical Center. J Bone Joint Surg (Am) 68(2):226–234
13. Hagemann, WF, Woods GW, Tullos HS (1978) Arthrodesis in failed total knee replacement. J Bone Joint Surg (Am) 60(6):790–794
14. Hood RW, Insall JN (1983) Infected total knee joint replacement arthroplasties. In; Surgery of the musculo-skeletal system. Eds; McCollister, Evarts. Churchill Livingstone Edimburgh, 1983; 4:173–188
15. Insall J, Ranawat CS, Scott WN et al (2001) Total condylar knee replacement: preliminary report. 1976. Clin Orthop Relat Res (388):3–6
16. Insall JN, Lachiewicz PF, Burstein AH (1982) The posterior stabilised condylar prosthesis. A modification of the total condylar design. J Bone Joint Surg (Am) 64(9):1317–1323
17. Insall JN, Ranawat CS, Aglietti P et al (1976) A comparison of four models of total knee-replacement prosthesis. J Bone Joint Surg (Am) 58(6):754–765
18. Irvine R, Johnson BL, Jr, Amstutz HC (1974) The relationship of genitourinary tract procedures and deep sepsis after total hip replacement. Surg Gynecol Obstet 139(5):701–706
19. Johnson D, Bannister GC (1986) The outcome of infected arthroplasty of the knee. J Bone Joint Surg (Br) 68(2):289–292
20. Johnson DP (1993) Infection after knee arthroplasty: the incidence of infection following knee arthroplasty. Acta Orthop Scand Suppl 252:5
21. Lidwell OM, Lowbury EJL, Whyte W et al (1983) Ventilation in operating rooms. Br Med J(Clin Res Ed) 286(6372):1214–1215
22. Lynch AF, Bourne RB, Rorabeck CH et al (1988) Deep vein thrombosis and continuous passive motion after total knee arthroplasty. J Bone Joint Surg (Am) 70(1):11–14
23. Masquelet AC, Romana MC, Wolf G (1992) Skin island flaps supplied by the vascular axis of the sensitive superficial nerves: anatomic study and clinical experience in the leg. Plast Reconstr Surg 89(6):1115–1121
24. McKenna R, Bachmann F, Kausal SP et al (1976) Thromboembolic disease in patients undergoing total knee replacement. J Bone Joint Surg (Am) 58(7):928–932
25. Petty W (1999) Knee arthrodesis in the treatment of failed total knee replacement. Med Gen Med 1(1) [formerly published in Medscape Orthopedics and Sports Medicine Journal 1998 2(3)]
26. Ponten B The fasciocutaneous flap: its use in soft tissue defects of the lower leg. Br J Plast Surg. 1981 Apr;34(2):215–220
27. Rand JA, Bryan RS (1983) Reimplantation for the salvage of an infected total knee arthroplasty. J Bone Joint Surg (Am) 65(8):1081–1086
28. Rose HA, Hood RW, Otis JC et al (1982) Peroneal nerve palsy following total knee arthroplasty; A review of the Hospital for Special Surgery experience. J Bone Joint Surg (Am) 64(3):347–351
29. Shaw AD, Ghosh SJ, Quaba AA (1998) The island posterior calf fasciocutaneous flap: an alternative to the gastrocnemius muscle for cover of knee and tibial defects. Plast Reconstr Surg 101(6):1529–1536
30. Shim JS, Kim HH (2006) A novel reconstruction technique for the knee and upper one third of lower leg. J Plast Reconstr Aesthet Surg 59(9):919–26; discussion 927
31. Stone MH, Wilkinson R, Stother JG (1989). Some factors affecting the strength of the cement metal interface. J Bone Joint Surg (Br) 71(2):217–221

32. Walker RH, Schurman DJ (1984) Management of infected total knee arthroplasties. Clin Orthop Relat Res (186):81–89
33. Whiteside LA (1997) Surgical exposure in revision total knee arthroplasty. Instr Course Lect (46):221–225
34. Wiedel JD (2002) Salvage of infected total knee fusion: the last option. Clin Orthop Relat Res (404):139–142.

Novel Applications and Perspectives

The Management of the Shoulder Prosthesis Infection

L.A. Crosby

Department of Orthopaedic Surgery, Wright State University Boonshoft School of Medicine, Dayton, Ohio, USA

Historical Perspective

Infection following total shoulder arthroplasty, although uncommon, can be a devastating complication. The established incidence ranges from 0 % to 3.9 % [1]. Patients commonly present with pain; many show radiographic evidence of loosening. Unlike management of total knee and hip arthroplasty, management of these infections has limited description in the literature. Treatment options include: suppressive antibiotics, combined joint debridement and antibiotic therapy, resection arthroplasty, primary exchange arthroplasty, and two-stage reimplantation [4].

Reports dedicated to infection following shoulder arthroplasty are limited. Recently, Sperling, et al [2]. reported their results of 32 patients diagnosed with deep shoulder periprosthetic infections. The highest rates of recurrent infection were seen in those with debridement and retention of the components (50 %), and in those with a one-stage revision (50 %). Six patients who underwent prosthesis removal and debridement with subsequent two-stage reimplantation developed no recurrent infection. Their conclusion was that a two-stage reimplantation offered the best chance at a satisfactory outcome.

Mileti et al [3] reported the results of four resection arthroplasties who were reimplanted at a mean of 7.4 years and reported no recurrent infection. Two patients each reported satisfactory and unsatisfactory outcomes. Their conclusion was that while resection arthroplasty yielded a low risk of infection, reimplantation following resection arthroplasty was especially challenging due to the potential for significant bone and soft tissue deficits.

Two-stage revision shoulder arthroplasty with the use of an antibiotic spacer has also been addressed in the literature [4, 5]. Recently, Loebenberg and Zuckerman [6] described an articulating interval spacer as their treatment both to address the infection and to maintain satisfactory range of motion until reimplantation. Their patient suffered limited pain and had excellent range of motion three months after the first revision.

The purpose of the present article is to describe a technique for an articulating shoulder hemiarthroplasty with antibiotic impregnated cement for treatment of deep shoulder infection following arthroplasty and the early results of this treatment regimen.

Indications/Contraindications

Acute and chronic infection of the postoperative shoulder arthroplasty, whether it be a total shoulder arthroplasty or hemiarthroplasty, are primary indications for removal of implants with insertion of an antibiotic coated spacer. Included are primary shoulder sepsis with humeral head involvement and osteomyelitis as an indication [5].

Preoperative Management

A thorough history and physical examination is obtained in all patients. Preoperative physical examination including range of motion and wound status are documented. A thorough neurovascular examination is completed and documented as well. Preoperative laboratory studies include a complete blood count, basic metabolic profile, an erythrocyte sedimentation rate and C-reactive protein.

Under sterile conditions in the office setting, arthrocentesis of the shoulder is performed. The fluid is sent for standard laboratory evaluation including cell count, Gram stain, and aerobic and anaerobic cultures. If the studies indicate infection is present, the patient is then admitted to the hospital and prepared for surgery. Antimicrobial therapy is delayed until intraoperative cultures and biopsies have been obtained. Infectious Disease consultation is highly recommended.

Standard radiographs are made in the office. These include: 1. anteroposterior radiograph in the scapular plane; 2. axillary view; and 3. lateral radiograph of the scapula. The radiographs are evaluated for any evidence of loosening or lucency. If the diagnosis is not obvious from the patient presentation, the work-up may require nuclear medicine studies.

Technique

Patient Positioning

Place the patient in the modified beach chair position with the head of the bed elevated 30–45 degrees after general anesthesia has been administered. The patient should be positioned to enable hyperextension of the extremity off the side of the table.

Approach

An extended deltopectoral approach is undertaken, typically through the patient's previous skin incision. Care is taken to avoid detachment of the proximal deltoid origin. If the rotator cuff is intact, then standard take down of the subscapularis tendon is required. Intraoperative fluid and tissue cultures are taken. A first generation cephalosporin is administered after the intraoperative cultures have been taken.

Removal of Components

The humeral head is removed per manufacturer protocol. The glenoid, while often loose secondary to the infection, is then removed with care taken to preserve as much glenoid bone stock as possible. If the prosthesis was cemented, all remnants are thoroughly debrided.

Removal of the humeral component is then completed. Again, secondary to infection, the component typically is loosened to the point that standard revision/removal instrumentation is sufficient.

Removal of Humeral Cement

Removal of cement from the humerus is completed with the aid of arthroplasty revision instrumentation. Ultrasonic cement removal equipment aids in removal of the distal cement without the need for corticotomy. If needed, a corticotomy is performed to adequately remove all cement from the humeral canal.

Irrigation and Debridement

A thorough irrigation and debridement is then completed with nine liters of pulsatile lavage. The entire shoulder cavity is explored to ensure no loculated fluid collections are present. A biopsy of the greater tuberosity is then sent for frozen section to evaluate for the presence of osteomyelitis.

Humeral Stem Preparation and Insertion

The antibiotic cement is prepared by adding one gram of vancomycin powder to Palacos® cement after removing an equivalent amount of cement powder. Utilizing the smallest humeral stem available (6 mm × 130 mm), the vancomycin impregnated cement is then mixed and applied to the prosthesis and a humeral head is fashioned. The humeral canal and glenoid cavity are evaluated to ensure that the antibiotic coated prosthesis will easily fit into the available space. The cement is allowed to dry around the prosthesis and the antibiotic coated stem is inserted into the humeral canal. Retroversion is applied as necessary to maintain reduction of the hemiarthroplasty.

The subscapularis is repaired with #5 nonabsorbable monofilament sutures. The deltopectoral interval is closed with prolene sutures to aid in identification of the interval at the time of revision surgery. The wound is then closed over a drain and the arm is placed in a sling and swathe.

Postoperative Management

The patient is maintained in the hospital on intravenous antibiotics until culture results and sensitivities are finalized. Physical therapy is instituted on the first postoperative day and includes passive range of motion of the shoulder and active elbow, wrist and hand exercises. The patient is discharged home when home antibiotic therapy has been finalized. Patients wear the sling for 3–6 weeks postoperatively. Outpatient physical therapy is continued with progression from passive to passive-assist and finally to active motion.

Home antibiotics are continued for four to six weeks postoperatively at the direction of the infectious disease consultant. Upon completion of the antibiotic program, clinical evaluation is undertaken. If the patient is progressing well, the antibiotic spacer may be left in place and the patient continues with their home rehabilitation program.

Materials and Methods

Fourteen consecutive patients referred to the shoulder service with deep shoulder infection following shoulder arthroplasty have been treated with the above protocol at our institution. Seven patients are men and seven are women. The average duration of follow-up was 22 months (range 12–40 months). Ten infections involved right shoulders and four were in the left shoulder.

Results

No patient had evidence of recurrent infection upon repeat irrigation and debridement with exchange of the antibiotic coated hemiarthroplasty. When bone biopsy and intraoperative cultures were negative at the second procedure, the patient was then scheduled for definitive reimplantation.

Nine patients (9/14) were converted to standard total shoulder arthroplasty, hemiarthroplasty, or reverse ball and socket prostheses. The remaining five patients (5/14) were satisfied with their functional level with the antibiotic coated hemiarthroplasty and wanted no further surgery. Their visual analog pain scale decreased from 9 to 2 postoperatively and their ASES score improved from 18 to 72. All repeat cultures and biopsies were negative for infection.

Complications

Potential complications mirror those associated with primary and revision shoulder arthroplasty, and include instability, rotator cuff tear, glenoid component loosening, intraoperative fracture, nerve injury and humeral component loosening [7, 8].

Possible Concerns, Future of the Technique

The cost of the prosthesis is a possible concern. Utilizing a prosthesis is meant to improve function and range of motion without sacrificing strength of the prosthesis. Our experience with fracture of isolated cement spacers led us to utilize a small diameter (6 mm × 130 mm) prosthesis as a solid core. Possible alternatives include several Kirschner wires within a cement spacer to provide some core strength. Antibiotic cement prostheses are being commercially manufactured and have been recently approved by the FDA (InterSpace Shoulder/Spacer-S – Exactech, Gainesville, FL, USA). The benefit of these prostheses would be a more concentrated elution of the impregnated antibiotic.

As no osteomyelitis was found on bone biopsy and no infection was present on repeat biopsy and culture at the time of exchange arthroplasty, we now recommend only one interval vancomycin coated hemiarthroplasty prior to definitive reimplantation.

References

1. Cofield RH, Edgerton BC (1990) Total Shoulder Arthroplasty: complications and revision surgery. Instr Course Lect (39):449–462
2. Sperling JW, Kozak TK, Hanssen AD et al (2001) Infection after shoulder arthroplasty. Clin Orthop Relat Res (382):206–216
3. Mileti , Sperling JW, Cofield RH (2004) Reimplantation of a shoulder arthroplasty after a previous infected arthroplasty. J Shoulder Elbow Surg 13(5):528–531
4. Ramsey ML, Fenlin JM Jr (1996) Use of an antibiotic-impregnated bone cement block in the revision of an infected shoulder arthroplasty. J Shoulder Elbow Surg 5(6):479–482
5. Seitz WH Jr, Damacen H (2002) Staged exchange arthroplasty for shoulder sepsis. J Arthroplasty 17(Suppl):36–40
6. Loebenberg MI, Zuckerman JD (2004) An articulating interval spacer in the treatment of an infected total shoulder arthroplasty. J Shoulder Elbow Surg 13(4):476–478
7. Wirth MA, Rockwood CA Jr (1994) Complications of shoulder arthroplasty. Clin Orthop Relat Res (307):47–69
8. Crosby LA Ed. *Complications in* Total Shoulder Arthroplasty. American Academy of Orthopaedic Surgeons: Chicago. 2000:39–46

39 Shoulder Spacer as a Definitive Solution?

A. Giraldi, A. Pellegrini, C. Romanò, E. Meani

Department for Treatment of Osteoarticular Septic Complications (COS) –
Director: Prof. Enzo Meani
Operative Unit for Septic Prosthesis – Responsible: Prof. Carlo L. Romanò
"G. Pini" Orthopaedic Institute, Milan, Italy

Introduction

Infection is a rare but severe complication in prosthetic surgery of the shoulder. Data collected from the literature reveals an incidence of about 0.5 % (0 – 3.95 % range) for non-cemented prostheses and about 2.9 % (0 – 15.4 % range) for cemented prostheses [15]. Due to the low statistical incidence and the low total number of cases, compared to the more common hip and knee prostheses, this experience is limited to few cases and few surgeons. We can, however, forecast that these cases, and possibly the incidence, will increase in future as the number of shoulder arthroplasties is increasing both for arthritis of the glenohumeral joint as well as proximal humeral fractures.

Review of the Literature

In 1996, Ramsey et al. [13] referred to a case treated with a two-stage revision inserting an antibiotic-loaded acrylic cement spacer which was prepared in the operating room. Two months later a second operation was performed with removal of the spacer, further debridement and implantation of a new, definitive prosthesis. 29 months after the second operation restoration of function was observed with no sign of infection. In 1997, Kozak et al. [10] reported 33 patients treated with a shoulder prosthesis infection. Five out of nine patients were treated with debridement or one-stage revision, and later required prosthesis removal ("resection arthroplasty"). In 2000, Sperling et al. [19] published data on 2,512 shoulder prostheses implanted at the Mayo Clinic between 1972 and 1994. Patients with a prosthetic infection were divided into groups on the basis of the treatment received. Group I (20 patients, 21 shoulders) were treated with prosthesis removal, soft tissue debridement and resection arthroplasty. Six patients had reoccurrence of infection. Group II (6 patients) was treated with debridement alone without removal of the implant. Three patients were had reoccurrence of their infections. Group III (2 patients) were treated with removal of the implant and a one-stage reimplantation. After nine months, one patient had reoccurrence of the infection and required resection arthroplasty. In Group IV, three patients were treated with two-stage reimplant. No patient had an infection relapse after an average follow up of 4.8 years (2.2 – 8.9 % range) with good functional results. In 2002, Seitz et al. [16] reported their experience with eight cases of infection of prostheses treated with two-stage revision. After an average follow up of 4.8 years all patients were free from infection and had no pain. The functional evaluation using the Univ. of Pennsylvania Shoulder Score revealed an average score of 68.4/100 for subjective evaluations and 63/100 for objective evaluation. In 2004, Ince et al. [7] referred to their experience with 16 consecutive patients, treated with one-stage revision and an average follow up of 5.8 years. Four patients were lost to follow up, nine patients are free from infection and three required further surgery secondary to complications that cannot be contributed to infection. According to Constant-Murley, the functional evaluation was 33.6/100 while for U.C.L.A. the score was 18.3/35. Proubasta et al. [12] report a case of sepsis that occurred two years after the implant of a hemiarthroplasty secondary to four-part fracture. The patient, treated with a two-stage revision, was satisfied with the pain relief and joint function. The patient refused further treatment and has the antibiotic spacer in place. After five years, the clinical and radiological evaluation has not changed. Coste et al [2] reported on a multi-center study of 2342 shoulder prostheses with 42 patients (49 shoulders) treated for infection of the prosthesis. In this report, the three patients treated with a one-stage revision were free of infection and the 10 patients treated with a two-stage revision, the infection reoccurred in four patients out of ten.

Classification

Sperling et al. [19] classified infections of shoulder prosthesis into acute (< 3 months), subacute (3 months – 1 year) and late (> 1 year). For hip and knee arthroplasty infections, Insall et al. have been subdivided in a similar fashion [5, 6, 8]. On the basis the literature that was reviewed and our personal experience, we agree to classify shoulder prosthetic infections into early (< 4 months), delayed (4 – 12 months) and late (> 12 months).

Bacteriology

Staphylococcus aureus is the most common bacteria causing prosthetic infections of the shoulder [9, 11, 12, 13, 16, 19], followed by *Staphylococcus epidermidis* and *Propionibacterium* bacteria [17]. All the authors report rare cases in which it was impossible to identify any bacteria, not only in the pre-operation specimens but also in intra-operation specimens. In order to reduce the impact of false negative results to the minimum, it is necessary to obtain multiple intra-operation specimens. A useful precaution is to send at least a fragment of the cement to the laboratory, membrane from cement bone interface, as well as one or two specimens collected from the joint capsule.

Treatment

Possible treatments for an infected shoulder prosthesis are: suppressive antibiotic therapy, debridement, one-stage or two-stage revision, resection arthroplasty or amputation.

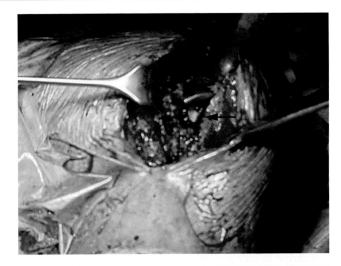

Fig. 1. The arrow indicates the purulent material in the back of the prosthetic head

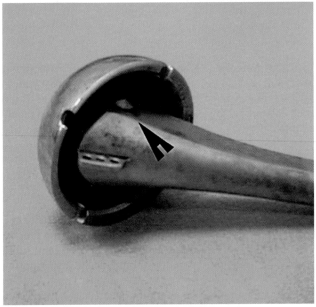

Fig. 2. The arrow indicates purulent material in the blocking screw of the prosthetic head

- Suppressive antibiotic therapy. In the elderly or patients who are at high risk for surgery, a long-term antibiotic therapy can be applied. This must be directed and monitored by the infectious disease specialist.
- Debridement. Removing all non-vital tissues with an aggressive removal of all non-viable tissue and aggressive irrigation of the soft tissue envelope. All the components need to be removed to enable an adequate wash-out and then reimplanted after sterilization in the autoclave or even replaced. Specific sponges of reabsorbable material soaked in slow-release antibiotic (Septocoll) can be left *in situ*.

- Amputation. This is used in very rare cases of local infection with multiresistant bacteria and/or in the event of a more seriously compromise of the soft tissue of the entire extremity.
- Arthrodesis. It is technically difficult to arthrodesis a glenohumoral joint after removal of a prosthesis. Bulk allograft tissue with or without autogenous bone graft is often required.
- Resection Arthroplasty. The British use the term "resection arthroplasty" to indicate the removal of the prosthesis and an accurate wash-out of the soft tissue and the bone. From a functional standpoint, the results are poor
- One-stage and two stage revision. This technique provides a rigorous debridement of soft tissue and an accurate debridement of the bone. The one-stage revision implant is replaced after the initial irrigation and debridement with antibiotic-loaded cement. The two-stage revision places the antibiotic-loaded cement spacer, which is then removed and replaced with a definite prosthesis after a period of intravenous antibiotics and the laboratory parameters have returned to normal. The spacer has a two-fold function: it releases antibiotic locally and it keeps the right tension in the soft tissues, particularly in the deltoid, preventing contractures of the soft tissue. It also enables the execution of passive range of motion exercises that keeps some muscle tone as well as promotes the formation of an articular pseudo-capsule, which is useful during the reconstruction phase. The antibiotic spacer used to be hand-made in the operating room utilizing a metal core (Kirschner, Steinmann, Rush) and coating it with antibiotic-loaded cement and shaping it into a prosthesis (Fig. 3). The cement is pre-loaded with Gentamicin but additional antibiotics can be included, according to the pre-operation culture test, provided that it is heat stable. Pre-formed spacers have recently been made available. These offer the advantage of having a regular shape with a smooth surface that is less destructive to the remaining joint surface (Fig. 4). If possible, it is advisable to have the head 20 %-50 % larger with respect to the removed prosthesis. The spacer is then fixed with antibiotic-loaded cement around as a collar and introduced at an advanced polymerization stage to facilitate its subsequent removal. Remaining parts of the rotator cuff can be sutured around the spacer. In rare cases, the spacer can be used as a final prosthesis (elderly patients or associated pathologies that make subsequent surgery impossible).

Choosing the Definitive Implant

It is generally understood that for shoulder prostheses, soft tissues play a critical role. The rotator cuff ensures not only the prosthesis's mobility but more importantly its stability. Most often, the rotator cuff is seriously damaged or totally absent. It is therefore not possible to be able to use a "normal" prosthesis for the revision. The alternatives were to utilize a prosthesis with a large head, a bipolar prosthesis, or a CTA-modified head prosthetic, as proposed in the past for arthropathy with rotator cuff deficiency [14]. Reverse ball and socket prostheses (semi-constrained) have been recently introduced. The reverse prosthesis is theoretically the ideal solution in these cases to establish stability in the absence of the rotator cuff since only the deltoid is functional. The use of this prosthesis is, however, advised only for low

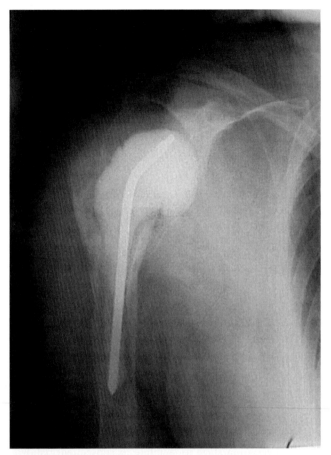

Fig. 3. Intra-operatively made spacer

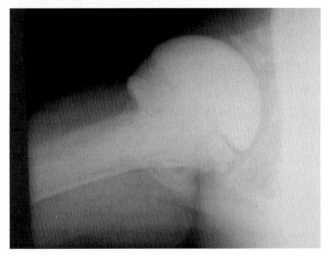

Fig. 4. Preformed spacer (Spacer-S – Tecres Spa, Italy)

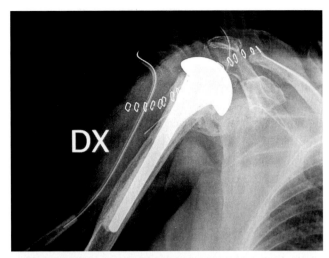

Fig. 5. CTA prosthesis

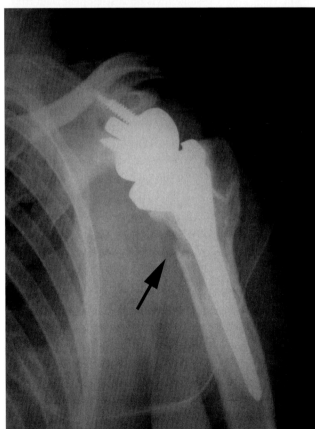

Fig. 6. Delta prosthesis: the arrow indicates the trans-osseous fistula of the previous prosthesis

demand patients. In our recent experience, we used a CTA prosthesis in the presence of some rotator cuff remnants and a reverse prosthesis in the absence of the rotator cuff.

Conclusions

Infections in prosthetic surgery of the shoulder are a rare complication, but they are very serious if not devastating for its function. The experience is limited as few surgeons have much experience. However, the experience gained by infection of the hip and knee prostheses has enabled the establishment of guidelines for diagnosis, antibiotic therapy and surgical treatment which can be generally applied to the shoulder. Very encouraging results have been reached in early infections (with an aggressive debridement of the soft tissue), in late infections (with one-stage and two-stage prosthesis revision surgery). For delayed infections, cases need to be evaluated individually on the basis of clinical, diagnostical, laboratory and radiological tests. The debate on one-stage and two-stage revision is still open. Data from the literature generally highlight a more reliable control of the infection with two-stage revision, with the exception of the work published by Coste et al. [2]. Meticulous debridement and handling of the soft tissue with bacterial identification and appropriate use of antibiotics to eradicate the infection is crucial. Reconstruction with appropriate use of antibiotic cement is then effective.

References

1. Burkhead WZ, Hutton KS (1994) Biologic resurfacing of the glenoid in young patients with post-traumatic arthritis, post reconstruction arthritis or ostearthritis. Tech Orthop 8:163–170
2. Coste JS, Reig S et al (2004) The management of infection in arthroplasty of the shoulder. J Bone Joint Surg (Br) 86(1):65–69
3. De Lima Ramos PA, Martin–Comin J, Bajen MT et al (1996) Simultaneous administration of 99Tcm-HMPAO labelled autologous leukocytes and 111-In labelled non specific polyclonal human immunoglobulin G in bone and joint infections. Nucl Med Commun 17(9):749–757
4. Demirkol MO, Adalet I et al (1997) 99Tc(m)-polyclonal IgG scintigraphy in the detection of infected hip and knee prostheses . Nucl Med Commun 18(6):543–548
5. Drobny TK, Munzinger U (1991) Problems of infected knee prosthesis. Orthopade 20(3):239–249
6. Harle A (1989) Infection management in total hip replacement. Arch Orthop Trauma Surg 108(2):63–71
7. Ince A, Seemann K, Frommelt L et al (2005) One-stage exchange shoulder arthroplasty for periprosthetic infection. J Bone Joint Surg (Br) 87(6):814–818
8. Insall JN, Thompson FM, Brause BD (1983) Two-stage reimplantation for the salvage of infected total knee arthroplasty. J Bone Joint Surg (Am) 65(8):1087–1089
9. Jerosch J, Schneppenheim (2003) Management of infected shoulder replacement. Arch Orthop Trauma Surg 123(5):209–214
10. Kozak TKW, Hanssen AD, Cofield RH (1997) Infected shoulder arthroplasty. J Shoulder Elbow Surg 6(3):177–185
11. Petersen SA, Hawkins RJ (1998) Revision of failed total shoulder arthroplasty. Ortho Clin North Am 29(3):519–533
12. Proubasta IR, Itarte JP, Lamas CG et al (2004) Permanent articulated antibiotic-impregnated cement spacer in septic shoulder arthroplasty. J Orthop Trauma 19(9):666–668

13. Ramsey ML, Fenlin JM (1996) Use of an antibiotic-impregnated bone cement block in the revision of an infected shoulder arthroplasty. J Shoulder Elbow Surg 5(6):479–482
14. Rockwood CA, Matsen FA (1990) The Shoulder, W.B.Saunders , Philadelphia
15. Sawyer JS, Estheray JL (1997) Shoulder infections. In: Warner JP, Iannotti JP,Gerber C (eds) Complex and Revision Problems in Shoulder Surgery, Lippincott-Raven, Philadelphia
16. Seitz WH, Damacen H (2002) Staged exchange arthroplasty for shoulder sepsis. J Arthroplasty 17(4):36–40
17. Settecerri JJ, Pitner MA, Rock MG et al (1999) Infection after rotator cuff repair. J Shoulder Elbow Surg 8(1):1–5
18. Spangehl MJ, Masri BA, O'Connell JX et al (1999) Prospective analysis of preoperative and intraoperative investigations for the diagnosis of infections at the sites of two hundred and two revisions total hip arthroplasties. J Bone Joint Surg (Am) 81(5):672–683
19. Sperling WJ, Kozak TK, Hanssen Ad et al (2000) Infection after shoulder arthroplasty. Clin Orthop Relat Res (382):206–216

The Gentamicin-Vancomycin Spacer: A Pharmacological Study

E. Bᴇʀᴛᴀᴢᴢᴏɴɪ Mɪɴᴇʟʟɪ, A. Bᴇɴɪɴɪ

Department of Medicine and Public Health, Pharmacology Section, University of Verona, Italy

Introduction

Gentamicin-loaded spacers are used in two-stage revision prosthesis to deliver high local antibiotic concentrations for the treatment of prosthetic infections [6, 18]. The concentration of antibiotics released largely exceeds the minimum inhibitory and bactericidal concentration of susceptible bacteria.

With the emergence of resistant bacteria, the addition to bone cement of two antibiotics potentially synergistic has became a frequent practice [9]. The antibiotics utilised in spacer preparation should be carefully selected and should respond to ideal characteristics, such as wide spectrum of activity against the majority of microorganisms, bactericidal activity, good release from cement at inhibitory concentrations for prolonged periods, low interference with mechanical properties of the cement, high biocompatibility, low hypersensitivity and adverse drug reactions, capacity and maintenance of antimicrobial activity at the site of infection. The combination of two or more antibiotics in PMMA cement should consider the inhibitory [11] or synergistic [12] effects on drug release. In addition, when mixed in combination, antibiotics should maintain their antimicrobial activity and possibly exerting a synergistic antimicrobial effect.

The combination of two antibiotics with PMMA may result in modified release kinetics, or in inactivation of drug or in reduced drug release [11, 16]. Consequently, the antimicrobial activity of the mixture may result in an unpredictable effect. The release of vancomycin is modified by the presence of imipenem, and the amount released depends on type of cement [5].

Vancomycin and an aminoglycoside are often combined for their potential synergistic effect in the treatment of severe infections. Vancomycin is a bactericidal glycopeptide antibiotic with a primary spectrum of activity against Gram-positive cocci, such as *Staphylococcus aureus* – including methicillin-resistant –, *Staphylococcus epidermidis, Enterococcus faecalis*, etc.

The elution characteristics of antibiotic-loaded spacers and their antimicrobial activity *in vivo* is poorly known. Few data are available for the comparison of spacers made with a single antibiotic or with antibiotic combinations both *in vitro* and *in vivo* [2, 7, 8, 10, 14]. In two-stage revision of infected THA, spacers are either hand moulded from bone cement, fabricated in a teflon mould, or preformed.

A new spacer has been studied to respond the demand of surgeons and the increasing infection rate due to gentamicin-resistant pathogens. Preformed industrial spacers incorporating gentamicin and vancomycin made with high porosity resin which provides a long-lasting release were tested. This preformed spacer exhibits adequate properties such as good mechanical resistance and compatibility of drugs in PMMA cement. The release of antibiotics *in vitro* from this new spacer is described.

Material and Methods

Spacers prepared with a high porosity PMMA-based resin (HP Cemex, Tecres Spa, Italy) incorporating gentamicin (1.15 g) and vancomycin (1.15 g) were obtained from a mould under aseptic conditions (sterile chamber). The amount of each antibiotic in the fully formed device is equivalent to a final concentration of 1.9 % (3.8 % total antibiotic). Spacers prepared with the same resin incorporating gentamicin alone (1.15 g) were studied for comparison.

The tested spacers were sterile (ethylene oxide).

Spacers' surface area was 122.21 cm^2.

Elution of Antibiotics

As previously described [3], the spacers were immersed in pyrex tubes with 600 ml of phosphate buffer (0.2 M, pH = 8.0, phosphate buffer [PB]) at 37 °C for 30 days. The PB was removed and replaced with the same volume of fresh PB after 24, 48, 72, 240, 480 and 720 hours of immersion. The removed buffer was subdivided into small aliquots and frozen at –24°C. The PB samples from each prosthesis were analysed in the same experiment.

Drugs

Gentamicin and vancomycin (powder, EP grade) were utilised for the preparation of standards. Stock solutions of antibiotic were prepared in PB. Standard concentrations of antibiotics were processed along with samples.

Antibiotic concentrations in eluted samples and standards were processed in parallel using two methods, namely, bioassay and fluorescence polarization immunoassay.

Bioassay

Concentrations of gentamicin and vancomycin were determined using the standard large-plate agar-well diffusion method [4] according to the NCCLS guidelines [15]. Briefly, *Bacillus subtilis* spore suspension ATCC 6633 (final concentration 0.02 %) in Isosensitest Agar (Oxoid Unipath Ltd, Basingstoke, England) was used as the test-microorganism. After overnight incubation at 37°C, the diameters of the inhibition zones were measured. Antibiotics concentrations were determined in relation to the diameters of the inhibition zones yielded by a standard series of known concentrations of antibiotics. All samples and standard concentrations were assayed in duplicate or triplicate.

The assay for gentamicin and vancomycin was linear over a range of 0.6–20.0 mg/L ($R^2 = 0.98$). The assay for the combination was linear over a range of 1.25–40.0 mg/l

($R^2 = 0.99$). The between-day coefficients of variation were 0 % and 2.2 % for the highest and lowest concentrations, respectively, for both drugs alone and in combination.

Fluorescence Polarisation Immunoassay (FPIA)

Concentrations of gentamicin and vancomycin in the PB samples were also determined by FPIA (TDx, Abbott). Vancomycin and gentamicin can be measured separately by the FPIA method even when used in combination. The method was calibrated and applied according to the manufacturer's recommendations (TDx, Abbott). The lowest measurable level of drug concentration was 0.27 mg/L for gentamicin and 2.0 mg/L for vancomycin [1]. All tests were carried out in duplicate.

Results

The release of gentamicin and vancomycin in combination from PMMA spacer is reported in Figure 1.

Gentamicin and vancomycin are released from spacer in high amounts, 31.2 mg and 13.1 mg, respectively, in the first 24 hours. This initial peak is followed by a high and constant release over the next days. The amount of gentamicin released from spacer is higher than that of vancomycin.

Gentamicin and vancomycin in combination 1:1 are released from spacer in different amounts, 63.2 mg and 29.3 mg, respectively, after 30 days of elution. The ratio of gentamicin to vancomycin in the eluate corresponds to 2:1. The elution of gentamicin (mg 31.2) in presence of vancomycin is higher than that recorded for the elution of

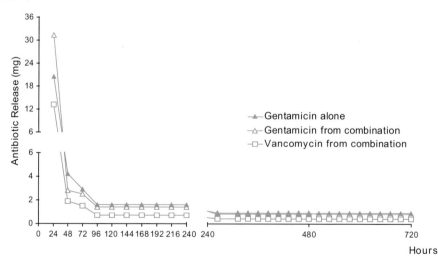

Fig. 1. Release (mg) of Gentamicin and Vancomycin in combination (G+V 1:1) and Gentamicin alone from PMMA hip spacers. Values of antibiotics release from 72 to 720 hours are extrapolated as mg/day of elution. (FPIA method).

Table 1. Release of gentamicin (G, 1.9 %) and vancomycin (V, 1.9 %) in combination (1:1) from HP-PMMA spacer (HP Cemex ®) and gentamicin (1.9 %) alone evaluated with FPIA and microbiological method. Results determined after 24, 240 and 720 hours of elution.

Elution time after	Antibiotics	Methods			
		FPIA			Microbiological
		Gentamicin (mg)	Vancomycin (mg)	Total calculated (mg)	(mg)
24 hours	G alone	20.4	–	20.4	30.6
	G + V	31.2	13.1	44.3	59.3
10 days	G alone	40.1	–	40.1	51.1
	G + V	46.3	21.9	68.2	92.6
30 days	G alone	56.8	–	56.8	68.5
	G + V	63.2	29.3	92.5	117.2

Table 2. *In vitro* activity of gentamicin and vancomycin in combination against multi-resistant clinical isolates. Checker-board method [13].

* Oxacillin Resistant
° Methicillin Resistant
R   = Resistant
I   = Intermediate
FIC ≤ 0.5 Synergism S
FIC = 1 Additivity   A
FIC ≥ 2 Antagonism Ant

Vancomycin + Gentamicin			
Strain	FIC Index	MIC (mg/L)	
		Vanco-mycin	Genta-micin
S. epidermidis (8/28)	1.00 A	2.5	R
S. haemolyticus (8/28)	1.00 A	1.25	R
* S. haemolyticus (82/26)	1.00 A	1.25	R
S. haemolyticus (70/26)	1.00 A	1.25	R
* S. epidermidis (137/25)	0.50 A	2.5	R
° S. hominis (126/26)	1.02 A	1.25	I
S. aureus (3A10)	0.15 S	2.5	I
S. aureus (9A28)	0.48 S	1.25	1.25
E. coli (7A27)	0.25 S	156.25	5
P. aeruginosa (4/28)	0.12 S	1250	5

gentamicin alone (mg 20.2) in the first 24 hours, thereafter the release of gentamicin shows similar values.

The determination with microbiological method allows to evaluate a good antibacterial activity, represented by higher values in comparison with those determined by immunoenzymatic method at any time considered (Table 1). The antimicrobial activity of the combination is higher than expected from the sum of amounts of gentamicin and vancomycin determined separately (59.3 mg versus 44.3 mg calculated amount by FPIA at 24 hours, respectively).

Gentamicin and vancomycin are released from spacers in bactericidal amounts in the first ten days of elution, maintaining high bioactivity. In the following period (20 days) the release (extrapolated as mg/day) corresponds to 1.4 – 1.6 mg/day after 30 days of elution (Fig. 2). Considering the spacer area, this equals 11.5 – 13.1 µg per cm², an amount which is highly inhibitory against multi-resistant clinical isolates. The antimicrobial activity of the combination is higher than gentamicin alone (Figure 2 and Table 1). This effect is defined as summatory or synergistic as shown in Table 2, according to FIC method [13].

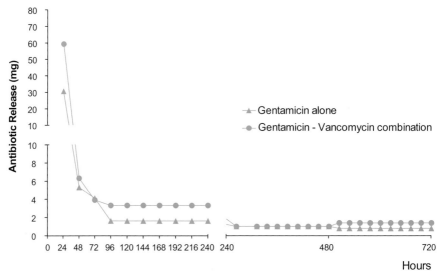

Fig. 2. Release (mg) of Gentamicin and Vancomycin in combination (1:1) and of Gentamicin alone from PMMA hip spacers. Values of antibiotics release from 72 to 720 hours are extrapolated as mg/day of elution. (Microbiological method)

Discussion and Conclusions

The release kinetics of the combination show that: i- high initial peak is followed by sustained constant release of both antibiotics; ii- the release profile of gentamicin and vancomycin is superimposable; iii- gentamicin release seems enhanced by the presence of vancomycin.

The antibiotics maintain their bactericidal activity once they have been released from cement and show synergistic effect in these experimental conditions. Anagnostakos et al [2] demonstrated a synergism between vancomycin and gentamicin against MRSA and *S. epidermidis*, and autonomy against *E. faecalis* and *S. aureus*. The antimicrobial activity is maintained at the site of infection. Kelm et al [10] showed that spacers loaded with gentamicin and vancomycin (1 g + 4 g / 80 g PMMA), can release both antibiotics in different amount ratio exhibiting an inhibitory activity *in vitro* for two weeks after removal. These data seem to confirm the potential efficacy of such combination *in vivo* in two-stage revision infection treatment. These results are in agreement with Anagnostakos et al [2] where the combination vancomycin-gentamicin (ratio 2:1) shows superior percentage elution of gentamicin compared to vancomycin and good antimicrobial activity against Gram-positive microorganisms. In this study vancomycin showed a peak concentration on day 2 of elution. Differently, the release of both gentamicin and vancomycin from the preformed tested spacer showed peak concentrations on day 1. Gentamicin confirms very favourable release characteristics from bone cement.

Further investigations are warranted in order to determine if an optimal ratio of gentamicin to vancomycin is needed to obtain inhibitory synergistic effect. Moreover, the optimal concentrations of both antibiotics in spacer cement should be defined ranging from 1.25 % to 10 % [2, 10, 16, 17]. Compatibility with cement, interference with polymerization process and mechanical resistance are limitations for the use of vancomycin at too high concentrations.

The industrial preparation seems to overcome the limitations derived from hand-made spacers [3, 11, 17] such as the variability depending on hand-made mixture and preparations. The use of preformed spacers may be advantageous in terms of standardization of the device characteristics, mechanical resistance, uniform antibiotic-cement mixing and reproducible antibiotic release.

In conclusion, the new preformed spacer loaded with gentamicin and vancomycin exhibits *in vitro* favourable properties and release characteristics similar to those described for PMMA cements. The combination shows inhibitory activity against microorganisms responsible for prosthetic infections.

Acknowledgements

We thank Chiara Caveiari for her excellent technical assistance.

References

1. Abbott Laboratories Diagnostic Division. (1996). TDx FLx™ system assay I. North Chicago, IL; Abbott Laboratories
2. Anagnostakos K, Kelm J, Regitz T et al (2005) In vitro evaluation of antibiotic release from and bacteria growth inhibition by antibiotic-loaded acrylic bone cement spacers. J Biomed Mater Res B Appl Biomater. 72(2):373–378
3. Bertazzoni Minelli E, Benini A, Magnan B et al (2004) Release of gentamicin and vancomycin from temporary human hip spacers in two-stage revision of infected arthroplasty. J Antimicrob Chemother 53(2):329–334
4. Bertazzoni Minelli E, Caveiari C, Benini A (2002). Release of antibiotics from polymethylmethacrylate (PMMA) cement. J Chemother 14(5):64–72
5. Cerretani D, Giorgi G, Fornara P et al (2002) The in vitro elution characteristics of vancomycin combined with imipenem-cilastatin in acrylic bone-cements: a pharmacokinetic study. J Arthroplasty. 17(5):619–626
6. Cohen J (1999) Management of chronic infection in prosthetic joints. In "Infectious Disease" (Armstrong D. and Cohen J. Eds). Mosby, London. Vol. I, Section 2 – p 46.1–46.6
7. Gonzales Della Valle A, Bostrom M, Brause B et al (2002). Effective bactericidal activity of tobramycin and vancomycin eluted from acrylic bone cement. Acta Orthop Scand 72(3): 237–240
8. Holtom PD, Warren CA, Greene NW et al (1998) Relation of surface area to in vitro elution characteristics of vancomycin-impregnated polymethylmethacrylate spacers. Am J Orthop 27(3):207–210
9. Joseph TN, Chen AL, and Di Cesare PE. (2003). Use of antibiotic-impregnated cement in total joint arthroplasty. J Am Acad Orthop Surg 11(1):38–47
10. Kelm J, Regitz T, Schmitt E et al (2006) In vivo and in vitro studies of antibiotic release from and bacterial growth inhibition by antibiotic-impregnated polymethylmethacrylate hip spacers. Antimicrob Agents Chemother 50(1):332–335
11. Klekamp J, Dawson JM, Haas DW et al (1999) The use of vancomycin and tobramycin in acrylic bone cement: biochemical effects and elution kinetics for use in joint arthroplasty. J Arthroplasty 14(3):339–346
12. Kuechle DK, Landon GC, Musher DM et al (1991) Elution of vancomycin, daptomycin, and amikacin from acrylic bone cement. Clin Orthop Rel Res 264:302–308

13. Lorian V (1996) Antibiotic in laboratory medicine. Fourth edition. Williams & Wilkins Ed., Baltimore
14. Masri BA, Kendall RW, Duncan CP et al (1994) Two-stage exchange arthroplasty using a functional antibiotic-loaded spacer in the treatment of the infected knee replacement: the Vancouver experience. Semin Arthroplasty 5(3):122–136
15. National Committee for Clinical Laboratory Standards. Methods for dilution antimicrobial susceptibility testing for bacteria that grow aerobically, 5th ed. Approved standard. NCCLS document M7-A5. National Committee for Clinical Laboratory Standards, Wayne, PA 2000
16. Neut D, de Groot EP, Kowalski RS et al (2005) Gentamicin-loaded bone cement with clinda-mycin or fusidic acid added: biofilm formation and antibiotic release. J Biomed Mater Res A 73(2):165–170
17. Takahira N, Itoman M, Higashi K et al (2003) Treatment outcome of two-stage revision total hip arthroplasty for infected arthroplasty using antibiotic-impregnated cement spacer. J Orthop Sci 8(1):26–31
18. Toms AD, Davidson D, Masri BA, Duncan CP. (2006) The management of peri-prosthetic infection in total joint arthroplasty. J Bone Joint Surg (Br) 88(2):149–155

Rationale of Nail Antibiotic Clothing and *"in vivo"* Animal Study

R. Giardino[1], M. Fini[1], G. Giavaresi[1], V. Sambri[2], C. Romanò[3], E. Meani[3], R. Soffiatti[4]

[1] Department of Experimental Surgery, Rizzoli Orthopaedic Institutes, Bologna, Italy
[2] DMCSS – Microbiology, St.Orsola Hospital; University of Bologna, Bologna, Italy
[3] Department of Orthopaedic Surgery C.O.S.; "G.Pini" Orthopaedic Institute, Milan, Italy
[4] Research & Development; Tecres Spa, Sommacampagna, Verona, Italy

Introduction

Osteomyelitis is a severe complication of both fracture osteosynthesis and joint replacement surgery [2, 5, 30, 33]. While healthy bone is very resistant to infections, and bacteria alone will not necessarily cause osteomyelitis, other factors such as vascular stasis, soft tissue injuries, fracture instability and the presence of foreign materials are important pathogenetic factors [9]. Fracture instability, caused by inappropriate repair techniques or by implant failure, allows ongoing interfragmentary motion which impairs vascularization and promotes bone necrosis [9]. Fixation devices and prostheses may assist the bacterial colonization, because bacteria produce a mucoid polysaccharide biofilm which binds them to bone and metallic implants and protects them from host defences such as phagocytes and antibodies [2, 9]. Postoperative osteomyelitis is ususally treated by removal of the infected implanted device, surgical debridement of the implant bed and reimplantation of a new device [5, 25]. Antibiotic therapy is also necessary for a successful treatment [5, 25].

Since osteomyelelitis is predominantly a local problem, various studies have suggested also that the local application of antimicrobials clearly provides higher local antibiotic concentrations than those achieved with intravenous application and additionally avoids toxicity due to high plasma levels [14, 15, 24, 32]. In one-stage revision surgery antibiotic-loaded bone cements are generally used for the fixation of the new prosthesis and to provide a high local tissue concentration of antibiotics [4, 6, 12, 28, 29]. In two-stage revisions, the insertion of the new implant is postponed until the infection is treated with systemic antibiotics and/or local antibiotic-loaded beads as well as temporary spacers made of bone cements (poly-methylmethacrylate, PMMA) and antibiotics [1, 10, 11, 16, 17, 19, 21, 27, 29, 34, 35, 37, 38]. The use of a temporary antibiotic-loaded spacer avoids above all periarticular soft tissue shortening, keeps a correct limb positioning and sterilizing the infected areas without the risk of recurrent infections [6, 12, 22, 28, 35]. However, some problems still exist with the use of antibiotic-loaded bone beads/cements or spacers such as bone loss, generation of cement debris, inadequate dosing of cement with the appropriate antibiotic and biologic failure [13]. Despite the presence of antibiotic, they can be colonized with bacteria, allow persistence of the microorganism in the wound similarly to any foreign body, and can lead to a decreased function of immune cells and local immuno suppression [25, 26].

Aminoglycosides such as gentamicin are considered the most effective antibiotics to be used in combination with PMMA because of their high solubility, heat stability and bactericidal activity at low concentration. However, the increase in antibiotic-resistant bacteria with a prevalence of methicillin-resistant or gentamicin-resistant *Staphylococcus aureus*, has led surgeons to load cements and cement spacers with other antibiotics such as vancomycin and teicoplanin or antimicrobial peptides [3, 4, 14, 15, 21–24, 27, 30, 31, 34]. Vancomycin presents chemical characteristics similar to those of gentamicin, but it is considered the drug of choice in infections caused by methicillin-resistant staphylococci (MRSA) and *S. epidermidis*. Various researchers showed *in vitro* the excellent properties of the combination of gentamicin and vancomycin in PMMA as concerns synergistic antimicrobial activity against *Escherichia coli* and *Enterococcus faecalis* [3, 4], enterococci [20] and variable against *S.aureus* according to strains [18].

The aim of the present study was to investigate *in vivo* the efficacy of a new gentamicin-vancomycin impregnated cement nail for posttraumatic and postoperative intramedullary infections. An animal model of intramedullary bone infection was used to evaluate the capacity of such nail to reduce bacterial load and restore bone stock compared to bone debridement and systemic antibiotic therapy [3, 4, 27].

Materials and Methods

The study was performed in accordance with the European and Italian Law on animal experimentation. The animal research protocol was approved by the Ethical Committee of the "Istituti Ortopedici Rizzoli" and by the responsible public authorities as required by the Italian Law in accordance with EU regulations.

Twenty adult male New Zealand rabbits (Charles River SpA, Calco – Lecco, Italy), b.w. 3.15 ± 0.30 kg, were obtained 10 days prior to surgery to acclimatize, caged in individual cages and fed with standard pellet diet (Piccioni Settimo Milanese, Milano, Italia) and water *ad libitum*. General anaesthesia was induced by i.m. injection of 44 mg/kg ketamine (Ketavet 100, Intervet Productions Srl, Aprilia-Latina, Italy) and 3 mg/kg xylazine (Rompun, Bayer SpA, Milano, Italy) under assisted ventilation with O_2/N_2O (1/0.4 l/min) mixture and 2.5 % isofluorane (Forane, Abbott SpA, Campoverde di Aprilia-Latina, Italy). Postoperatively the functional activity of animals was not limited and they received only standard postoperative pain medication for three days (0.2 mg/kg meloxicam s.c., Metacam, Boehringer Ingelheim Italia SpA, Milano, Italy).

Intramedullary bone infection of the right femur was induced via inoculation of methicillin-resistant *S. aureus* (MRSA), by a modification of Rodeheaver at al. femoral models [2]. The MRSA strain used in this study was originally isolated from a patient suffering from chronic osteomyelitis and maintained in culture for several years. The antimicrobial susceptibility of this MRSA isolate was determined using an antibiotic 2-fold method performed in tubes containing Mueller Hinton Broth (MHB) [36] before using the strain to induce the experimental osteomyelitis in rabbits. The isolate used in this study was resistant, *in vitro*, to β-lactam antibiotics, erythromycin, tetracycline, quinolones and trimethoprim-sulfamethoxazole. The susceptibility to clindamycin, aminoglycosides, glycopeptides and rifampin was conserved. Bacteria were grown overnight in MHB starting from a frozen batch and aliquots were prepared. The number of viable CFU in each aliquot was determined by serial dilution and plating on horse blood agar. The number of colonies in each plate was counted by a blinded operator and the bacterial concentration was determined and adjusted to 5×10^6/ml of MHB and stored frozen at -80°C until inoculated into the rabbit.

Nails 4-mm in diameter and 50-mm in length with an inner core of 1.31-mm in diameter stainless steel wire (AISI316), each weighing 1.21 g (0.52 g inner core) were prepared from the polymerized PMMA cement (Cemex®, Tecres SpA, Sommacampagna-Verona, Italy) with PP molds 1.9 % of gentamicin (powder, USP grade, Shangai Fourth, China) and 1.9 % of vancomycin (powder, USP grade, Abbott Lab, Latina, Italy) were mixed with powder of PMMA (polymer) and liquid MMA (monomer) under laminar flow with a ratio 2 : 1 between powder and liquid. Each antibiotic-loaded PMMA nails contained a combination of 13 mg of active gentamicin and 13 mg of active vancomycin. Stainless steel (AISI316) nails of 4-mm in diameter and 50-mm in length were also prepared by turning lathe, cleaned in in Ethyl Alcohol 70 % and rinsed in distilled water. Both type of nails were sterilized with ethylene oxide.

The right knee area was shaven and washed with iodine solution. By using sterile conditions, the knee joint was opened via a parapatellar incision and exposed in flexion. Anterior to the insertion of the anterior cruciate ligament on femur, a small stab incision was made in the intercondylar region, and subsequently a 1-mm drill hole was made by means of a hand-held drill. Then, a 18-gauge needle was inserted into the femoral medullar cavity, the local bone marrow was suctioned and flushed with saline lavage. Subsequently, 0.2 ml (total load of 10^6 CFU) of MRSA was injected into the medullar cavity through the same needle. Finally, the defect created in the intercondylar region was filled with a small block of bone wax (Knochenwachs, B|Braun, Aesculap AG & CO.KG, Tuttlingen, Germany), and the joint capsule and skin wound sutured in layers.

Four weeks later, the animals underwent an X-ray of the operated femur and were treated according to one of four regimens. Five rabbits (Group 1) were treated with bone debridement and received an intramedullary stainless steel nail. Five rabbits (Group 2) were treated with bone debridement and received a gentamicin-vancomycin (1.9 % – 1.9 % w/w) loaded PMMA intramedullary nail. Five rabbits (Group 3) were left untreated for the duration of the study. The last five rabbits (Group 4) had only 1 week of intramuscular teicoplanine (Targosid 200 mg/3 ml, Aventis, Lainate-Milano, Italy) administration at a dose of 20 mg/kg twice daily [23, 30].

By using the previous surgical approach an access to the femoral medullar cavity was gained by using progressive diameter drills until 3.5 mm in groups 1 an 2, under general anaesthesia as described above. Before performing the debridement, a dacron swab was inserted for 3 cm into the femoral medullar cavity to verify the MRSA load. The femoral cavity was then debrided with a stainless steel reamer of 4-mm in diameter in order to remove as much infected and necrotic tissue as possible. Then, the intramedullary nail was inserted in the femoral cavity and the joint capsule and skin wound sutured in layers.

One ml of MHB was added to each swab and the tube was agitated for 3 minutes on a vortex to suspend the bacteria collected onto the swab. A serial ten-fold dilution of each suspension was used to evaluate the bacterial load: 10 μl of each dilution was plated onto horse blood agar and the plates were incubated at 37°C for 48 hours. At the end of the incubation period the number of MRSA colonies on each plate was counted and the total viable CFU load was determined.

At the experimental time of 7 weeks from inoculation, the animals were pharmacologically euthanized under general anaesthesia by an IV injection of a solution 1 ml/kg consisting of 200 mg N-[2-(m-methoxyphenyl)-2-ethyl-buthyl-(1)]-gamma-hydroxybutyramide, 50 mg 4,4'-methylene-bis(cyclohexyltrimethyl-ammoniumiodide) and 5 mg tetracaine hydrochloride (Tanax, Hoechst Roussel Vet, Milan, Italy). The right femur of each rabbit was explanted, cleaned of soft tissue by using sterile conditions, and placed in a sterile 50 ml Falcon tube for taking radiography with a small cabinet X-ray device (Faxitron® Cabinet X-ray System Model 43855A, Faxitron X-ray Corporation, Wheeling-IL,USA).

The radiographic signs of osteomyelitic bone changes were assessed on the basis of evidence (0 = absence; 1 = presence) of (a) periosteal elevation, (b) osteolysis; (c) presence of sequestra; (d) joint effusion; and (e) soft tissue swelling [32] Animals were considered to have radiological osteomyelitis when the severity score was 2 or more.

Then, the femurs were removed from the Falcon tube and always in sterile conditions the midshaft of each femur was cut with a bone saw. Only the distal part of the femurs were used for microbiologic and histological investigations: (a) the femoral canal sampling was repeated immediately after the removal of the intramedullary nail and the swab was processed as above reported in order to evaluate the response to the treatment; and (b) the remnant parts of the proximal femurs were fixed in 4 % paraformaldehyde and processed for histology.

The bone segments used for histology were dehydrated in alcohol series, and embedded in polymethylmethacrylate. Undecalcified transversal sections of femoral midshafts and longitudinal sections of distal epiphyses of 60 μm in thickness were yielded by means of the Leica SP 1600 diamond saw microtome cutting system (Leica SpA, Milano, Italy). Then, the sections were stained with Toluidine Blue and Acid Fuchsin and observed to an optic microscope (BX41, Olympus Optical Co. Europa GmbH, Germany). The disease severity score described by Smeltzer et al. was used to rate sign of infection [33]. This score is divided into four categories that are scored with 0 to 4 points: intraosseous acute inflammation, intraosseous chronic inflammation, periosteal inflammation and bone necrosis. The diagnosis of osteomyelitis was considered positive when the Smeltzer score was at least 4. The maximum score of 16 signifies severe osteomyelitis with intramedullary abscesses, fibrosis, and multiple foci of sequestra.

Results

All animals tolerated both operations well, displaying no signs of systemic infection, soft tissue swelling or fistulae. A rabbit of Group 1 was euthanized at the end of the second surgery for the fracture of treated femur.

The radiological score at 4 and 7 weeks after osteomyelitis induction are plotted in Figure 1. The severity score for the Group 3 increased from weeks 4 to 7, while it decreased significantly for Group 2 (50 %, $p < 0.001$) and Group 4 (24 %, $p < 0.01$). At 7 weeks, the lowest radiographic score was achieved by Group 2 which significantly differed from the other groups ($p < 0.01$).

Figure 2 reports the results of the bacterial load of swab specimens. The highest bacterial load in femoral canal at the sacrifice (10^5 CFU/ml) was found in Group 1

Fig. 1. Radiographic score at 7 weeks from bacterial inoculation (Mean ± SEM, n = 5). Mann Whitney U test: Group 2 *versus* other groups (*, $p < 0.01$); Wilcoxon test: 4 weeks *versus* 7 weeks for Group 2 ([a], $p < 0.001$) and Group 4 ([b], $p < 0.01$).

Fig. 2. Quantitative microbiological analyses of the cultured swab specimens at 4 and 7 weeks from bacteria inoculums. Mean ± SEM, n = 5. Mann Whitney U test: *, Group 1 *versus* Group 2 (the bacterial load was 0) and Group 4 ($p < 0.05$).

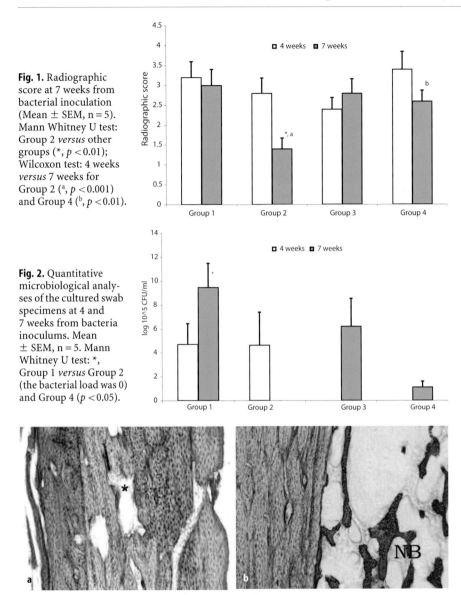

Fig. 3. Representative photomicrographs of longitudinal sections of the femoral midshaft at a magnification of 10 × (the left side of each picture shows the periosteal region): (**a**) a stainless steel intramedullary nail treated specimen (Group 1); (**b**) a gentamicin-vancomycin loaded PMMA intramedullary nail treated specimen (Group 2)

which resulted significant different with Group 2 and Group 4 ($p < 0.05$). No significant differences were observed between Group 3 and Group 4 (Fig. 2).

Figure 3 illustrates that disease severity varied considerable between animals and this variation is reflected in the disease severity scores reported in Figure 4. Group 2

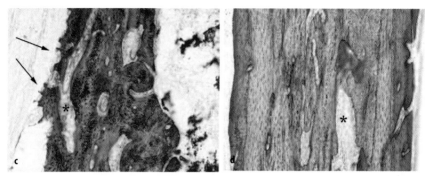

Fig. 3c. An untreated control specimen (Group 3); (**d**) a teicoplanine treated specimen (Group 4). The presence of bone necrosis with signs of bone resorption are still present in all groups, except for the Group 2 (*). A new bone formation towards the nail is visible in the medullary cavity of specimen of Group 2 (NB). Arrows indicate the important periosteal inflammation observed in Group 3.

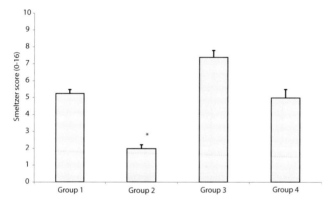

Fig. 4. Histopathologic results as scored using the score of Smeltzer et al. (Mean ± SEM, n=5). Mann Whitney U test: *, Group 2 *versus* other groups (*, $p < 0.01$).

significantly ($p < 0.01$) presented a reduction of the disease severity score compared to the other groups. A histological score 4 or more points was seen in all rabbits of Group 1, Group 3 and Group 4, and none in Group 2.

Conclusions

Antibiotic-loaded PMMA cements are considered as a safe method of delivering and antibiotic to the infection site, with a high initial release of drug followed by an elution that progressively diminishes over a period ranging from few weeks to several months. The gentamicin-vancomycin loaded PMMA nails used in this study have proved previously *in vitro* to maintain the antimicrobial activity with a synergistic effect [3, 4]. It has been showed that the gentamicin elution is not affected by the presence of vancomycin, while the elution of vancomycin from PMMA is reduced of 50 % by the presence of gentamicin, even if it is enough to exert good antimicrobial activity at the infection site for prolonged periods [4]. The microbiological and histological results of the current experimental study confirmed the potentially microbiological efficacy of gentamicin-vancomycin combination in treating local osteomyelitis caused by MRSA, when compared to surgical débridment and to systemic antibiotic therapy.

References

1. Abendschein W (1992) Salvage of infected total hip replacement: use of antibiotic/PMMA spacer. Orthopedics 15(2):228–229
2. An YH, Kang QK, Arciola CR (2006) Animal model of osteomyelitis. Int J Artif Organs 29(4):407–420
3. Bertazzoni Minelli E, Benini A, Magnan B et al (2004) Release of gentamicin and vancomycin from temporary human hip spacers in two-stage revision of infected arthroplasty. J Antimicrob Chemother 53(2):329–334
4. Bertazzoni Minelli E, Caveiari C, Benini A (2002) Release of antibiotics from polymethylmethacrylate cement. J Chemother 14(5):492–500
5. Brandt CM, Sistrunk WW, Duffy MC et al (1997) Staphylococcus aureus prosthetic joint infection treated with debridement and prosthesis retention. Clin Infect Dis 24(5):914–919
6. Buchholz HW, Elson RA, Heinert K (1984) Antibiotic-loaded acrylic cement: current concepts. Clin Orthop Relat Res (190):96–108
7. Callaghan JJ, Katz RP, Johnston RC (1999) One-stage revision surgery of the infected hip. A minimum 10-year follow-up study. Clin Orthop Relat Res (369):139–143
8. Carlsson ÅS, Josefsson G, Lindberg L (1978) Revision with gentamicin-impregnated cement for deep infections in total hip arthroplasties. J Bone Joint Surg (Am) 60(8):1059–1064
9. Cockshutt JR (2002) Bone infection. In: Summer-Smith G Bone in Clinical Orthopedics, 2nd edn., AO Publishing, Dubendorf CH
10. Cuckler JM (2005) The infected total knee: management options. J Arthroplasty 20(4 Suppl 2):33–36
11. Duncan CP, Beauchamp C (1993) A temporary antibiotic-loaded joint replacement system for management of complex infections involving the hip. Orthop Clin North Am 24(4):751–759
12. Elson RA, Jephcott AE, McGechie DB et al (1977) Antibiotic-loaded acrylic cement. J Bone Joint Surg (Br) 59(2):200–205
13. Evans RP (2004) Successful treatment of total hip and knee infection with articulating antibiotic components: a modified treatment method. Clin Orthop Relat Res (427):37–46
14. Faber C, Hoogendoorn RJ, Stallmann HP et al (2004) In vivo comparison of Dhvar-5 and gentamicin in an MRSA osteomyelitis prevention model. J Antimicrob Chemother 54(6):1078–1084
15. Faber C, Stallmann HP, Lyaruu DM et al. (2005) Comparable efficacies of the antimicrobial peptide human lactoferrin 1–11 and gentamicin in a chronic methcillin-resistant Staphylococcus aureus osteomyelitis model. Antimicrob Agents Chemother 49(6):2438–2444
16. Garvin KL, Hanssen AD (1995) Infection after total hip arthroplasty. Past, present, and future. J Bone Joint Surg (Am) 77(10):1576–1588
17. Hanssen AD, Rand JA (1998) Evaluation and treatment of infection at the site of a total hip or knee arthroplasty. J Bone Joint Surg (Am) 80(6):910–922
18. Hershberger E, Aeschlimann JR, Moldovan T et al (1999) Evaluation of bactericidal activities of LY333328, vancomycin, teicoplanin, ampicillin-sulbactam, trovafloxacin, and RP59500 alone or in combination with rifampin or gentamicin against different strains of vancomycin-intermediate Staphylococcus aureus by time-kill curve methods. Antimicrob Agents Chemother 43(3):717–721
19. Hofmann AA, Goldberg TD, Tanner AM et al. (2005) Ten-year experience using an articulating antibiotic cement hip spacer for the treatment of chronically infected total hip. J Arthroplasty. 20(7):874–879
20. Houlihan HH, Stokes DP, Rybak MJ (2000) Pharmacodynamics of vancomycin and ampicillin alone and in combination with gentamicin once daily or thrice daily against Enterococcus faecalis in an in vitro infection model. J Antimicrob Chemother 46(1):79–86

21. Hsieh PH, Shih CH, Chang YH et al (2004) Two-stage revision hip arthroplasty for infection: comparison between the interim use of antibiotic-loaded cement beads and a spacer prosthesis. J Bone Joint Surg (Am) 86(9):1989–1997

22. Hsieh PH, Shih CH, Chang YH et al (2005) Treatment of deep infection of the hip associated with massive bone loss: two-stage revision with an antibiotic-loaded interim cement prosthesis followed by reconstruction with allograft. J Bone Joint Surg (Br) 87(6):770–775

23. Ismael F, Bléton R, Saleh-Mghir A et al (2003) Teicoplanin-containing cement spacers for treatment of experimental Staphylococcus aureus joint prosthesis infection. Antimicrob Agents Chemother 47(10):3365–3367

24. Joosten U, Joist A, Gosheger G et al (2005) Effectiveness of hydroxyapatite-vancomycin bone cement in the treatment of Staphylococcus aureus induced chronic osteomyelitis. Biomaterials 26(25):5251–5258

25. Koort JK, Mäkinen TJ, Suokas E et al. (2005) Efficacy of ciprofloxacin-releasing bioabsorbable osteoconductive bone defect filler for treatment of experimental osteomyelitis due to Staphyloccocus aureus. Antimicrob Agents Chemother 49(4):1502–1508

26. Mader JT, Stevens CM, Stevens JH et al. (2002) Treatment of experimental osteomyelitis with a fibrin sealant antibiotic implant. Clin Orthop Rel Res (403):58–72

27. Magnan B, Regis D, Biscaglia R et al (2001) Preformed acrylic bone cement spacer loaded with antibiotics: use of two-stage procedure in 10 patients because of infected hips after total replacement. Acta Orthop Scand 72(6):591–594

28. Marks KE, Nelson CL, Lautenschlager EP (1976) Antibiotic impregnated acrylic bone cement. J Bone Joint Surg (Am) 58(3):358–364

29. Nijhof MW, Fleer A, Hardus K et al (2001). Tobramycin-containing bone cement and systemic cefazolin in a one-stage revision. Treatment of infection in a rabbit model. J Biomed Mater Res 58(6):747–753

30. Saleh Mghir A, Cremieux AC, Bleton R et al (1998) Efficacy of teicoplanin and autoradiographic diffusion pattern of [14C]teicoplanin in experimental Staphylococcus aureus infection of joint prostheses. Antimicrob Agents Chemother 42(11):2830–2835

31. Shirtliff ME, Calhoun JH, Mader JT (2002) Experimental osteomyelitis treatment with antibiotic-impregnated hydroxyapatite. Clin Orthop Rel Res (201):239–247

32. An YH, Friedmann RJ (1998) Animal models of prosthetic infection. In: An YH Animal models in orthopaedic research, CRC – Taylor & Francis, Boca Raton – FL

33. Smeltzer MS, Thomas JR, Hickmon SG et al (1997) Characterization of a rabbit model of staphylococcal osteomyelitis. J Orthop Res 15(3):414–421

34. Springer BD, Lee GC, Osmon D et al (2004) Systemic safety of high-dose antibiotic-loaded cement spacers after resection of an infected total knee arthroplasty. Clin Orthop Relat Res (427):47–51

35. Steinbrink K (1990) The case for revision arthroplasty using antibiotic-loaded acrylic cement. Clin Orthop Relat Res (261):19–22

36. Woods GL, Washington JA (1995) Antibacterial susceptibility tests: dilution and disk diffusion methods. In: Murray PR, Baron EJ, Pfaller MA et al Manual of clinical microbiology, 6th edn. American Society for Microbiology, Washington DC

37. Younger ASE, Duncan CP, Masri BA (1998) Treatment of infection associated with segmental bone loss in the proximal part of the femur in two stages with use of an antibiotic loaded interval prosthesis. J Bone Joint Surg (Am) 80(1):60–69

38. Zilkens KW, Casser HR, Ohnsorge J (1990) Treatment of an old infection in a total hip replacement with an interim spacer prosthesis. Arch Orthop Trauma Surg 109(2):94–96.

The Use of Antibiotic-loaded Spacers in Post-traumatic Bone Infection

F. Baldo, G. Zappalà, M. Ronga

Department of Orthopaedic and Traumatological Sciences "Mario Boni", University of Insubria, Varese, Italy

Introduction

Open fractures continue to be common, with a high risk of complications such as osteomyelitis and septic nonunion [17].

Current treatment of open fracture dictates the use of the methods that reduce risk of infection (urgent or emergent treatment, removal of all foreign materials, sharp debridement of devascularized host tissue etc), post-traumatic bone infection is still a common and serious problem [19].

Despite the use of new antibiotics and advances in surgical technique and soft tissue coverage procedures, the treatment of osteomyelitis is unsuccessful approximately in one of every five case [6].

Bone damage and bone loss suffered in the initial trauma, fibrotic soft tissue in the area of infection, and tenuous skin coverage, all contribute to the difficulty in clearing infection [4]. Generally, these are areas of poor vascular perfusion, which limits penetration of systemically administered antibiotics [17].

Once microorganism attach to bone , the bacteria become metabolically less active and cover themselves with biofilm, rendering them unresponsive to usual therapeutic antibiotic levels. To achieve pharmacologic kill of bacteria in a biofilm, antibiotic concentration must be from 10 to 100 times higher then the usual bactericidal concentration, which cannot be achieved by safe dose of parenteral antibiotics [5, 7, 16].

The use of a local antibiotic delivery system obtains a high local concentration of antibiotics and simultaneously minimizes their systemic toxicity. The most comprehensive information regarding drug delivery system in orthopaedic surgery is derived from the information provided by studies of antibiotic-loaded bone cement [11].

The historic use of antibiotic bone cement starts in the 1970s with the pioneering work of Buchholz and Engelbrecht [2] in which they established the principle of using antibiotic bone cement in the treatment of infected total joint replacement. In this study, a success rate of 77 % was obtained using cement removal, debridement, and replacement of implant with antibiotic-laden bone cement: it is important to note that the patients were not treated with systemic antibiotics. The success rate rose to 90 % using an association of systemic antibiotics [2].

Six years later, Marks [9] et al made the first confirmatory laboratory studies on the release of microbiologically active form from the various bone cements.

In 1977, Elson et al showed that if depot PMMA antibiotics are introduced next to the cortical bone, dense cortical bone is penetrated and the concentration in the bone is much higher than that can be achieved safely by systemic administration, revealing that antibiotic concentration surrounding the antibiotic-laden implant was many times greater than what could be achieved by safe intravenous administration [4]. In 1981, the same conclusion was reported by Hoff at al using penicillin G and gentamicin [8].

At the same time, a new way of local antibiotic delivery system was studied in the form of beads: size, number and pattern of elution from beads were collected in animal and clinical studies [1, 3, 12].

A multicenter randomized controlled study attempted to compare systemic antibiotic therapy to local therapy with Septopal beads in the treatment of osteomyelitis: no difference were reported in the recurrence rate in the Septopal group compared with the systemic antibiotic group [1].

A randomized controlled trial by Calhoun et al [3] compared 4 weeks of intravenous antibiotics with Septopal beads in 52 patients with infected non-union having debridement and reconstructive surgery. Patients in the antibiotic bead group also received perioperative systemic antibiotic therapy (2 to 5 days). The success rate for treating the infection was 83 % in the systemic antibiotic group and 89 % in the antibiotic bead group: local antibiotic therapy can be a useful alternative substitute instead of long-term systemic antibiotic therapy in treating infected non-unions.

Patzakis et al [12] compared Septopal beads (supplemented with as much as 5 days of systemic antibiotic) to systemic antibiotic therapy in 33 patients with chronic osteomyelitis and bone defects. The infection control rate was 100 % in the Septopal group and 95 % in the systemic antibiotic group. Bony union was achieved in all patients.

Nowadays, there are few reports about the use of spacer blocks in the treatment of post-traumatic infections [14]. We report the use of antibiotic-loaded spacers in post-traumatic bone infection in selected cases.

Materials and Method

Our series included 4 patients, 3 male and 1 female, with an average age of 37 years (range: 30 – 44 years) (Table 1, 2). One septic non-union of distal tibia, 1 chronic osteomyelitis of distal tibia (Fig. 1), 1 septic non-union of ankle arthrodesis, 1 chronic osteomyelitis of femoral diaphysis were treated. The patients had undergone an average of 6 (range: 3 – 12) operations before being referred to our institution. All patients had a history of infection of more than 6 months, clinical signs of infection (purulent drainage from fistulas), radiographic findings consistent with infection (lytic lesion, bone resorption, bone sequesters, sclerosis, soft tissue swelling) and positive bone bacterial culture. The initial fracture were classified using the Gustilo classification: 3 cases had a Gustilo 3A fracture and 1 case had a Gustilo 3B fracture.

All patients had a draining sinus tract without soft tissue defects at the time of surgery. We obtained in all patients bone bacterial cultures from the draining sinus.

Our treatment was performed in two stages: the first was to treat the infected bone and the second to realize the bony consolidation. After an initial thorough soft tissue debridement, we resected the infected bone until a free margin of bleeding bone was observed. The bony defect was filled with gentamicin-impregnated cement spacer.

Table 1. Clinical data at the time of first stage of reconstruction. DMET: distal meta-epiphysis of tibia; MDF: meta-diaphysis of femur; ORIF: open reduction internal fixation; EF: external fixator.

Case	Age	Diagnosis	Site	Month from trauma	Delay since bone infection	Number of previous treatment	Previous treatment	Smoke status
1	39	chronic osteomyelitis	DMET	245	6 years	13	(incomplete anamnesis) Nailing Nailing exchange Nailing removal External fixator + bone Grafting	> 10
2	30	septic nonunion of ankle arthrodesis	DMET	37	2 years	7	EF EF exchange EF exchange + bone grafting EF removal Ankle arthrodesis with retrograde "Russel Taylor" Nail Nailing Removal + debridement + EF Debridement + antibiotic beads + EF	> 10
3	38	septic nonunion of distal tibia	DMET	42	4 years	5	ORIF Bipedicle flap Plate removal and EF Debridement Debridement	> 10
4	44	chronic osteomyelitis	MDF	26	6 months	4	EF Debridement Debridement + EF exchange Debridement	> 10

Table 2. Procedures and follow-up

Case	Bone defect	Bone transport time	Union (from the last surgery)	Duration of oral antibiotic therapy (from the last surgery)	Return to pre-trauma activity level (from the last surgery)
1	7 cm	6 months	11 months	7 months	15 months
2	3 cm	–	6 months (failure) Amputation	6 months	–
3	3 cm	–	11 months	5 months	16 months
4	5 cm	9 months	8 months	5 months	11 months

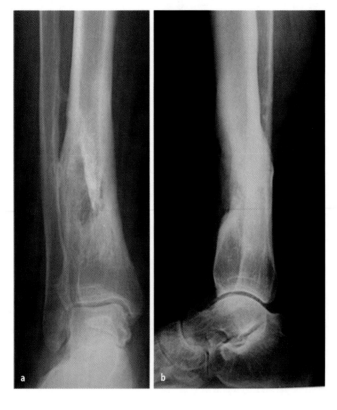

Fig. 1. Case 1: Chronic osteomyelitis at the time of the first surgery (**a, b**)

We use Cemex® Genta (Tecres Spa, Sommacampagna VR, Italy), a gentamicin-impregnated bone cement, equivalent to 1 g gentamicin base in 40 g unit. We shaped the cement into a cylindrical spacer sufficient to fill the entire bone defect, with an attempt to make a seal with the bone surface.

The bone segment was then fixed with a monoaxial external fixator. Deep swab cultures were taken and then parenteral antibiotic were administred until patients was dismissed (mean 6 days: range 5 to 8 days). At the moment of discharge the patient was given high dose oral antibiotics continued for 8 weeks.

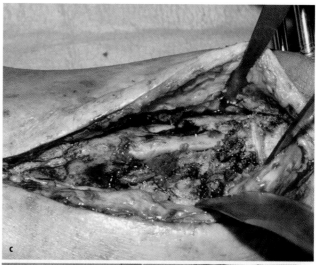

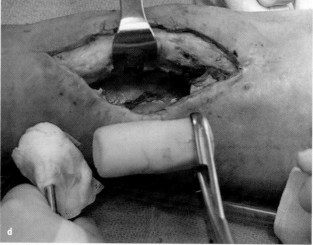

Fig. 1c. Intra-operative details: before debridement (**c**) and just before antibiotic-loaded spacer implant (**d**)

We performed the second surgical procedure after completion of the antibiotics consisting of cement spacer removal. In two cases (cases 1 and 4) we utilized an autologous bone grafting form iliac crest to promote direct bone healing without bone transport. In the other two cases, we utilized an antegrade bone transport. At the end of lengthening we performed a surgical procedure to stimulate the union of the docking site using autologous cancellous bone grafting from iliac crest. In all cases no external fixation exchange was performed at the time of second surgery. In all case we used Osteogenic Protein-1 (OP-1-Osigraft®, Stryker Biotech, Limerik, Ireland) at the time of bone grafting to enhance bony union. CRP and ESR laboratory values every two weeks were repeated for two months and then monthly until 6 months from bone healing, to determine if there was a significant change. Patients continued oral antibiotic therapy for a minimal of 6 weeks and then discontinued if no clinical and radio-

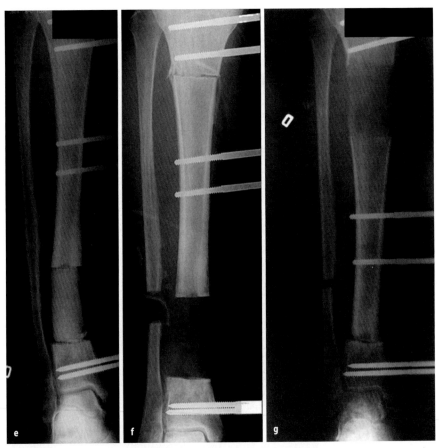

Fig. 1d. Post-operative X-ray control after antibiotic-loaded spacer implant (**e**). Post-operative control eight weeks later, at the time of the second surgery: we have performed cement removal, fibulectomy, high tibial osteotomy to begin the bone transport (**f**). Radiological control 6 months from the second surgery: at this time we have performed the third surgical step consisting in treating docking site using autograft with iliac crest cancellous bone and Osigraft implant (**g**)

logical signs of infection were present, CRP less than 5 mg/L, and ESR less than 20 mm/h after a minimal period of three months.

Results

At the time of the initial surgery, cultures taken from the sinus tract and deep swab were positive in all patients and revealed the presence of Staphylococcus aureus (cases 1, 2 and 4) and Enterococcus faecalis (case 3). All patients received antibiotic therapy pre-operatively and post-operatively for 8 weeks.

In all patients white blood cell count (WBC) count, C-reactive protein (CRP), erythrocyte sedimentation rates (ESR), clinical and surgical site signs of infection did

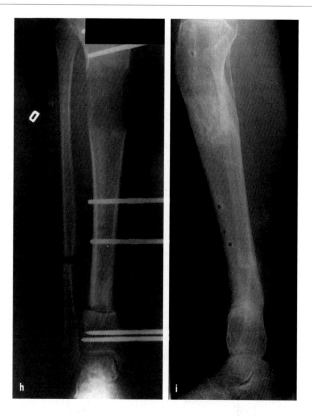

Fig. 42.1. (*cont.*) Radiological union at 12 months after grafting of docking site (**h, i**)

not reveal active infection at the time of second surgery (8 weeks after first operation).

Two of the patients have consented for bone transport and the other two patients rejected this option. In the last two cases, we performed fixation using a mono-axial external fixation and autologous bone grafting from iliac crest.

In the former two cases, we began antegrade bone transport using mono-axial rail external fixator to restore 7 cm of bone defect in case 1, and 5 cm in case 4. At the and of lengthening (case 1: 6 months; case 2: 9 months) we added autogenous bone graft to facilitate fusion at docking site.

At the time of bone grafting, in all patients we used two units of Osigraft® to enhance bony union.

Patients have continued oral antibiotic therapy for a mean period of 5.7 months (range: 5 – 7) after the last surgical procedure.

In cases 1 (Fig. 1), 3 and 4 the external fixators were removed after respectively 9, 6 and 6 months after bone grafting. Case 1 and 3 required a supplementary weight bearing casting for two months after external fixator removal. Union was achieved at a mean period of 10 months (range 8 – 11).

Case 1, 3 and 4 returned to their prefracture activity level and no patients had any sign of recurrence of the osteomyelitis after 2 year follow-up.

Case 4 required amputation for a recurrence of the osteomyelitis at sixth months after the cement spacer was removed.

Discussion

Post-traumatic infection continues to be a formidable challenge for the clinician [1].

Septic non-union and post-traumatic osteomyelitis are very difficult to treat, especially when they are complicated by significant bone and soft tissue defects [18].

Meticulous debridement is the hallmark of treatment. Well established colonies of bacteria may be impossible to eliminate in any other way [17] Antibiotics eradicate any bacteria that are not removed from debridement. However there are microbiological factor that contribute to treatment failure [17]. One of these is that bacteria that are attached to surface of metallic fixation devices or dead bone and become resistant to the action of antibiotic by covering themselves with biofilm [5, 7, 11, 16].

High doses of antibiotic is necessary to achieve a pharmacologic kill of bacteria in a biofilm [5, 7, 11, 16]. Another factor is that antibiotic in systemic circulation penetrate healthy tissue in effective concentration and this concentration should reach the bacteria in normal tissue. If bacteria are isolated in avascular bone it may no be possible for systemic antibiotics to achieve critical local concentration. Therefore systemic antibiotic treatment of sessile bacterial infection is not possible by using a safe doses [5, 7, 16].

Local antibiotic delivery seems to be a useful and safe component in the armamentarium of the physician, by maximizing the local concentration of antibiotic while minimizing their systemic toxicity [19].

From the pioneering work of Buchholz and Engelbrecht [2] investigators have studied the properties of PMMA as delivery vehicle. Elution, pharmacokinetic properties and tissue penetration have been evaluated. The most common antimicrobial agents have been successfully incorporated into PMMA cement and nowadays on the basis of bacterial culture we can select the appropriate antibiotic to be administered [11].

Whereas a lot of literature have been released on the use of antibiotic spacers in the treatment of infected arthroplasty and antibiotic impregnated beads in the treatment of osteomyelitis, infected non-union and osteomyelitis, few reports on the use of a block spacer in the treatment of septic non-unions and osteomyelitis are available.

Our experience with use of antibiotic therapy with spacer in based on the observation of very difficult removal of the beads [13]. In addition, antibiotic-impregnated spacers fill the dead space that results after debridement and facilitate subsequent reconstruction.

Controversies regarding local antibiotic therapy include the length of implantation [19].

Although these concerns have not been shown to translate into clinical problem, beads removal within 4 to 6 weeks has been recommended because the beads progressively get enclosed in fibrous tissue or even incorporated in to the callus, resulting in reduced elution, and complicated or incomplete removal [13]. We prefer to wait 8 weeks between cement spacer implantation and removal to obtain a complete soft tissue healing.

Conclusion

The safety of local antibiotic therapy has been well documented in clinical studies [19]. PMMA is the standard material used as delivery vehicle for depot antibiotics in orthopaedic surgery [19].

In our experience cement spacer is easily placed, easily removed, patient friendly and inexpensive and we prefer it over beads.

Drawbacks associated with the use of PMMA delivery system is the necessity of secondary debridement, lack of osteoconductivity, and foreign body reaction. PMMA also appears to be surface friendly to biofilm-forming bacteria [10].

Bioabsorbable delivery vehicles seem to be a promising alternative and are currently being investigated [18]. Collagen sponge, calcium sulphate, morcelized bone and PLA-PGA have considerably potential for successful development to clinically usable products [10]. A biodegradable vehicle would eliminate the need for a secondary procedure to remove the PMMA and not only obliterate the dead space but aid in bone healing as well.

Until appropriate data is available, clinical use of these materials as delivery vehicles for antibiotic must be approached with caution [10, 19].

Even with extensive historic, clinical and outcome data that proves the effectiveness of antibiotic-laden cement, the ideal drug delivery system is neither agreed upon or available at this time, but the use of antibiotic-loaded spacers in post-traumatic bone infection seems to be a useful and safe component in the armamentarium of the physician.

References

1. Blaha JD, Calhoun JH, Nelson CL et al (1993) Comparison of the clinical efficacy of gentamicin PMMA beads on surgical wire versus combined and systemic therapy for osteomyelitis. Clin Orthop Relat Res (295):8–12
2. Buchholz HW, Engelbrecht H (1970) Ueber die Depotwirkung einiger Antibiotica bei Vermischung mit dem Kunstharz Palacos. Chirurg 41(11):511–515
3. Calhoun JH, Henry SL, Anger DM et al (1993) The treatment of infected nonunions with gentamicin-polymethylmethacrylate antibiotic beads. Clin Orhop Relat Res (295):23–27
4. Elson RA, Jephcott AE, McGechie DB al (1977) Antibiotic-loaded acrylic cement. J Bone J Surg (Br) 59(2):200–205
5. Garvin KL, Evans BG, Salvati EA et al (1994) Palacos gentamicin for the treatment of deep periprosthethic hip infection. Clin Orthop Relat Res (298):97–105
6. Haas DW, Mc Andrew MP (1996) Bacterial osteomyelitis in adult: evolving consideration in diagnosis and treatment. Am J Med 101(5):550–561
7. Hanssen AD, Osmon DR, Nelson CL (1997) Prevention of deep periprosthethic joint infection. Instr Course Lect (46):555–567
8. Hoff SF, Fizgerald Jr RH, Kelly PJ (1981) The depot administration of penicillin G and gentamicin in acrylic bone cement. J Bone Joint Surg (Am) 63(5):798–804
9. Marks KE, Nelson CL, Lautenschlager EP (1976) Antibiotic-impregnated acrylic bone cement. J Bone Joint Surg (Am) 58(3):358–364
10. Mc Laren A (2004) Alternative materials to acrylic bone cement for delivery of depot antibiotics in orthopaedic infections. Clin Orthop Relat Res (427):101–106
11. Nelson CL (2004) The current Status of material used for depot delivery of drugs. Clin Orthop Relat Res (427):72–78
12. Patzakis MJ, Mazur K, Wilkins J et al (1993) Septopal beads and autogenous bone graft for bone defects in patients with chronic osteomyelitis. Clin Orthop Relat Res (295):112–118

13. Salvati EA, Callaghan, Brause BD et al (1986) Reimplantation in infection. Elution of genta-micin from cement and beads. Clin Orthop Relat Res (207):83–93
14. Schöttle PB, Werner CML and Dumont CE (2005) Two-stage reconstruction with free vascu-larized soft tissue transfer and conventional bone graft for infected nonunions of the tibia. Acta Orthopaedica 76(6):878–883
15. Simons RK, Hoyt DB (1994) Immunomodulation. In Maull KI (ed.). Advance in Trauma and Critical Car. Vol 9. St Louis, CV Mosby 135–157
16. Trampuz A, Osmon DR, Hanssen AD (2003) Molecular and antibiofilm approaches to pros-thetic joint infection. Clin Orthop Relat Res (414):69–88
17. Tsukuyama TD (1999) Pathophysiology of post-traumatic osteomyelitis. Clin Orthop Relat Res (360):22–29
18. Ueng WN, Wei FC, Shih CH (1999) Management of femoral diaphyseal infected nonunions with antibiotic beads based local therapy, external skeletal fixation, and staged bone graf-ting. J Trauma (461):97–103
19. Zalavras GC, Patzakis MJ, Holtom P (2004) Local antibiotic therapy in the treatment of Open Fracture and Osteomyelitis. Clin Orthop Relat Res (427):86–93.

The Use of Antibiotic-impregnated Cement in Infected Reconstructions after Resection for Bone Tumors

M. MERCURI, D. DONATI, C. ERRANI, N. FABBRI, M. DE PAOLIS

5th Department of Oncologic Orthopaedics and Traumatology, Rizzoli Orthopedic Institutes, Bologna, Italy

Introduction

Significant advances in chemotherapy, radiography, and surgical techniques over the past two decades have made limb salvage surgery procedure of choice for most malignant tumours of the extremities. Massive segmental skeletal reconstruction after resection of bone tumours has become increasingly popular [24]. Endoprosthetic replacement and massive bone allograft transplantation following bone tumour resection are common [15]. However, complications are frequent, resulting in reoperation and, at times, even amputation. The relatively high frequency of complications is not unexpected, given the length and nature of the surgical procedures and the high demand placed on the implants [27]. Infection is the major cause of early failure and the most challenging for both surgeon and patient [5, 18, 24]. In literature the infection rate with endoprosthesis or massive bone allograft is between 2.9 and 30 % of cases [18, 21].

The pathophysiology and clinical implications of infection associated with allograft and endoprosthesis are similar [24]. The most common cause of an early infection is skin necrosis. Other causes of deep infection include intraoperative contamination and haematogenous infection. The endoprosthesis and bone allograft are a large foreign body capable of harbouring bacterial and fungal infections. The clinical signs and symptoms of a deep infection are highly variable, haematological parameters likewise may not be helpful and radiographic signs are frequently delayed. Osteosarcoma and Ewing sarcoma are the most frequent primary bone tumours and the most commonly affected site is around the knee [4, 25]. After the resection of bone tumours, prosthesis or bone allograft is usually implanted. Infection rates are highest in the tibia and pelvic reconstructions (Fig. 1). Clearly, the extensive surgery involved with resection of malignant neoplasm as well as the adjuvant use of chemotherapy and radiation therapy contribute to higher incidence of all complications, including infection, following limb salvage surgery [15, 24].

The risk factors include diabetes, obesity, pathologic fracture, operating time, blood loss, adjuvant chemotherapy, type of reconstruction, postoperative complications as haematoma and thrombophlebitis [15]. In more than 50 % of cases infection develops immediately or within three months after surgery; in the remaining cases it is evident after a mean of ten months. Infection is usually clinical evidence with draining sinus, fever, local warmth, swelling and inflammation, and wound slough. Laboratory tests can show alteration of the ESR, C-reactive protein, WBC, fibrinogen

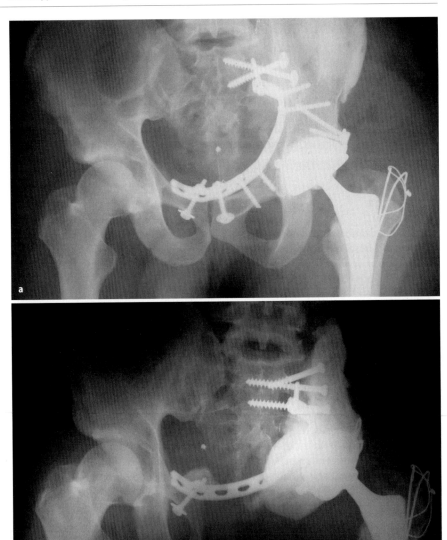

Fig. 1a, b. Antero-posterior radiographs showing **a** massive bone allograft and prosthesis for pelvic reconstruction **b** antibiotic-PMMA spacer after resection of the massive bone allograft

and gamma proteins. The commonest organisms are coagulase-negative *Staphylococcus*, *Staphylococcus aureus* and Group-D Streptococci; sometimes there is a bacteria association and in rare case the colture samples could prove sterile [6, 15].

Once a diagnosis of delayed (> 3 months) infection is made, there are four options. The first is to perform an initial debridement followed by chronic antibiotic treatment, but often the result in cure is unlikely. The second option is a one stage

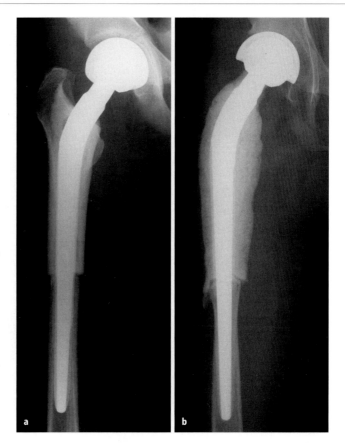

Fig. 2a, b. Antero-posterior radiographs show **a** allograft composite prosthesis after resection of right proximal femur **b** antibiotic-impregnated cement around the prosthesis

procedure with antibiotic impregnated cement around the prosthesis (Fig. 2) and systemic antibiotic treatment. The third option, associated with better success in long-term control, is initial debridement and removal of the implant, which is replaced with an antibiotic-impregnated polymethylmethacrylate (PMMA) "spacer", and a long-term (6 weeks) systemic treatment with intravenous antibiotics. Repeated debridement is recommended, and cultures are followed sequentially. Once sterile, a prosthesis may be implanted with antibiotic cement and additional postoperative antibiotics (Fig. 3). This option obviously requires a great deal of time, operative procedures, hospitalization, and disability, but is associated with ultimate salvage of extremity in about one half of cases [24, 27]. The final option is to proceed with an amputation, which is curative of the infection and is indicated particularly for patients requiring additional cytotoxic chemotherapy or for patients with a second prosthetic infection.

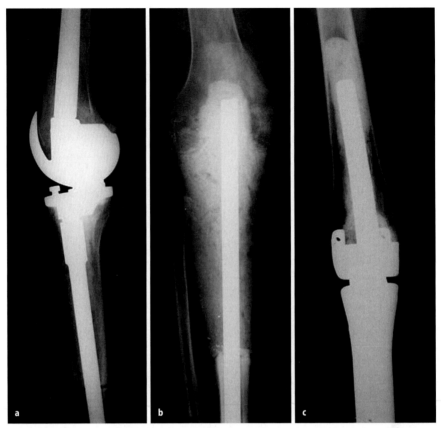

Fig. 3a. Latero-lateral radiograph showing an allograft composite prosthesis implanted for recon-struction of the proximal tibia. Antero-posterior radiographs show **b** antibiotic-impregnated cement spacer in place **c** reimplantation of HMRS cemented-modular system

Discussion

Local antibiotic therapy using chains of gentamicin PMMA beads is an established technique in septic bone surgery [1, 11]. Buchholz et al. [2, 3] reported the efficacy of antibiotic-loaded bone cement in the management of infected total hip arthroplasties and this is confirmed in further pharmacokinetic studies by Wahlig et al. [28]. They reported local levels of antibiotic 200 times higher than those achieved by systemic administration.

Walenkamp et al. [29] showed that the serum and the urine concentrations of gen-tamicin after the implantation of gentamicin PMMA beads were much lower than those after systemic use. The clinical efficacy of this method has been validated in post-traumatic, postoperative and haematogenous osteomyelitis and in infected con-ventional total hip and knee arthroplasty [8, 9, 22].

Since 1981 we have been using gentamicin-PMMA beads in infected reconstruc-tions after resection of bone tumours. Rotation of muscle flaps [7, 12, 19] can be used to heal the infection with or without removal of the prosthesis. When the prosthetic component is to be removed, however, a two-stage procedure has to be considered [23]. Since 1992 we have used antibiotic-impregnated acrylic cement as a block spacer. This technique has proved to be successful in infected conventional knee and hip prostheses [10, 13, 14], preserving length and space for later reinsertion of an implant.

Use of systemic antibiotics and surgery are the best therapy. The only satisfactory operation is a revision with antibiotic cement and debridement. Two different regimes of treatment are employed both of which entailed debridement and the use of cement impregnated with antibiotic. It is possible to use gentamicin-PMMA beads or antibiotic-impregnated cement spacer, but better results are achieved with the use of second procedure in terms of cases healed, the number of operations, time of healing, time of recovery and the functional score. The use of vancomycin in the cement spacer gave better local control [6].

The surgery consists in resection of allograft or prosthesis, placement of an antibiotic-impregnated polymethylmethacrylate (PMMA) spacer (Fig. 4), and intravenous antibiotics for at least five days during the perioperative period. As much cement is used as is necessary to fill the whole space left by the retrieved implant. Usually the cement is reinforced by a Kuntscher nail. Vancomycin is the antibiotic of choice mixed with cement in quantities varying between 3 and 9 g per cement pack, but cefamandole (2 g) or gentamicin (3 g) can also be used. Koo et al. [16] recommend using the combination of these 3 antibiotics in the cement spacer for 2-stage reconstruction in infected arthroplasty when the causative organism is not identified in the coulture of preoperative aspiration.

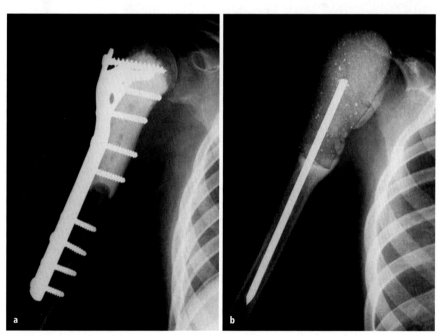

Fig. 4a, b. Antero-posterior radiographs showing **a** massive bone allograft for reconstruction of the right proximal humerus **b** antibiotic-impregnated PMMA spacer in place

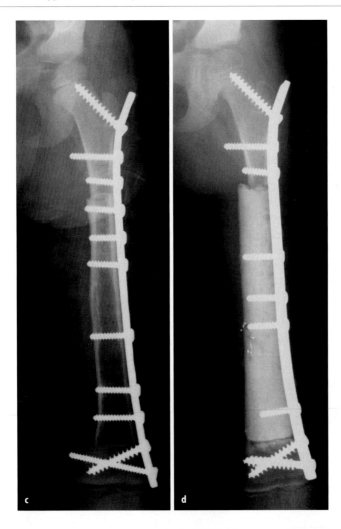

Fig. 4c, d. Antero-posterior radiographs showing **c** intercalary massive bone allograft after resection of diaphisyal left femur **d** antibiotic-impregnated PMMA spacer

After a mean interval of 10 months and between two and seven operative procedures, the infection is eradicated in the majority of the cases. Sometimes amputation is necessary because of persistent clinical signs of infection in the presence of the spacer. In the patients treated with postoperative chemotherapy the only notable feature is a higher rate of amputation [6].

There are significant correlation between successful eradication of the infection and infecting organism, duration of antibiotic treatment with effective bactericidal serum levels, and surgical management with particular regard to soft tissue coverage [20, 24]. Attempts at a one-stage procedure have resulted in a rate of reinfection of up to 30 % [14, 17, 22, 26].

Conclusion

Infection is a serious complication after segmental resection for bone tumours. The treatment of deep infection after limb salvage surgery remains controversial. In early infection several methods can achieve success in 50 % to 70 % of the cases, while for the remainder or in late infection, the removal of the implant and a high local concentration of antibiotic are needed. Revision with antibiotic-impregnated cement is the only reliable method for limb salvage following deep infection. Although deep infection after resection for bone tumours continues to result in a high rate of failure, this method of management results in successful limb salvage in more of the half of the patients [6, 15, 24]. Considering the complexity of patients with malignant disease, this method of attempted limb salvage in the presence of deep infection appears warranted. The combination of antibiotics and an improved cement is advisable for a better elution and higher and faster concentration of local antibiotics. Reliable and reproducible laboratory and image-based tests are needed to diagnose more accurately the early onset of the infection and to monitor the outcome. The total implant resection, microbiology, and correct antibiotic are crucial factors to obtain possible good outcome. Prevention is the key to reducing the incidence of this serious complication [15].

References

1. Blaha JD, Calhoun JH, Nelson CL et al (1993) Comparison of the clinical efficacy and tolerance of gentamicin PMMA beads on surgical wire versus combined and systemic therapy for osteomyelitis. Clin Orthop Relat Res (295):8–12
2. Buchholz HW, Engelbrecht H (1970) Depot effects of various antibiotics mixed with palaos resins. Chirurg 41(11):511–515
3. Buchholz HW, Gartmann HD (1972) Infection prevention and surgical management of deep insidious infection in total endoprosthesis. Chirurg 43(10):446–453
4. Campanacci M (1999) Bone and soft tissue tumors. 2nd Edition, Springer-Verlag Wien
5. Capanna R, Casadei R, Bettelli G et al (1992) Infection in limb salvage surgery. J Bone Joint Surg Br 74(Suppl 1):106
6. Donati D, Biscaglia R (1998) The use of antibiotic-impregnated cement in infected reconstructions after resection for bone tumours. J Bone Joint Surg Br 80(6):1045–1050
7. Eckardt JJ, Lesavoy MA, Dubrow TJ, et al. (1990) Exposed endoprosthesis: management protocol using muscle and myocutaneous flap coverage. Clin Orthop Relat Res (251):220–229
8. Evans RP, Nelson CL (1993) Gentamicin-impregnated polymethylmethacrylate beads compared with systemic antibiotic therapy in the treatment of chronic osteomyelitis. Clin Orthop Relat Res (295):47–53
9. Georgiadis GM, De Silva SP (1995) Reconstruction of skeletal defects inthe forearm after trauma: treatment with cement spacer and delayed cancellous bone grafting. J Trauma 38(6):910–914
10. Gusso MI, Capone A, Civinini R, et al. (1995) The spacer block technique in revision of total knee arthroplasty with septic loosening. . Chir Org Mov 80(1):21–27
11. Henry SL, Hood GA, Seligson D (1993) Long-term implantation of gentamicin-polymethyl-methacrylate antibiotic beads. Clin Orthop Relat Res (295):47–53
12. Horowitz SM, Lane JM, Otis JC et al (1991) Prosthetic arthroplasty of the knee after resection of a sarcoma in the proximal end of the tibia: a report of sixteen cases. J Bone Joint Surg Am 73(2):286–293
13. Hofmann AA, Kane KR, Tkach TK et al (1995) Treatment of infected total knee arthroplasty using an articulating spacer. Clin Orthop Relat Res (321):45–54

14. Ivarsson I, Wahlstrom O, Djerf K et al (1994) Revision of infected hip replacement. Two-stage procedure with a temporary gentamicin spacer. Acta Orthop Scand 65(1):7–8
15. Jeys L, Suneja R, Grimer RJ (2004) Deep infection in orthopaedic oncology prostheses. Am Acad of Orthop Surg, San Francisco; Vol 5: p622
16. Koo KH, Yang JW, Cho SH et al (2001) Impregnation of vancomycin, gentamicin, and cefotaxime in a cement spacer for two-stage cementless reconstruction in infected total hip arthroplasty. J Arthroplasty 16(7):882–892
17. Lieberman JR, Callaway GH, Salvati EA et al (1994) Treatment of the infected total hip arthroplasty with two-stage reimplantation protocol. Clin Orthop Relat Res (301):205–212
18. Lord CF, Gebhardt MC, Tomford WW et al (1988) Infection in bone allografts: incidence, nature, and treatment. J Bone Joint Surg Am 70(3):369–376
19. Manfrini M, Capanna R, Caldora P et al (1993) Gastrocnemius flaps in the surgical treatment of sarcomas of the knee. Chir Organi Mov 78(2):95–104
20. Manoso MW, Boland PJ, Healey JH et al (2006) Limb salvage of infected knee reconstructions for cancer with staged revision and free tissue transfer. Ann Plast Surg 56(5):532–5; discussion 535
21. McDonald DJ, Capanna R, Gherlinzoni F et al (1990) Influence of chemotherapy on perioperative complications in limb salvage surgery for bone tumors. Cancer 65(7):1509–1516
22. Nelson CL, Evans RP, Blaha JD et al (1993) A comparison of gentamicin-impregnated polymethylmethacrylate bead implantation to conventional parenteral antibiotic therapy in infected total hip and knee arthroplasty. Clin Orthop Relat Res (295):96–101
23. Peterson SA, Fitzgerald RH (1994) Complications of musculoskeletal infections. In: Epps CH ed, Complications in Orthopaedic Surgery. Vol 1.Philadelphia: J.B. Lippincott;155–182
24. Quinn RH, Mankin HJ, Springfield DS et al (2001) Management of infected bulk allografts with antibiotic-impregnated polymethylmethacrylate spacers. Orthopedics 24(10):971–975
25. Roberts P, Chan D, Grimer RJ et al (1991) Prosthetic replacement of the distal femur for primary bone tumours. J Bone Joint Surg Br 73(5):762–769
26. Scott IR, Stockley I, Getty CJM (1993) Exchange arthroplasty for infected knee replacements: a new two-stage method. J Bone Joint Surg Br 75(1):28–31
27. Simon MA, Springfield D (1998) Surgery for bone and soft-tissue tumors. Lippincott-Raven Publishers, Philadelphia
28. Wahlig H, Buchholz HW (1972) Experimental and clinical studies on the release of gentamicin from bone cement. Chirurg 43(10):441–445
29. Walenkamp GHIM, Vree TB, Guelen PJM et al (1983) Pharmacokinetic and nephrotoxicologic study to the use of gentamicin-PMMA-beads. Proceedings to 13th Int Congress Chemotherapy, Vienna;43:20
30. Willenegger H (1970) Clinical aspects and therapy of pyogenic bone infections. Chirurg 41(5):215–221.

Local Antibiotic Therapy: Present and Future

E. Meani, C.L. Romanò

Department for Treatment of Osteoarticular Septic Complications (COS) –
Director: Prof. Enzo Meani
Operative Unit for Septic Prosthesis – Responsible: Prof. Carlo L. Romanò
"G. Pini" Orthopaedic Institute, Milan, Italy

Historical Overview

Since ancient times, physicians and healers have been aware of the anti-infective and anti-spoilage properties of certain substances. Egyptian embalmers used resins, naphtha and liquid pitch, along with vegetable oils and spices. Persian laws instructed people to store drinking water in bright copper vessels. The ancient Greeks and Romans recognized the antiseptic properties of wine, oil, and vinegar. The use of wine and vinegar in the dressing of wounds dates back to the Greek physician Hippocrates (460–357 BC). Human use of honey is traced to some 8000 years ago as depicted by stone age paintings. Different traditional systems of medicine have elaborated the role of honey as medicinal product. Sumerian clay tablets (6200 BC), Egyptian papyri (1900–1250 BC): Vedas (5000 years); holy Koran, Bible and Hippocratic methods (460–357 BC) have described the uses of honey. Camphor is said to have been first used as a drug in the Arabian Peninsula around AD 600, and, eventually came to be used as a sacred panacea in Greece and Egypt. Balsam, an antiseptic of both southeast Asia and Peru, was introduced to Europe in medieval times and remained in use through the 1800s.

The first concept of antisepsis was introduced by Genevieve Charlotte d'Arconville who introduced the use of chloride of mercury as an antiseptic in 1766. After Bernard Courtois (1777–1838) discovered iodine in 1811, it became a popular antiseptic treatment for wounds. None of these antiseptics, however, was sufficient to prevent the almost certain infection of wounds, particularly following surgery. The introduction of anesthesia in 1846 made the problem worse. It permitted more complicated and lengthy surgical operations, greatly increasing the likelihood of infection.

Another deadly form of infection was puerperal (occurring at the time of childbirth) fever, a streptococcus infection of the uterus that struck women who had just given birth.

Until the relationship between bacteria and disease was discovered by Louis Pasteur (1822–1895), doctors paid little attention to surgical cleanliness.

English surgeon Joseph Lister (1827–1912) applied this new knowledge of bacteria to develop a successful system of antiseptic surgery. Lister studied wound healing with the use of a microscope. After reading Pasteur's work, Lister concluded that microorganisms in the air caused the infection of wounds. He sprayed a wound and surrounding areas with carbolic acid to destroy infectious organisms and also protected the area from new invasion by bacteria by using multiple-layer dressings (1965).

A final obstacle to surgical antisepsis were the human hands. Although surgical instruments and dressings can be sterilized, surgeons' and nurses' hands can only be washed with antiseptics. An American doctor, William Halsted, solved this problem in 1890. There, he pioneered the use of rubber gloves in surgery to protect his head nurse from the antiseptic that was irritating her hands. Today sterile gloves are required during all surgical procedures.

The generalization of antiseptic procedures allowed in the fist decades of the 20th century to face with fewer problems amputations and generally surgical interventions, today classified as "clean", whereas general surgery was still at high-risk of post-operative infection. The discovery of antibiotics by Sir Alexander Fleming (1928) changed the course of medicine.

In particular in the orthopaedic field the combined medical and surgical treatment increased enormously the possibility to provide a solution to bone and joint infection.

Local and Systemic Antibiotic Therapy

Today antibiotic therapy plays an essential role in any kind of surgery and has allowed the reduction of post-operative infection enormously. In particular the orthopaedic field has seen a great development of the local antibiotic therapy as adjunct to systemic antibiotic therapy.

The addition of antibiotics to bone cement, used for the fixation of joint prosthesis has been shown to have a positive effect on the reduction of deep infection following surgery [12].

In the last decades research has been done towards the possibility of finding the "perfect" carrier for the local release of antibiotics, both for prophylaxis and treatment.

This is because systemic antibiotic therapy has limits:

1. poor bone penetration is reported for many antibiotics [10, 21, 32, 33];
2. side effects can be as high as 22 % related to antibiotic suppression [31];
3. eventually "the race for the surface" of bacteria described by Gristina in 1983 [17] cannot be stopped.

Self-defending implants with anti-adhesive surfaces and local antibiotic release (antibacterial coating) may be a tool to reduce as much as possible this terrible complication [4, 9].

Local antibiotic therapy has been shown to be effective: animal and clinical studies have shown that high effective local concentration may be achieved and maintained over a prolonged period [6, 38]. Data from the Norwegian register have shown that the the combination of systemic and local antibiotic therapy (antibiotic-loaded bone cement) is effective in reducing prosthetic deep infection [12].

Nonetheless local antibiotic therapy as well has its own limits:

1. it cannot cure alone bone infections and it must be associated to a) an accurate and radical debridement; b) general antibiotic therapy; c) the filling of bone defect and dead spaces; d) soft tissue covering; e) vascular support.

2. the slow release and concentrations below the MIC may determine the selection of resistant strains and the selection of small colony variants [18, 28, 36, 37].

Local Antibiotic Delivery Today

In the application of a local antibiotic therapy variuos aspects should be considered: a) delivery technique; b) type of antibiotic that can be used; c) pharmacokinetics; d) possibility of application to a coating and to fillers; e) possibility of combination with osteoconductive and osteoinductive factors; f) use as prophylaxis and/or therapy; g) drawbacks (Table 1).

Today local antibiotic therapy can be performed with:

1. antibiotic-loaded PMMA in the form of cement, beads and spacers;
2. local infusion (micropumps);
3. bone grafts;
4. collagen;
5. calcium sulphate and carbonate;
6. demineralized bone matrix

PMMA is used for the fixation of primary and revision prosthesis, in one-stage procedures [7, 33] and in two-stage infection treatment in the form of spacers [11, 43]. PMMA beads can be used in the treatment of osteomyelitis [39]. Many different antibiotics can be admixed to PMMA. Antibiotics must be thermally stable and water soluble, with bactericidal effect at the tissue levels attained; furthermore, it must be released gradually over an appropriate time period, evoke minimal local inflammatory or allergic reaction. Finally, the antibiotic must not significantly compromise mechanical integrity, especially if the cement is used for implant fixation [19].

Infusion micropumps are used in the treatment of osteomyelitis. The device can be internally or externally portable [24, 27]. Unfortunately the clinical efficacy of these device has still to be confirmed.

Collagen sponges (gentamicin) have been used in a clinical setting since 1986 [5]. No clinical long-term follow-up studies have been published. They are used in primary and revision surgery.

Bone grafts are an interesting tool, with limited availability, which show a fast release are used in primary and revision surgery, in osteomyelitis and in clean surgery [8, 29, 41, 42].

Calcium sulphate and carbonate might be used in revision surgery and osteomyelitis. In a goat model four treatment groups were evaluated: no treatment, hand-made tobramycin-impregnated PMMA beads, commercially-available tobramycin-impregnated calcium sulphate pellets and commercially-available tobramycin-impregnated PMMA beads. Three weeks after intraosseous inoculation with streptomycin-resistant *Staphylococcus aureus* tissue cultures showed no evidence of infection in any of the antibiotic-treated groups. All of the cultures were positive in the untreated group. These results show that effective local antibiotic delivery can be obtained with both commercially-available products and with hand-made PMMA beads. The calcium sulphate pellets have the advantage of being bioabsorbable, thereby obviating the need for a second procedure to remove them [40].

Table 1

	PMMA	Infusion micropump	Bone graft	Collagen sponge	Calcium sulphate or carbonate	Demineralized bone matrix
Antibiotic delivery	Non-resorbable carrier	Local catheter	Resorbable carrier	Resorbable carrier	Resorbable carrier	Resorbable carrier
Antibiotic type	Aminoglycosides; Glycopeptide, other	Amikacin, vancomycin, etc (stable ATB)	Gentamicin, vancomycin	Gentamicin	Tobramycin	Teicoplanin
Pharmacokinetics	Slow, long-lasting release	Infusion rate and concentrations chosen for each case	Fast release	Fast release	Slow release	Fast release
Coating	See future application	–	–	–	–	–
Filler	Yes	–	Yes	No	Yes	No
Osteoconduction	No	–	Yes	–	Yes	Yes
Osteoinduction	No	–	Yes	–	No	Yes
Prophylaxis	Yes	No	Yes	Yes	–	Yes
Therapy	Yes	Yes	Yes	Yes	Yes	Yes
Drawbacks	Small colony variant Cement fragilization Non resorbable	Logistically demanding Not clinically proven Costs	Limited availability Viral contamination (homologous) Costs	Resistant strain Limited clinical studies Costs	Long time to resorption	Low consistency of the material Costs

Aminoglycosides = gentamicin, tobramycin, amikacin,..
Glycopeptides = vancomycin, teicoplanin
Other = clindamycin, erythromicin, colistin, imipenem, meropenem,...

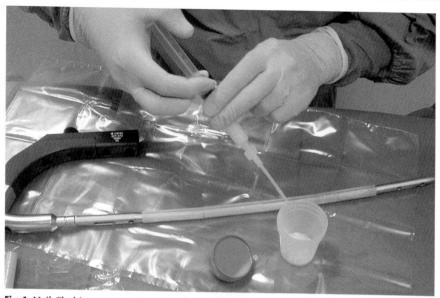

Fig. 1. Nail Clothing preparation: once all the metamers have been placed, a gentamicin PMMA glue is used to fix the metamers to the nail

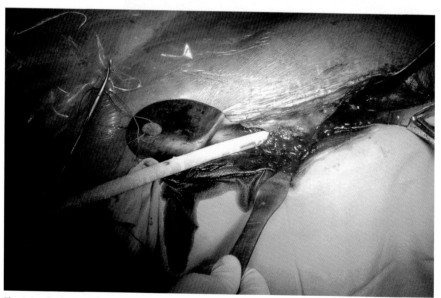

Fig. 2. Nail Clothing insertion in the femur

Demineralized bone matrix might be used in revision surgery and osteomyelitis. The combination of tricalcium phospate (Calcibon®) and bone demineralized matrix (Targobone®) has been used for the treatment of bone defects after debridement of bone infection (Fig. 3). The preliminary results after 1-year of follow-up have shown

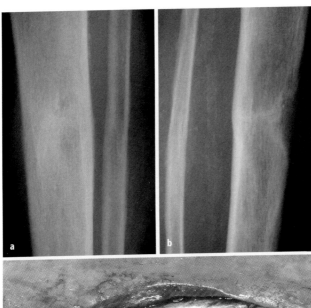

Fig. 3a, b. Chronic osteomyelitis of the tibia. Pre-operative X-rays

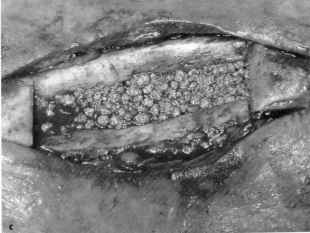

Fig. 3c. Filling of the bone defect with Calcium phospate (Calcibon®) and bone demineralized matrix (Targobone®)

the absence of infection recurrence or draining in all the 16 patients: Radiographic findings showed at the latest available follow-up new bone formation, but incomplete bone substitutes resorption (Figures 4–5) [30].

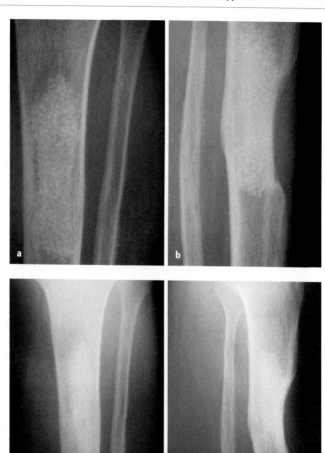

Fig. 4a, b. X-rays showing the 3 months follow-up

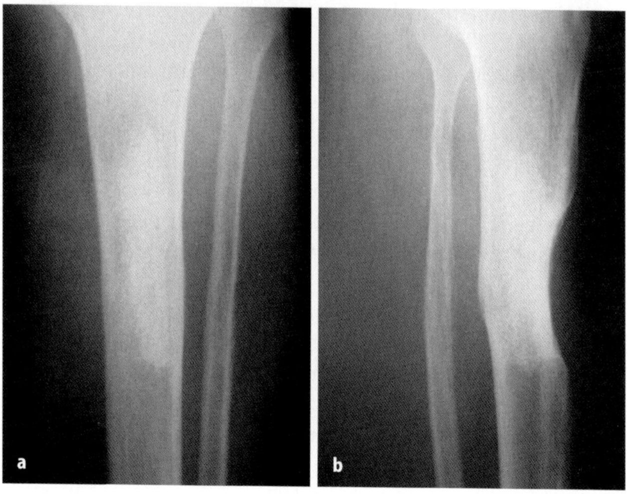

Fig. 5a, b. X-rays showing the 15 months follow-up

Local Antibiotic Therapy in the Future

The future of local antibiotic therapy is directed towards the use of:

1. PLLA and other polymers;
2. hydrossyapatite (HA);
3. PMMA coating;
4. covalent binding;
5. silver and new peptides.

1. Polylactic acids and other polymers are used in some hardware materials (screws, etc.), suture wires and coating of metallic hardware. Such material has been shown

to be able to deliver incorporated antibiotics (gentamicin and teicoplanin) for prolonged time (96 hours) and could offer new perspectives in preventing biomaterial-associated infections. Combinations with other drugs to formulate custom-tailored surfaces are also feasible [16]. A study in rabbits has shown that PLLA loaded with antibiotic and used as a coating to osteosynthesis material has the capacity to reduce the infection rate [20].

Polylactide-polyglycolide antibiotic implants might provide an absorbable system for localized antibiotic delivery: *in vitro* studies have shown promising results of antibiotic elution from bioresorbable microspheres and beads; animal studies have shown that induced osteomyelitis can be treated [14] therefore human trials should be planned to assess the efficacy of such devices.

2. Hydroxyapatite is used for the coating of metallic hardware. Various antibiotics (cephalotin, carbenicillin, amoxicilin, cefamandol, tobramycin, gentamicin and vancomycin) have been incorporated and the release and antibiotic efficacy have been positively tested and might be used to prevent post-surgical infections and to promote bone bonding of orthopaedic devices [34] Animal studies have shown that gentamicin-hydroxiapatite coating are able to reduce the infection rate [3]

3. PMMA coating is another alternative (intramedulary nail, IM): animal studies have shown the effectiveness of such procedure for the eradication of infection [15]. The clinical application of such devices, extemporaneously made in the OR [25] or preformed (Nail Clothing, Figures 1–2) is promising. In particular preformed PMMA coating offers the possibility to maintain a mechanical function, while providing a high local release of antibiotics for a prolonged period. Moreover such a system may be applied to all types of cylindrical IM nail.

4. Vancomycin covalent binding is a new route being studied: it has been shown that vancomycin covalently bound to a metal (titanium) surface has effective bactericidal activity [26]. This technology holds great promise for the manufacturing of "smart" implants that can be self protective against peri-prosthetic infection, or can be used for the treatment of periprosthetic infections when they occur.

5. Silver has known antiseptic properties [22]. Recently nano-silver particulate bone cement was shown to have antibacterial properties (high effectiveness against multi-resistant bacteria, MRSE and MRSA) and free from cytoxicity effect [1, 2]. Should the reults be confirmed *in vivo*, NanoSilver might have an interest in joint arthroplasty.

6. Peptides: some peptides have been shown to have antibacterial properties comparable to some antibiotics. In particular in an animal study hLF1–11 (human lactoferrin 1) incorporated into Ca-P bone cement has been shown to be effective in the treatment of osteomyelitis, an effectiveness comparable to that of gentamicin. Therefore, the results of this study warrant further preclinical investigations into the possibilities of using hLF1–11 for the treatment of osteomyelitis [13].

Conclusion

The new local antibiotic technologies should therefore be focused on effectiveness, proper pharmacokinetics, antibiotic resistant strains, effects on osteointegration and callus formation.

The ideal local antibiotic therapy should provide:

- Antibiotic choice based on antibiogram
- High local antibiotic concentrations
- Programmable and complete release
- Ostoconductive and/or osteoinductive carrier completely resorbable
- No interference with osteointegration
- Act as a filler when needed

References

1. Alt V, Bechert T, Steinrucke P et al (2004) An in vitro assessment of the antibacterial properties and cytotoxicity of nanoparticulate silver bone cement. Biomaterials 25(18):4383–4391
2. Alt V, Bechert T, Steinrucke P et al (2004)Nanoparticulate silver. A new antimicrobial substance for bone cement Orthopade 33(8):885–892
3. Alt V, Bitschnau A, Osterling J et al (2006) The effects of combined gentamicin-hydroxyapatite coating for cementless joint prostheses on the reduction of infection rates in a rabbit infection prophylaxis model.Biomaterials 27(26):4627–4634
4. Anagnostakos K, Kelm J, Tegits T et al (2005) In vitro evaluation of antibiotic release from and bacteria growth inhibition by antibiotic-loaded acrylic bone cement spacers. J Biomed Mater Res B Appl Biomater 15;72(2):373–378
5. Ascherl R, Stemberger A, Lechner F et al (1986) Treatment of chronic osteomyelitis with a collagen-antibiotic compound--preliminary report Unfallchirurgie 12(3):125–127. German
6. Bertazzoni Minelli E, Benini A, Magnan B, Bartolozzi P (2004)Release of gentamicin and vancomycin from temporary human hip spacers in two-stage revision of infected arthroplasty. J Antimicrob Chemother 53(2):329–334
7. Buchholz HW, Elson RA, Englebrecht E et al (1981) Management of deep infection of total hip replacement. J Bone Joint Surg (Br) 63(3):342–353
8. Buttaro MA, Pusso R, Piccaluga F (2005) Vancomycin-supplemented impacted bone allografts in infected hip arthroplasty. Two-stage revision results. J Bone Joint Surg (Br) 87(3):314–319
9. Cordero J, Garcia Cimbrelo E (2000) Mechanism of bacterial resistance in implant infection. Hip International 10(3):139–144
10. Cunha BA, Gossling HR, Pasternak HS et al (1977) The penetration characteristics of cefazolin, cephalothin and cephradine into bone in patients undergoing total hip replacement. J Bone Joint Surg (Am) 59(7):856–860
11. Duncan CP, Beauchamp C (1993) A temporary antibiotic-loaded joint replacement system for management of complex infections involving the hip. Orthop Clin North Am 24(4): 751–759
12. Espehaug B, Engesaeter LB, Vollset SE et al (1997) Antibiotic prophylaxis in total hip arthroplasty. Review of 10,905 primary cemented total hip replacements reported to the Norwegian arthroplasty register, 1987 to 1995. J Bone Joint Surg (Br) 79(4):590–595
13. Faber C, Stallmann HP, Lyaruu DM et al (2005) Comparable efficacies of the antimicrobial peptide human lactoferrin 1–11 and gentamicin in a chronic methicillin-resistant Staphylococcus aureus osteomyelitis model. Antimicrob Agents Chemother 49(6):2438–2444
14. Garvin K, Feschuk C (2005) Polylactide-polyglycolide antibiotic implants. Clin Orthop Relat Res (437):105–110
15. Giadino R, Fini M, Giavaresi G et al (2006) Rationale of nail antibiotic clothing and "in vivo" animal study (this book)

16. Gollwitzer H, Ibrahim K, Meyer H et al (2003) Antibacterial poly(D,L-lactic acid) coating of medical implants using a biodegradable drug delivery technology. J Antimicrob Chemother 51(3):585–591

17. Gristina AG (1987) Biomaterial-centered infection: microbial adhesion versus tissue integration. Science 237(4822):1588–1595

18. Hendriks JG, Neut D, van Horn JR et al (2005) Bacterial survival in the interfacial gap in gentamicin-loaded acrylic bone cements. J Bone Joint Surg (Br) 87(2):272–276

19. Joseph TN, Chen AL, Di Cesare PE /(2003) Use of antibiotic-impregnated cement in total joint arthroplasty. J Am Acad Orthop Surg 11(1):38–47. Review

20. Kalicke T, Schierholz J, Seybold D et al (2004) Influence on local infection resistance of the local antibacterial coating of titanium plates in osteosynthesis. An experimental study in rabbits. Proceedings to EBJIS 2004 Milan

21. Kutscha-Lissberg F, et al (2003) Linezolid penetration into bone and joint tissues infected with methicillin-resistant staphylococci. Antimicrob Agents Chemother 47(12):3964–3966

22. Lansdown AB (2002) Silver I: Its antibacterial properties and mechanism of action. J Wound Care 11(4):125–130

23. Magnan B, Regis D, Biscaglia R et al (2001) Preformed acrylic bone cement spacer loaded with antibiotics. Use of two-stage procedure in 10 patients because of infected hip after total replacement. Acta Orthop Scand 72(6):591–594

24. Meani E, Romanò CL (1994) Traitement de l'ostéomyelite par antibiothérapie locale utilisant une micropompe électronique portable. Rev Chir Reparatrice Appar Mot 80:285–290

25. Paley D, Herzenberg JE (2002) Intramedullary infections treated with antibiotic cement rods: preliminary results in nine cases. J Orthop Trauma 16(10):723–729

26. Parvizi J, Wickstrom E, Zeiger AR et al (2004) Frank Stinchfield Award. Titanium surface with biologic activity against infection. Clin Orthop Relat Res (429):33–38

27. Perry CR, Davenport K et al (1988) Antibiotic administration using an implantable drug pump in the treatment of osteomyelitis. Clin Orthop Relat Res (226):222–230

28. Proctor RA, Peters G (198) Small colony variants in staphylococcal infections: diagnostic and therapeutic implications. Clin Infect Dis 27(3):419–422

29. Rhyu KH, Jung MH, Yoo JJ et al (2003) In vitro release of vancomycin from vancomycin-loaded blood coated demineralised bone. Int Orthop 27(1):53–55

30. Romanò C, Trezza, Zavaratelli et al (2006) Tricalcium phospate and teicoplanin-added demineralized bone matrix for the treatment of bone defects in infections. A minimum one-year follow-up. Proceedings to EBJIS 2006 Budapest

31. Segreti J, Nelson JA, Trenholme GM (1998) Prolonged suppressive antibiotic therapy for infected orthopedic prostheses. Clin Infect Dis 27(4):711–713

32. Smilack JD, Flittie WH, Williams TW Jr (1975). Bone concentrations of antimicrobial agents after parenteral administration. Antimicrob Agents Chemother 9(1):169–171

33. Steinbrink K (1990) The case for revision arthroplasty using antibiotic-loaded acrylic cement.Clin Orthop Relat Res (261):19–22. Review

34. Stigter M, Bezemer J, de Groot K et al (2004) Incorporation of different antibiotics into carbonated hydroxyapatite coatings on titanium implants, release and antibiotic efficacy. J Control Release 99(1):127–137

35. Summersgill JT, Schupp LG, Raff MJ (1982). Comparative penetration of metronidazole, clindamycin, chloramphenicol, cefoxitin, ticaricillin and moxalactam into bone. Antimicrob Agents Chemother 21(4):601–603

36. Thomes B, Murray P, Bouchier-Hayes D (2002) Development of resistant strains of Staphylococcus epidermidis on gentamicin-loaded bone cement in vivo. J Bone Joint Surg (Br) 84(5):758–760

37. van de Belt H, Neut D, Schenk W et al (2000) Gentamicin release from polymethylmethacrylate bone cements and Staphylococcus aureus biofilm formation. Acta Orthop Scand 71(6):625–629

38. Wahlig H, Buchholz HW (1972) Experimental and clinical studies on the release of gentamicin from bone cement Chirurg 43(10):441–445

39. Walenkamp GH, Kleijn LL, de Leeuw M (1998)Osteomyelitis treated with gentamicin-PMMA beads: 100 patients followed for 1–12 years. Acta Orthop Scand 69(5):518–522

40. Wenke JC, Owens BD, Svoboda SJ et al (2006) Effectiveness of commercially-available antibiotic-impregnated implants. J Bone Joint Surg (Br) 88(8):1102–1104

41. Winkler H, Janata O, Berger C et al (2000) A. In vitro release of vancomycin and tobramycin from impregnated human and bovine bone grafts. J Antimicrob Chemother 46(3):423–428
42. Witso E, Persen L, Loseth K et al (2000) Cancellous bone as an antibiotic carrier. Acta Orthop Scand 71(1):80–84
43. Zilkens KW, Casser HR, Ohnsorge (1990) Treatment of an old infection in a total hip replacement with an interim spacer prosthesis. J Arch Orthop Trauma Surg 109(2):94–96

Printing and Binding: Stürtz GmbH, Würzburg